D1716169

CLINICALLY APPLIED ANTHROPOLOGY

CULTURE, ILLNESS, AND HEALING

Studies in Comparative Cross-Cultural Research

VOLUME 5

CLINICALLY
APPLIED
ANTHROPOLOGY

Anthropologists in Health Science Settings

Edited by

NOEL J. CHRISMAN

University of Washington, Seattle

and

THOMAS W. MARETZKI

University of Hawaii, Honolulu

D. REIDEL PUBLISHING COMPANY

DORDRECHT : HOLLAND / BOSTON : U.S.A.

LONDON : ENGLAND

Library of Congress Cataloging in Publication Data

Main entry under title:

Clinically applied anthropology.

    (Culture, illness, and healing ; 5)
    Includes index.
    1. Social medicine. 2. Medical anthropology. 3. Medicine
and psychology. I. Chrisman, Noel J., 1940–   . II. Maretzki,
Thomas. III. Series. [DNLM: 1. Anthropology. 2. Medicine.
W1 CU445 v. 5 / GN 296 C641]
RA418.C64   1982   362.1′042   82–12301
ISBN 90–277–1418–5
ISBN 90–277–1419–3 (pbk.)

Published by D. Reidel Publishing Company,
P.O. Box 17, 3300 AA Dordrecht, Holland.

Sold and distributed in the U.S.A. and Canada
by Kluwer Boston Inc.,
190 Old Derby Street, Hingham, MA 02043, U.S.A.

In all other countries, sold and distributed
by Kluwer Academic Publishers Group,
P.O. Box 322, 3300 AH Dordrecht, Holland.

D. Reidel Publishing Company is a member of the Kluwer Group.

TABLE OF CONTENTS

PREFACE

Like other collections of papers related to a single topic, this volume arose out of problem-sharing and problem-solving discussions among some of the authors. The two principal recurring issues were (1) the difficulties in translating anthropological knowledge so that our students could use it and (2) the difficulties of bringing existing medical anthropology literature to bear on this task. As we talked to other anthropologists teaching in other parts of the country and in various health-related schools, we recognized that our problems were similar. Similarities in our solutions led the Editors to believe that publication of our teaching experiences and research relevant to teaching would help others and might begin the process of generating principles leading to a more coherent approach. Our colleagues supported this idea and agreed to contribute.

What we agreed to write about was 'Clinically Applied Anthropology'. Much of what we were doing and certainly much of the relevant literature was applied anthropology. And our target group was composed mostly of clinicians. The utility of the term became apparent after 1979 when another set of anthropologists began to discuss 'Clinical Anthropology'. They too recognized the range of novel behaviors available to anthropologists in the health science arena and chose to focus on the clinical *use* of anthropology. We see this as an important endeavor, but very different from what we are proposing. Clinically applied anthropology is oriented toward clarification and expansion of perspective – a teaching, research, and consulting role. If the anthropologist is, or subsequently becomes, prepared to be a clinician, the clinical activities are genuinely nursing, medicine, alcohol and drug abuse counseling, or the like, but not anthropology. As anthropologists, we are not educated to intervene; nor is the legal, ethical, or supervisory structure set up to allow it.

The nearly simultaneous development of similar new directions in medical anthropology highlights a decade of rapid change in this subfield that promises to continue. Significantly, medical anthropology's focus is shifting away from its roots in the anthropology of religion – health related beliefs and rituals – and traditional physical anthropology – describing biological variation. Research is directed toward understanding the cultural underpinnings of genetic diseases, population dynamics, nutrition, healing practices, health care organization, and patient choices among health care alternatives in complex societies. The proliferation of journals related to anthropological study of health issues and the accelerated development of medical anthropology programs for graduate study are further evidence of growth.

These changes in medical anthropology have increased its relevance for the health science professions of medicine, nursing, public health, pharmacy, dentistry, and social work. Thus, we have the opportunity to contribute in health related academic, clinical, and research settings. What remains is to take advantage of that opportunity. We see this volume as one step in that direction.

The Editors wish to acknowledge the important typing and editorial assistance provided by Donna Van Winkle. In addition, we benefitted from many helpful suggestions offered by colleagues at the Universities of Washington and Hawaii. The most significant support came from Arthur Kleinman. As series editor and friend, he has helped with advice, ideas, and rewriting throughout the entire process. Our families, too, deserve recognition for relinquishing some family activities that would have occurred except for our work on this book.

THE EDITORS

NOEL J. CHRISMAN AND THOMAS W. MARETZKI

ANTHROPOLOGY IN HEALTH SCIENCE SETTINGS

THE NEED FOR THIS BOOK

The explosive expansion of anthropology is startling when held against the short span of time it has existed as a discipline. Numerically it appears to attract a disproportionately large number of interested individuals to its medically focused sub-discipline. Less than two decades old as a recognized distinct area within anthropology, medical anthropology has taken an independent and vigorous course of its own. Its roots in anthropology and its continuing ties with the theoretical formulations and important general data base of biological, linguistic, and social anthropology are not in question. New areas of investigation are generated and tested with theories central to anthropology, and with reliance on interdisciplinary thinking. The core activities within medical anthropology are social science brought to bear on issues that relate to the universal human challenge of health maintenance and response to sickness.

Clinically applied anthropology is one special emergent direction within medical anthropology, found within the context of health science schools. The move to that setting happened long ago, but only recently have the implications for the field and for our professional behavior emerged as interesting enough to stimulate sharing information. The recent interest stems from the existence of larger numbers (though still not very large) of anthropologists in health science settings and the likelihood that these numbers will grow as the anthropological job market changes. Working alone for the most part, anthropologists in health science settings have developed their own approaches for doing anthropology in novel environments. They endured the problems and celebrated the successes by themselves, but sometimes shared them in conversation at the meetings of the American Anthropological Association, the Society for Applied Anthropology, or the Association for the Behavioral Sciences and Medical Education.

The need to more formally communicate what we have learned — to ourselves and to anthropologists who hope to work in the health sciences — is what stimulated this volume. Although clinically applied anthropology is no exception to the notion that new interest areas arise through coffee and cocktail table talks, a time comes for putting pen to paper. Steps in this direction began in 1980 with the preliminary discussions of clinical anthropology and the debate on that subject in the Medical Anthropology Newsletter (MAN 1980). More will appear through this decade. Rather than debate the format of an interest area, we have chosen to exchange information — about teaching strategies, about research relevant to our clinical audiences, about the nature of where we work. These issues deserve communication if only to create a sense of community among those of us who buck anthropological

1

N. J. Chrisman and T. W. Maretzki (eds.), Clinically Applied Anthropology, 1–31.
Copyright © 1982 by D. Reidel Publishing Company.

tradition by working outside anthropology departments. There is, however, a broader need. It appears unlikely, even with the funding crises apparent for the 80's, that all anthropologists will leave health science schools. In addition, we believe that anthropology can benefit from the expansion of some of its members into a new niche. Growth, analogous to that in medical anthropology and urban anthropology, is possible. This expansion will depend on two qualities: close adherence to the established norms of anthropology and clear translation and communication of these norms to members of other disciplines who work with us.

We see clinically applied anthropology as a specialized focus within the discipline that clusters the data, theory, and methods of anthropology in ways that serve to clarify specific clinical issues in health maintenance and response to sickness. To some extent, this view contrasts with the notion that what happens in health science schools is the medical anthropology of anthropology departments. It is true that clinically applied anthropology like medical anthropology is concerned with the anthropological issues surrounding health and sickness. Yet the professional thrust differs and the difference is most strikingly seen in the nature of the intended audience. The readers of literature in medical anthropology are predominantly anthropologists who hope to expand knowledge of their field. The audience for clinically applied anthropologists is primarily constituted by clinicians of various sorts. Thus the presumed recipients of our social science skills do not automatically share the professional assumptions that sustain discourse within a discipline.

We believe that this lack of congruence in professional assumptions is the fundamental challenge and source of excitement in the field. It permeates the daily life of an anthropologist in a health science setting. An experienced anthropologist, working for a year in a health science school, said that the most bothersome aspect of his new position was the constant need to justify his existence. Academic anthropologists are accustomed to teaching graduates and undergraduates taking courses with established content and to debating disciplinary perspectives on various subjects with colleagues from their own and other departments. But the persistent need to legitimize a claim to be there in the first place is beyond the experience of most of us.

This book was explicitly designed to aid anthropologists in health science settings as we attempt to justify our existence in a novel territory. And the most important topographical feature of this territory is the service mandate of clinicians. This mandate is an essential element in the professional assumptions of health scientists. It also contrasts strongly with the thrust toward 'understanding' common within anthropology. In this volume, we hope to present some examples of how anthropologists have attempted to translate the understandings of anthropology for health professionals so that their services to patients can be more humanistic, holistic, or culture-sensitive. This is a difficult task: the basic perspectives of the two fields differ; educational experiences are dissimilar; the personality types and personal interests of people drawn into anthropology are probably different from those drawn into the health sciences. Yet both fields stand to gain. And, more importantly to the health scientist and applied anthropologist, the clientele stands to benefit.

Why anthropologists are included among the faculty and research scientists of health science schools is a complex question. Currently, the answer may be phrased in terms of the need to make medical care more responsive to the needs of consumers and the need to promote humanistic rather than veterinary standards in medical care (Young 1981). These needs are very much the result of social movements extraneous to medical care, but with significant impact: e.g., the civil rights, consumer, ethnic, and women's movements. These currents of social change have stimulated attention to the varying perspectives and needs of American minority groups, to people's desires that medical care take family, community, and life style patterns into account, and to the taken-for-granted, but sometimes harmful, effects of bureaucracy on the interpersonal nature of health care. In all these areas, anthropology can make its contribution — both through describing the social lives of patients and their families and through its client-based, relativistic perspective. Yet the presence of anthropologists in health science settings began to be felt prior to these contemporary needs and anthropological contributions form a continuity to the present day.

ANTECEDENTS

Antecedents to clinical medical anthropology reflect several themes of separate though related topics. Lasting contributions were made in each of these areas. A few selected examples follow, though they are in no way exhaustive of the precursory work to the present. Awareness of historical background for clinically applied anthropology gives perspective on the present and may help in avoiding duplication of efforts. It also highlights long term obstacles and attempts to remove or circumvent them.

Culture and Behavior

Culture and behavior is a major theme that predates others in terms of both clinical and anthropological interest. The clinical problem is related to varying definitions of normal and abnormal cross-culturally. Associated with the culture and personality school of anthropology, the focus is on cultural explanations of behavior. The definition and functional understanding of normality and abnormality were considered in abstract terms by anthropologists. These ideas assumed practical dimensions in psychiatry as diversity in the range of behaviors began to emerge from anthropological and psychiatric investigations throughout the world. Questions raised by this expanding awareness concerned individual behavior and psychological functioning: what links could be sought in the cultural environment in which individuals grew up to the nature of the adult world in which they matured, and how could these linkages be related to behavioral expressions and cultural labeling of behaviors? To what extent could normal and abnormal dimensions of behavior be explained by cultural variations in environments as well as specific cultural meanings and definitions of what is appropriate and what is inappropriate behavior? Is madness (psychosis) universally viewed the same, regardless of culture? Are there commonalities in its phenomenology, course, and treatment response? Are there cultural illnesses? Are there effective cultural treatments? Do they share universal features of healing with psychotherapy? These questions remain central to psychiatric practice in different parts of the world in spite of modern psychiatric classifications that are universal in their claims; although in the United States, culture is explicitly recognized. Anthropology, in contrast with psychiatry, leans towards relativistic explanations that allow for cultural construction of normality as well as pathology, and was influenced by the anthropologists who debated these puzzling questions earlier (Sapir 1949a, 1949b; Mead 1939; Benedict 1934). More recently, the recognized thresholds of behavior and acknowledgment of psychological problems in different (non-Western) cultures has attracted anthropological research attention (Edgerton 1966).

Cultural Diagnoses

A second theme concerned cultural constructions of and cultural variables related to diagnostic categories. As a medical specialty, psychiatry emphasized universal scientifically or at least systematically developed criteria for diagnostic and interventive purposes. Anthropologists served chiefly as interpreters of the cultural role in psychological functioning as reflected in human behavior and pathology. Several anthropological approaches addressed to this topic were directed toward anthropological readers, to psychiatric specialists, or to both (e.g., Linton 1956; Devereux 1956; Opler 1967). The anthropological emphasis continues on the side of theoretical development and conceptual clarification. For example, Langness raised the question of the logical classification of certain behaviors in non-Western cultures (Langness 1967). In so doing, he considered several important points: the need, on the one hand, to separate behavioral styles that are characteristic in certain populations and described in the literature as "culture bound disorders (or syndromes)" from, on the other hand, the more general psychiatric necessity to classify psychiatric disorders independent of a specific cultural environment in which behavior style has taken on a specific form of expression. This remains a significant focus of concern in clinical psychiatry in the development of a workable diagnostic classification system which is general, yet incorporates specific expressions of behavior.

The emergence of cultural psychiatry as a sub-specialty of general psychiatry in the West, and its identity as a medical professional activity rather than a social or behavioral science, is a natural response to the situation in which there is a direct need for translation of concepts into care of patients and establishment of mental health services. In the United States the newly formed group of cultural psychiatrists grapples with these issues. But more importantly, these matters are of immediate and practical concern to psychiatrists practicing in non-Western countries. Although not a major focus for anthropological explorations in the past, one can see linkages with past research and the possibilities for developing continued and future ties to clinical psychiatry. This is especially so because of the natural complementarity of the anthropological orientation to meanings and the psychiatric orientation to behavioral description. Overlap occurs in concerns with social relations and psycho-dynamics (Maretzki 1981).

Ethnographic Data

Taking a retrospective view of these developments, it seems that anthropologists have thought at great length about problems of human functioning and have tied these ideas to ethnographic data generated by them or their colleagues. But they had only limited familiarity with the nature of clinical psychiatric and other medical practice and the nature of clinical problem solving. There are, of course, exceptions to this statement among individual anthropologists. At least some should be mentioned here as forerunners of the present important role of anthropologists providing relevant ethnographic data to their clinician colleagues.

Jules Henry, a representative of the culture and personality school in anthropology, assumed the role of an ethnographer in looking at the nature of schizophrenia as experienced in families with an identified child patient (Henry 1972). These naturalistic observations were carried out during one week which Henry spent with each of the five families from early morning until just before everyone retired at night. The work required of the anthropologist insights into the nature of a disease which, to this day, is not well understood. Henry met the challenge with unusual clinical sensitivity that he joined with his fine anthropological skills of observation and interviewing while participating in the daily life of each of the families as a companion/researcher.

Ethnographic exploration of the role of treatment institutions, and within each clinic, the specific roles of health care staff, was considered, even before Goffman's classic publication (Goffman 1961) as an important area for anthropological investigation by William Caudill. His study of the patient experience in a mental health in-patient institution required insights and skills different from those developed by anthropologists for fieldwork in small non-Western (indigenous) societies (Caudill 1958). Otto von Mering subsequently explored further the cultural premises that had an influence on the process of disease as it developed and became expressed in institutions, beginning with the family (von Mering 1970a), and extended to out-patient clinics, hospital settings, and other parts of the community. Edgerton (1967) in a study which became known among his anthropological colleagues only long after it was first published, probably because it was not considered to be "anthropology", focused on the coping styles of mentally retarded patients who showed abilities to function inside and outside institutions that exceeded the expectations and broad stereotypes about limitations, even among professionals.

We can gain a feeling of the activities during this period of thirty years ago and the relevance for subsequent events by reading Caudill's summary statement. It suggests that some of the activities and some of the issues flowing from them retain a sense of continuity over many years:

Social anthropologists and other social scientists have recently been doing some unusual things:

participating with physicians and in conferences on social medicine, teaching in medical schools, working with public health services in Peru, studying the social structure of hospitals and the flow of life on the wards, interviewing patients about to undergo plastic surgery, and doing psychotherapy with Plains Indians (Caudill 1953: 773).

Many changes took place during the intervening years, but Caudill's concluding observations reveal amazingly the continuity of unresolved points:

Just where anthropology might fit into the scheme of things is a complex problem. Medicine is itself in a state of flux: old definitions of disease and health are being called into question; there are many competing concepts of comprehensive medicine, environmental medicine, psychosomatic medicine, preventive medicine, etc . . . . There is much discussion of how the social sciences are to find their place in an already overcrowded medical curriculum. It is not, then, a simple matter to determine where applied anthropology fits into the maze that now constitutes the field of science in medicine (Caudill 1953:799).

To develop what Caudill considered a mutually desirable close collaborative relationship between medicine and anthropology would turn out to be, as he predicted, an arduous task. In his own career, Caudill maintained a close working relationship and personal ties to many physicians, mostly psychiatrists, who seem to have absorbed much valued knowledge from this association. Caudill had developed effective ways of communicating, both in the face to face contacts and in his publications which are widely read by psychiatrists.

Von Mering's work, in particular his position as a faculty member in a Department of Psychiatry, had similar effects. Actively associated with clinical health care settings since the early 1950's, von Mering combined a commitment and rootedness in the relevant theories of psychological anthropology and their application. He was holistically oriented to his own discipline, linking biological and social phenomena. Von Mering's perspective is Euro-American, and marked by an intimate knowledge and understanding of medicine as a social and scientific system, practiced by a profession with a strong historical tradition. For von Mering "the formal relationship between anthropology and medicine began one hundred years ago when the pathologist Rudolf Virchow helped found the first anthropological society in Berlin" (von Mering 1970b).

Cultural Experience of Illness

So overwhelming was the intitial impact of the modern science of medicine on thinking about health and sickness among physicians, that the anthropological theme concerning the cultural experience of illness and its important links with ethnicity was left out of awareness until much later. At a time when medical anthropology had not yet emerged as a separately identifiable sub-discipline of anthropology with a body of knowledge directly relevant to the modern health care professions, there was work done by individuals which illustrated the cultural nature of illness phenomena. In Mark Zborowski's studies, pain was shown to differ along lines of ethnicity as part of shared cultural experiences with different meanings and interpretations (Zborowski 1969). This work was carried out in hospitals through patient interviews and observations. It challenged the biomedically oriented medical approaches. In focusing on ethnic variation in symptom presentation, anthropological and sociological research, largely influenced by Talcott Parsons' eminent role at Harvard, proceeded side-by-side. Examples are the important studies by Zola (1966, 1973) on ethnic variations in symptom expression, and the work by Renée Fox, which is anthropological in orientation and methods (Fox 1959). Fox documented the clinical activities of medical specialists in a hospital unit that treated metabolic disorders, a field on the forward edge of medical knowledge of that time. These examples of research illustrate an almost dramatic quality of some patient experiences. Also, especially in the work of Fox, it can be shown how a researcher who approaches problems in clinical medical settings without negative bias can establish working relationships and therefore a research climate which permits unusual results and insights.

Human Relationships

Another consistent theme has been the microcosmic examination of human relationships found for example, in the work of Gregory Bateson. His ideas developed from a distinct theoretical position in which the nature and logic of relationships and their effect on individual interactions was the focus. Bateson traced these phenomena by contrasting the different implications of symmetrical and hierarchical relationships and the problems arising when one type of relationship was confounded by inappropriate communications (Bateson 1972). The theoretical foundations emerged in Bateson's early field studies in New Guinea and Bali. Their relevance for clinical psychiatric and general medical services was developed later in conjunction with psychiatrists. This work by Bateson in direct association with psychiatrists anticipated much of today's interest in role relationships among medical anthropologists, yet it never became a topic for self reflexivity. Later, Linda Alexander analyzed relationship problems arising in hemodialysis treatment for patients with failure in kidney functioning. In her work we find the clearest example of Bateson's influence on others in clinical medical anthropology (Alexander 1977).

Sociocultural Change

Yet another set of issues linking anthropology to health emerged earlier as a result of anthropological concern with change. Two separate developments can be traced. On the one hand, anthropologists like Anthony Wallace investigated change as a universal phenomenon affecting individuals and groups. Wallace developed a cognitive model that he linked to psychiatric phenomena (Wallace 1961). On the other hand, events after World War II presented American anthropologists with opportunities to study similar dimensions of theoretical significance related to areas of change in health conditions throughout the world. In Benjamin Paul's work the relevance of cultural conditions and social change for health behavior assumed a central place for Public Health teaching. The case studies prepared by Paul remain useful in teaching health officials until the present (Paul 1955). These examples illustrate the relationship of culture to practices that perpetuate infectious and communicable diseases. No longer was that a problem only for individual communities and small populations, but because of increasing communication through travel, it had become a world-wide concern. Public health and aid-oriented programs in the developed countries drew on anthropology for a better understanding of the cultural basis of health paractices and the appropriate leverage for change. Sanitation and other basic aspects of daily life as they are affected by varying styles of relating to the environment were the focus then, and continue. Changing them was seen as a matter of "introducing" superior practices and techniques but there were few tangible results. What has changed today is the awareness that community participation is the key to modifications in health-related behavior (see Anderson et al. this volume). What has often not changed sufficiently are the policy and administrative approaches to the problems, although there is now a broad appreciation of the cultural dimensions.

Community Psychiatry

Finally, and importantly, the work of anthropologists Jane Murphy, Charles Hughes, and others with Alexander Leighton, a psychiatrist, has been of great importance in the development of anthropological involvements with aspects of community psychiatry and epidemiology (Murphy 1976; Murphy and Leighton 1965). The ties to current challenges for psychiatry related to the community in various ways is quite apparent, and directly pursued, for example by Jane Murphy's continued work.

TRENDS

These prior concerns and related research projects continue as central themes in the work of the clinically applied anthropologists represented in this volume. Gaines shows how anthropologists in departments of psychiatry confront the issues of defining normal and abnormal in cross-cultural perspective and attempt to provide knowledge of specific cultures when diagnostic categories are in question. Blumhagen and Estroff provide ethnographic data on patients' experiences with illness in community contexts. Anthropological views of health care institutions and the impact of unexamined cultural assumptions on the nature of health care are of central concern in the Goods' exploration of patient requests and in the plan to increase the fit of patient and provider needs discussed by Anderson, Toledo, and Hazam.

A focus on ethnicity and its impact on understanding illnesses or the health care system persists in the work of many clinically applied anthropologists. Anderson and her colleagues found that a wide range of Mexican-American cultural patterns needed to be understood to work with cardiac patients and their families. Weidman's contributions at the University of Miami—Jackson Memorial Medical Center are founded on an extensive study of ethnic minorities. Yet the concepts and health care strategies deriving from this long-standing project can be generalized to many groups, including WASPs.

Examination of social relationships in health care settings and those underlying pathological conditions have also become an important part of clinically applied anthropology. Stein deftly uses knowledge of the former in his teaching of residents. Alexander follows Bateson in her contribution to this volume as she illustrates interactions among interpersonal relationships inside and outside health care settings. The strong anthropological link with public health, originated in the post-war period, is found here in the Byerly and Molgaard contribution in which a distinctive life style and its impact on the spread of disease is discussed. Finally, the continuing interest of community psychiatry may be found in Sue Estroff's contribution in which she documents current problems in implementing this treatment strategy.

If there were an impact of the earlier anthropological ventures into the culture of clinical medicine and health care, the effects were negligible. Whether the contributions of the current and larger group of clinically applied anthropologists will result in more remains to be seen. In the past, the negative evaluation by the majority of anthropologists of doing "applied" work raised barriers which were penetrated only by a few anthropologists who had a primary basic research identification, such as Caudill. Caudill's hospital study was probably the least generally known among his publications. The same applies to Robert Edgerton's remarkable study of the adaptation of mentally retarded patients.

BRIDGES TO THE HEALTH SCIENCES

If there is an increase of interest, and an incipient resonance, in academic anthropology related to work that builds bridges into applied areas, the reasons for it may have a variety of explanations. On the theoretical side, the growing interest in comparative studies of health systems as part of medical anthropology is a late, but important acknowledgement that attention to studies of Western phenomena related to health and health care are of anthropological relevance (Kleinman et al. 1975; Leslie 1976). Another set of factors can be traced to critical public reactions to health care, the increased emphasis on technological approaches in Western medicine, and the quest for a more humanistic, broadly based delivery of care. Within anthropology, a third factor is a shift in the employment situation. These new employment opportunities include not just medicine, but also primary medical care, aging, and community mental health, and research on the social aspects of diseases such as cancer, hypertension, diabetes, epilepsy, and the like.

The search for funding of academically based anthropological research, and a need to respond to growing pressure towards "relevance", brought about conferences and the publication of their results, partly at the initiative of the disciplines, partly because of the sponsoring funding agencies. Margaret Mead, throughout her career, communicated effectively to non-anthropologists (including health professionals) in positions of influence and decision making, how anthropology could contrbibute effectively to human problem solving. She was the most vocal proponent of applied and problem focused anthropological research. Laura Nader, in legal anthropological research by her and her students, provides another example of a combination of widely recognized scholarship with attention and contribution to problem areas in society. Bela Maday, through his personal commitment and his professional role as an anthropologist in the National Institute of Mental Health, assisted anthropologists in developing and carrying out basic research that could have an impact on the development of mental health policies and programs. These and other anthropologists assumed realistic and supportive positions in struggles with the realities of research support. Relevance of research for specific health and mental health problems, as it is understood outside anthropology, had to be dealt with and balanced against the need for freedom from the constraints of specific institutional interests and health professional dominance.

Because we worked for so long as anthropologists in what seemed to be non-reactive field situations, we assumed naively and unrealistically the purity of anthropological research. Acting as though such work were immune from community and broader institutional social and political concerns, anthropologists were awakened by events in the 1960's to the fact they lived in a real world to which they owed more than research reports and monographs. Valuable lessons were learned, more slowly perhaps than in other social science disciplines. Culture as a concept, and as part of social and political realities, has been accepted broadly, more often in spite of anthropology's reluctance to become involved, than with the help of anthropologists. The issues raised directly and indirectly in this book cannot be separated from the general professional values and the ideals of the discipline as a whole. Medical settings as field situations are not only subjects of research, they are institutions that have specific tasks, specific requirements for all participants; the "neutral" observer role is useful and sometimes tolerated or even requested by such institutions. In effect, hoever, it is never neutral, never without reactivity.

The growing number of anthropologists in health care settings could be taken as good evidence for an increasing need and openness of medical institutions for anthropological contributions. Yet, without adidtional systematic assessments of the situation such as that provided by Logan (1979), this remains a speculative and probably discipline-centered sanguine view. In fact, there are more anthropologists in health science settings today than there were a decade ago. But their number is still so small and their professional profile so low, that there is an almost daily necessity for anthropologists in health science schools to explain their role to those in the health professions and to patients — and often to themselves. The fact is that there is no general job description for a medical anthropologist in hospitals and other health care institutions. The title "clinical anthropologist" sounds good to many, but strikes clinicians as a threat to their control over therapy. The general ideas of systems analyst or cultural specialist are too vague to convey any practical significance. Individual struggles to define positions for anthropologists as teachers, researchers, or administrators in health settings have occasionally been won, but frequently they have been lost because of uncertainty over what they would actually do. In addition, in these times of budget cuts, there is a sense that whatever they do is marginal, not a central activity.

If there were job descriptions or visible and successful role models for anthropologists in health care, major public and private institutions would more likely respond positively. As it is, for most anthropologists the exploration of opportunities in clinical settings is left to personal initiative. This results in low visibility and idiosyncratic examples without much generalizability. It is hard to imagine that medical institutions will reach out to anthropologists without more concentrated and relevant effort on our part.

Yet there have been, and continue to be, opportunities. There is the growing recognition that health care systems are overinvested in biomedically based, organ pathology medicine. This has resulted in limited and highly specialized curing, but does not always eventuate in humanistic caring in which prevention and health maintenance are linked to the complex interactions among organic and psychosocial systems. George Engle's biopsychosocial systems model has gained wide attention in medicine, for example (Engle 1977). Change will occur if constructive approaches are tried within the system. Frontal attacks such as those of Illich (1975) and others could hardly be expected to accomplish more than a defensive closing of ranks.

Bringing the new and growing awarenesses of health professionals closer to ongoing and expanding medical anthropology is more likely to occur if we can show that anthropology can make a cost effective contribution. The challenge is to build bridges between clinical and academic emphases. The basis for these links can be found now in the publications of clinician anthropologists, anthropologically oriented health professionals, and clinician-anthropologist teams. These obvious bridge builders include Kleinman (1980), Fabrega (1974), and Eisenberg (1977) among the physicians and Brink (1976) and Leininger (1978) among the nurses. But their significant statements tend to get lost unless they are frequently reiterated and backed by practical demonstrations. Anthropological publication in clinical journals is essential and can reach large numbers of readers (e.g., Kleinman et al. 1978). When followed by others and by case illustrations, the basis can be laid for acknowledgement, interest, and possibly greater receptiveness to anthropological participation in clinical care. More often, though, the easier thing to do has been to publish for our own in anthropology journals, ignoring the challenging medical and popular audiences.

It is also important to recognize the most receptive audiences within the health professions. These tend to be those more marginal to high prestige medicine — or, stated positively, those central to comprehensive and personal care: Public Health, Nursing, Community and Social Medicine, Family Medicine, and Psychiatry. These specialties are highly aware of ever growing patient care problems concerned with social and psychosomatic issues, ethnic differences, compliance, and chronicity. Surgery and subspecialty internal medicine seem impermeable to anthropological input. Yet as Renée Fox regularly notes (Fox 1979), these core disciplines are of special importance precisely because they are at the center of medical teaching and research.

To build bridges with any of these disciplines, anthropologists need to adequately understand the culture of the clinical medical setting. This understanding requires an appreciation for shared responsibilities and therefore for constant accountability to the system itself and to the individuals with whom there is professional contact in solving a problem, including the patient. Yet anthropological experience varies. The style of learning and communication in medical settings is markedly different from that of liberal arts departments where anthropologists spend many of their formative years. In health science settings, verbal presentations center around problems presented in a structured fashion, usually in the form of cases that are followed by discussions in which alternative options are considered, but viable solutions, not intellectual debate, are the objective. A key problem for the anthropologists is posed by the paradox that theory in clinical settings is often negatively valued, yet anthropological contributions frequently center on critiques of tacit theory and values. These contributions are necessary, *but they must be made practical*. Self reflexive examination and consideration of alternative perspectives, so central to anthropological discourse, are foreign to most clinicians; but these too can be taught if they are made relevant to core clinical tasks.

Most importantly, anthropologists usually do not participate in the most valued and central activity: *taking responsibility for the care of the patient*. They are outsiders, not recognized members of the health care team. The symbolic activity with direct practical consequences in this respect is the authority to make written entries in the patient chart. The legal responsibility that goes with the general role and specific charting activities of health care team members is a further complication. For the clinician, the practitioner-patient relationship and the responsibility that goes with it, is central to the clinical task, no matter how this relationship is defined and shaped by individuals. It is the basic and major ideological basis for practicing medicine. There is no parallel in anthropological ideology and activities, with the exception of a continuing search among those who do applied anthropology.

Anthropologists can point to virtually nothing in their professional training or experience that parallels the service objectives of health professionals and to the legal and ethical demands placed upon them. Only recently has there been much communication about how anthropologists fare in non-academic, service oriented positions. *Practicing Anthropology* is filling that needed gap. Practical strategies need to be developed in clinically applied anthropology to demonstrate how we can justify our existence in economic terms. The subject of ethics is amenable to anthropological discussion, particularly when populations with diverse values and beliefs are considered. Yet this area remains underdeveloped in the anthropological literature. Anthropological approaches, carrying well founded conviction that would penetrate the health sciences, would serve us well as we attempt to exert stronger influences on the decision making processes in which health professionals engage.

These basic differences between anthropologists and health practitioners make it difficult for clinicians to view anthropologists as collaborators. The locus of power in decisions about how to use anthropological information and analyses remains with the clinicians. There is thus the tendency for health professionals to learn only what they believe is relevant about culture, health beliefs and practices, life style, ethnic identity, and the like. The translations to clinical practice under these conditions are likely to be made in the context of biomedical frameworks, reducing the potential for the humanizing and holistic influences of anthropology. An example is the recent separate emergence of transcultural psychiatry within psychiatry. It is too new as a specialty to predict whether it will invite direct participation by anthropologists. It is more likely, however, that cultural dimensions of clinical care, as understood by these psychiatrists, will be incorporated into their own direct and familiar clinical activities and research. The danger is that this translation may reduce cultural analysis from a robust relativist critique to a handmaiden of clinical universalism. Here we touch on the very sensitive area of professional territoriality and maintenance of professional niches, the most practical and vigorously defended interest in all health care professional specialties. If anthropology has so far succeeded anywhere, especially in the perception of physicians, it is in the low saliency, low profile, and low power position of anthropologists when they are compared to other social science based clinicians, psychologists, social workers, and lately, nurse clinicians.

Given these discrepancies between anthropologists and clinicians, what should anthropological contributions be? How can they be presented in ways that complement and expand the contributions made currently by health practitioners? The authors of chapters in this volume were invited to share their knowledge and experiences to provide anthropologists with role models for some of the activities going on now. Other kinds of positions are possible as more anthropologists attempt to enter the academic medical establishment and, beyond that, other clinical arenas. Whatever develops, we strongly believe that anthropologists must function as social scientists who are involved in contributions that directly and indirectly affect patients even though we do not directly assume treatment responsibilities. We can point to Linda Alexander's position in a School of Medicine in which she created collaborative relationships with clinicians, while making an independent contribution that she describes as potentially self supporting (Alexander 1979: 7). Another significant possibility is the consultant position. Most of us engage in informal consultations as part of normal collegial interactions. These might be expanded into full time slots, particularly when they can be linked with some teaching and research in clinical settings.

The key element in these and other scenarios for the future will be the abilities of clinically applied anthropologists to remold our discipline's knowledge base and unique perspectives into forms that aid our clinician colleagues in their central patient care tasks and make clear to patients that our activities contribute to their receipt of more humanistic care. In essence, we must modify — popularize — our exotic and esoteric findings and perspectives in ways that help practitioners and patients understand themselves and each other better. In carrying out these services, we promote practitioner and patient understanding of us. This is a useful first step in the even longer process of solving the problem of who should pay for what we do, and how. In sum, we need to acknowledge the realities of health science settings and to attempt to fit into this environment with the same kind of cultural sensitivity, awareness, and adaptability that we have been attempting to teach for these many years.

NATURE OF THE HEALTH SCIENTIST AUDIENCE

Medical and other health science schools have had anthropologists on their staffs for a relatively long period of time, particularly in departments of psychiatry. For introductions, it is "our" anthropologist; yet medical and other health care specialists have, in most instances, no clear sense of what to think or expect of an anthropologist. The gap of real awareness and understanding of anthropology by health professionals is something for anthropology to ponder and patiently endure. If there is any notion at all, it harks back to some introductory course in the past which covered everything from early hominids to contemporary pygmies, but nothing that could explain the presence of an anthropologist in a health care institution. The same is true for patients. One at the University of Washington wondered whether her family doctors considered her to be a "cave woman" after the anthropologist visited her in the hospital room.

There are cultural gaps that only effective and appropriate communication skills on the part of the anthropologist can hope to bridge. The basic science background and orientation of most health practitioners widens the gap. As scientists, clinicians are trained to rely on "hard" facts, often quantified and coveyed in a concrete and concise manner. The amount of hard data which is assimilated and expected to be remembered in medicine and nursing has no parallel in the social sciences. Anthropologists soon discover other cultural aspects of clinical medical settings. Technical language, the jargon of clinical interactions, and the various symbolisms in professional-to-professional and practitioner-patient interactions are all evident. The meaning and use of *time* contrast with experiences in both academic and community settings. Resident and attending physicians on the same medical service must know each other's whereabouts at all times. This heightened sensitivity to the location of significant professionals in the system may extend to others, including the anthropologist. Availability, an instant response to a beeper or phone call, are second nature in such an environment. Unavailability, even if there is no real professional urgency, can set up negative communication potentials. Examples in this area are endless, and decisions regarding style of response are complex and challenging for the anthropologist.

Among nurses in hospitals, much of this urgency is to be found, partly as a reflection of the demands of their physician colleagues. Nursing schools, however, seem to differ from medical schools in at least one important respect. A higher proportion of the faculty have Ph.D. degrees — at least in schools found in university health science centers. This means that the anthropologist is likely to work with peers with similar advanced degrees. Yet here another difference emerges. In contrast with schools of medicine wherein most anthropologists are not clinicians, virtually all anthropologists in nursing schools are nurses (Brink 1979).

As "natives", these anthropologists know the subculture in which they are enmeshed, have engaged in patient care, and practice and teach in clinical settings. Yet they are evidently not released from the common frustrations of anthropologists in other health science schools. They too note the frustrations with their colleagues' lack of understanding of anthropology. In comparison to the biological science orientation predominating in medical schools (and clearly evident in nursing schools), the behavioral sciences are strongly represented in schools of nursing. However, doctoral preparation in behavioral science tends to be in education, social psychology, or sociology, all of which frequently take a "hard data" approach to their research on social behavior. Hence, pursuit of meanings, values, and qualitative ethnographic issues is viewed as alien and pseudoscientific.

The situation is somewhat different in schools of public health. The increasing numbers of anthropologists who have completed degrees in public health (usually the M.P.H.) indicates the affinity between the two fields; not merely the potential practicality for the Ph.D. anthropologist of carrying a health-oriented label (Schreiber and Scrimshaw 1979). The disciplines represented in public health schools complement anthropology and most have compatible philosophies. As a profession, Public Health has a social orientation. It is directed toward communities, toward health as a goal rather than illness as a condition requiring intervention, and toward international perspectives. Well established schools of public health are academically rigorous in their approaches to health-related phenomena, much like highly ranked centers of anthropological training. Of all the health sciences, including social work, public health is most likely to give anthropologists a feeling of kinship.

With all their variability, the different health science schools share a most important feature: a culture whose most significant element is biomedicine. (This is also true in the more multidiciplinary field of public health since most programs have disease-prevention at least as a basic premise.) A second fundamental feature is the clinical or service mandate of the practitioners (or soon to be practitioners) — the mandate to care for and help cure patients. Even though American anthropologists were raised going to. the doctor and thus have a patient's-eye-view and acceptance of the system, the professional beliefs, assumptions, and behaviors of health practitioners are different from those of anthropologists in a number of key ways. There are also important similarities and clinically applied anthropologists have learned the value of stressing similarities in order to make ironing out the difficulties easier.

Anthropologists and health practitioners both approach the same subject matter (people) in highly descriptive ways; the case study is a fundamental element for both. Moreover, a biological conception of people — the basic approach· of health practitioners — is a strong traditional element in anthropology. Although stereotypic biomedicine is frequently seen to ignore patterns of behavior and the importance of social relationships — the key areas of interest for anthropologists — the behavioral consequences and correlates of sickness are strongly lodged in biomedical thought and practice. This is more true in nursing than in medicine, given nurses' mandate to aid people to cope with everyday life. Thus, biology and behavior as critical interest areas are shared, but with very different emphases among the health sciences and anthropology, and with cultural norms and social structure only a late arrival and marginal biomedical concern.

Although there are these basic similarities in descriptive, biological, and behavioral approaches, anthropologists and health scientists differ substantially in how they handle the information and what they do with it. These data gathered by a health practitioner are collated into a pattern and concretized into a diagnosis. Anthropologists engage in a similar task. However, the analysis rarely stops with the assessment of an individual pattern and even more rarely is this pattern phrased at the biological level. Anthropologists attempt to work comparatively to fit the individual into a cultural setting, and further to compare across cultures. Moreover, anthropologists are highly attuned to multiple, alternative (and sometimes competing) analytic models, a significant contrast with the predominant focus on biomedical explanations in the health sciences. Our ecological and systems approaches are only now becoming important in the health sciences, particularly in nursing, family and community medicine, and psychiatry. In general, clinicians perceive our appreciation and use of alternative models and perspectives as a source of analytic "weakness".

What is done with the information also differs when anthropologists are compared with health practitioners. With their more expansive analysis of behavior patterns, anthropologists hope to achieve understanding and perhaps to produce generalizations relating to consistencies and inconsistencies in human behavior historically and cross-culturally. A psychiatrist remarked in conversation recently that academics have the freedom to sit and ponder — and that there was no real hurry. Health practitioners, on the other hand, have a therapeutic mandate to aid their clients now to solve the usually exigent problem that is the subject of the consultation. Diagnosis, and its implications for treatment, is the stopping place for understanding. Action in the form of treatment must follow. Assessment (understanding) must be thorough enough that a treatment mistake will be unlikely to occur, but treatment is the focus.

In order to even begin to adapt and to contribute in a health science school, the anthropologist must understand and work within the confines of the reductionist and action oriented clinical style of health practitioners. The pejorative stereotype of an anthropologist called to consult about the bizarre behavior of a foreign or ethnic patient includes the complaint that the anthropologist is fully able to discourse at length about the general cultural pattern in which the patient's behavior might fit (e.g., grieving, sullenness, carrying out healing ceremonies), but he or she is unable to "tell us what to do!" Telling practitioners what they should do — treatment — is foreign to anthropological styles.

One way to approach this problem, and thus facilitate the integration of the anthropologist into the clinical setting, whether teaching or clinical practice, is to recognize and reinforce the strengths of the clinician — i.e., positively appraise the role that is enacted and then to go further. First, the anthropologist must recognize that the clinician is working with an individual and that unique problems must be recognized. Then it is useful to differentiate what can be done to aid diagnosis versus help that can be provided in management of the case.

Medical diagnosis is a process in which symptoms (both behavioral and biological) are seen as manifestations of internal biological processes — an empiricist model of clinical reasoning (Good and Good 1981) in which the fleeting phenomena related to sickness can be related to the absolute reality of hard biological science. As the Goods point out, clinicians are reluctant to accept the anthropological fact that symptoms are culturally constructed. Cases such as those presented in the Good and Good paper (1981) and in the Kleinman chapter in this volume may aid in lending credibility to anthropological suggestions about diagnosis. But nothing surpasses successful experiences with clinicians. Another approach is the appeal to current attempts to restructure clinical practice from within the professions, such as Engle's perspective (Engle 1977). The anthropologist can argue that specific sociocultural factors can be included in the biopsychosocial model.

The second area in which anthropological insight can be directly relevant is in the management of a case after a diagnosis has been made. This is far easier to do since clinicians recognize that compliance is a fundamental clinical problem and many are ready to accept the proposition that social and cultural features of a person's life have a major effect on compliance. Anthropological contributions can be far-ranging in this area and are less likely to conflict with clinicians' convictions than is true in the diagnostic phase. For example, the patient's explanatory model, which may have been seen merely as a source of invalidity during diagnosis, can be presented as the cornerstone for negotiation during the management phase of therapy. In addition, attention to the patient's illness problems, effects of the sickness on the daily life of the patient (see Kleinman in this volume), may provide the means for a clinician to motivate a person to follow through with the regimen in order to reduce these problems and an opportunity to demonstrate anthropology's benefits to the clinician.

A third sphere in which anthropologists might contribute is related to both prevention and curative therapy. This possibility exists in aiding health practitioners to work with their clients' social networks. Vivian Garrison, for example, points out that the maintenance of schizophrenics in community settings can be facilitated by involving members of the natural support network in the therapy (1978). Disease prevention, an area receiving much more attention by health practitioners recently, might also benefit from a social network approach. For example, insofar as supportive social networks may confer protection from either the occurrence or severity of disease (Brown et al. 1975), clinicians who are helped to identify networks with anthropologist help or by using anthropological techniques may be interested in strengthening supportive networks of social relationships. This could be done either directly – working with a whole family for example – or indirectly through teaching clients how to maintain appropriately strong social ties.

In all cases, the clinically applied anthropologist should be able to begin with the practical constraints facing the health practitioner. Working within the heavily biological diagnosis and management paradigm as above is critical. But it is also important to expand this biological perspective in ways that *do not seem* to conflict with the professional style of the clinician. However, one of the major goals of anthropology in health science settings is in fact to introduce and maintain a contrasting approach to patient care. Chrisman (this volume), Kleinman (1980), Fabrega (1974), and others call for the addition of a complementary sociocultural paradigm. Kleinman (1980) notes that the integration of ethnomedicine with biomedicine would ultimately provoke a restructuring of medicine as currently constituted — and no discipline takes a sanguine view of its own internal change. If a paradigm shift (toward a meaning centered ethnomedical approach) were to take place in medicine, nursing, and public health, it might have the further salutory effect of strengthening the conceptual integration among these professions.

The role of an anthropologist, once established and accepted, usually includes introducing more and more sociocultural material into biomedicine, material that is not always complimentary. Conflict in ideas neither can nor should be avoided. But such open disagreement, and consequent opportunities for change in both parties, can probably be achieved only by working within biomedicine as a known, trusted, and valued colleague. Dispelling stereotypes and the fears that may underpin them does not imply that the anthropologist must become a conformist member of "their team". But with collegial team relationships, one can more effectively engage and instruct colleagues on cultural analysis, including the exploration of cherished professional values and behaviors, provided that this analysis can be demonstrated to contribute to clinical teaching and patient care.

ANTHROPOLOGIST ROLES

The two basic and interdependent tasks facing an anthropologist in a health science school are (1) establishing a recognizable position or role in the social system and (2) contributing to the education of students. The teaching obligation usually constitutes the reason the anthropologist was hired, though a number take research positions and teach as they are able. Teaching also "makes sense" as a job description; it is what anthropologists tend to do. However, health science schools do not replicate the previous undergraduate and graduate educational experiences of the anthropologist. This is particularly true of the clinical and resident years in a medical school, in which time is not organized into quarters or semesters and regularly scheduled 50 minute class segments. The Kleinman and Stein contributions to this volume indicate that meetings with residents or medical students in clerkships frequently take place on clinical units. In addition, topics cannot be planned in advance.

Schools of nursing and public health and the preclinical medical school curriculum are more structured around regular class times and classrooms, but anthropological content is usually introduced into the curriculum in a different way than that found in an anthropology department. For example, as Ness points out in his paper, the anthropologist may take responsibility for some number of hours of instruction in large introductory behavioral science courses given in the preclinical medical curriculum. This same phenomenon is found in nursing and public health: guest lectures on either cross-cultural theoretical perspectives or ethnic and overseas health practices. In addition, anthropologists may offer elective courses (e.g., Ritenbaugh in this volume; Kay 1978) for health science and/or anthropology students on special topics in medical anthropology.

Although Chrisman's paper in this volume depicts a nearly traditional class and classroom type of teaching situation, this is atypical. Brink (1979) points out that schools of nursing that hire anthropologists do so because of their clinical background in nursing and they are expected to teach nursing practice. Thus, pediatric, obstetrical, psychiatric, or community health nursing taught by a nurse-anthropologist, like Kleinman's psychiatric clerkship, is clinical content modified by an anthropological perspective. This is similar to the presence of anthropology in schools of public health. Most of the courses listed by Schreiber and Scrimshaw (1979) are on traditional public health topics. Thus, in the health science schools reviewed here, the aspect of anthropological participation most familiar to the anthropologist — contributing to the education of student — is constructed differently from the anthropologist's past experience. The anthropologist cannot just *be* a professor.

What the anthropologist *should* be in terms of the multitude of roles possible simply cannot be predicted. The individual adaptations of a number of us are outlined or implied in our contributions. Each has been the result of relatively unique personal histories with overlapping areas determined in large measure by our common anthropological backgrounds. (Although most of us are sociocultural anthropologists, Ritenbaugh is a physical anthropologist.) It is true, however, that the set of decisions that underlie the anthropologist's presentation of self in the health science schools is (a close) second only to competence in anthropology in determining acceptance and thus productivity.

Anthropologists have all faced and solved the problem of establishing a role in a novel context when we carried out ethnographic fieldwork. In that process, the key was to have a brief role description that was all encompassing enough to allow elaboration in situations in which precision was needed. Frequently, the statement is something like: "I'm here to learn about your way of life so I can write a book." The same is needed in a health science school. There are some very important differences in the two contexts, however. One is that anthropology graduate students are required to know the ethnographic literature related to the focal area and group. Secondly, the research is usually accomplished away from one's own culture and thus away from one's own set of cultural meanings. Thirdly, the anthropologist usually does not intend to continue living in that culture so social relationships and sociopolitical position are not as major a concern as they otherwise would be, and as they certainly are to the clinically applied anthropologist.

We strongly recommend that anthropologists who intend to work in health science settings prepare well for the novel field. The most important element in this process is to know anthropology well — well enough to talk about it with conviction and precision, but in a way that is unlikely to be perceived as "talking down". This is easy to say, but very difficult to do. The issue of "jargon" is one of the most vexing. What is technical language for us is jargon for health practitioners; where jargon essentially means "language that obscures simple meanings that could be grasped by anybody if the speaker would just be clearer."

The simple issue of terminology sits astride one of the most infuriating problems of working in a health science setting: what anthropologists talk about is the patterning of life, and since health practitioners live their own lives, what we say sounds like common sense – *once we say it*. For example, the bit of information that family members are involved in the illness episode of one of their number seems to be frequently overlooked during patient care with its one to one style in America. Anthropological research forces the conclusion that the negative consequences of ignoring this fact – low compliance for example (see the Anderson, Toledo, and Hazam contribution), or inadequate care – should be remedied. Simply teaching about the importance of the family in health care can be seen as repeating common sense. Delivering a lecture on comparative family systems identifying variation in role relationships can be seen as jargon-filled irrelevancy. The middle ground lies in making the basic point, preferably using terms from the profession that constitutes the audience, and referring to research results that suggest that using this knowledge has been successful in similar (or the same) situations. What needs to be conveyed is understanding, a perspective of the phenomenon, not the intricacies of anthropology as a discipline. But that understanding must be conveyed convincingly, promoting the recognition that there is a conceptual and empirical basis for the ideas that could be reviewed if required.

A necessary, but not the only perspective to be advanced, is that clients of health practitioners need to be understood in the context of their life styles. Frequently, anthropological terminology (jargon) can be useful in helping to define a patient's life patterns in ways that illuminate the problem more clearly. It is up to the anthropologist to demonstrate that the clarity serves a purpose in patient care. Exotic cultural patterns are fun to know (for both anthropologists and others); but for this knowledge to have lasting impact, it should be relevant to helping patients to solve problems. The irony here is that very little anthropological knowledge of mainstream American culture is available, increasing our difficulties.

From this description, it is clear that the knowledge of anthropology referred to above is a transaction between anthropological knowledge and the needs of health practitioners. Anthropological understanding of those needs returns our attention to the relevance of anthropological fieldwork, presentation of self, and adaptation to the health sciences. First, knowledge of the culture of the group with whom one will work: there are two helpful types of literature. One contains behavioral science analyses of health practitioners and is useful in understanding the professions. The other is the clinical literature of the profession, which aids in discovering how they write about what they are interested in.

With a good foundation in this literature, the anthropologist is better prepared to understand one aspect of the culture with which he or she will work. However, there is another set of cultural variables that is frequently more difficult to surmount. This difficulty resides in the fact that the experience in a health science center occurs in one's own culture and thus one is embedded within existing, and sometimes unexamined, cultural meanings.

One of these meanings concerns anthropologists' perceptions and expectations of health practitioners, usually drawn from our experiences as lay consumers of care, though amplified by our knowledge of social science critiques of medicine. Like many other Americans we tend to be concerned with the impersonal, disease oriented approach of Western medicine and its lack of a holistic focus. Since practitioners also worry about these problems, the presence of the anthropologist may have been one attempt to introduce holism and humanism to the neophyte practitioners. We have a fine line to walk in this area. When anthropologists are perceived as strident and personal critiics of medical care, we run the risk of simply being ignored, because of having been offensive. On the other hand, the discipline of anthropology really can make contributions toward greater achievement of holism and humanism. The key seems to be the demonstration of a well founded professional and disciplined stance in which the objective, *shared* (and openly acknowledge as such) with our health science colleagues, is modification in contemporary patterns of health care delivery.

A second and closely related problem is the traditional anthropologist's desire to identify with, or root for the underdog — in this case, the patient who might well be us. This is especially true when the people in control, usually physicians, project an image of competent authority. Under these circumstances, anthropologists might be tempted to delight in pointing to the doctor's feet of clay (easily discovered when we share the backstage with physicians) and/or supporting an overly romanticized view of the strengths of folk healers or patients themselves. Again, since both these activities have a legitimate place in the education of health science students, it is necessary to develop a well argued framework for such criticism and deliver comments tactfully and appropriately. Moreover, a romantic view of alternative patterns of care — many of whose benefits for patients' welfare have been inadequately documented and whose injuries are little better known — is easily dismantled, particularly by our experienced and well traveled practitioner colleagues who have seen negative outcomes of folk treatment in their examination rooms.

A further word is necessary on the nature of power and its distribution in the health science school. Anthropologists, who are accustomed to the more egalitarian style of interaction and debate of an academic department, need to quickly learn how to work within the frequently rigid hierarchy of a health science school. As Atwood Gaines points out in his contribution, status differences between residents and attending physicians or local faculty and visiting dignitaries can determine the outcome of diagnostic debate. Gaines also suggests that the "gadfly" suggestions of an anthropologist, particularly if he or she is outside the line of authority, may be ignored or seen to be intrusive. Furthermore, Hazel Weidman has discussed the relative and time- or issue-bound merits of choosing a staff position (one of a group working together on common tasks) or a line position (accountable for actions in a chain of authority). The flexibility and freedom to roam that the staff anthropologist possesses carry with them some impotence in determining policy. It is evident that some of the activities Kleinman writes about in his paper in this volume would have been impossible except for his position as chief of the consultation-liaison service. In contrast, Chrisman's experiences in a school of nursing seem less bound by hierarchy.

One of the thorniest issues related to cultural meanings in a health science context influences both anthropological teaching and research: namely, biomedicine as a theoretical perspective. Young (1976) and others have shown that in our research, anthropologists have explicitly or implicitly drawn on clinical medicine as the standard for judging the "real" world of sickness. We have taken biomedicine as *the* etic view of sickness. In teaching too it is easy to over-adopt a biomedical view of sickness, especially since we were raised with respect for health practitioners' abilities to cure, and because most anthropologists do not know enough biomedicine to be critical of that part of health care delivery. A helpful antidote to this lack of knowledge is to be knowledgable about clinical praxis. Kleinman (1980) outlines five clinical functions that can be examined cross-culturally and thus can be applied in U.S. health science schools. It is also helpful – and soon may be essential – to be very well versed in biomedical theory and practice.

Some familiarity with biomedicine, and certainly knowledge about how practitioners perceive patients and their duties in respect to them, is valuable. A case can therefore be made to require basic knowledge (as it might be taught in two semesters) in anatomy and physiology for all clinically applied anthropologists. Just as anthropologists take it for granted that fieldworkers learn the language of the people in their field settings, so is the language of biomedicine a prerequisite to the clinical "field". Such bilingual and bicultural competence is desirable because strategies for patient care and reading about them in medical records are based on a biomedical model. From this perspective it is an easy step to argue that the best anthropologist in a health science school – other than public health schools which are composed of a strong mix of disciplines – should be a clinician with a degree in anthropology. As Brink (1979) shows, this is already the rule in schools of nursing. The advantages are manifold: the clinician would know both languages and be competent in the activities of both; the person would have a "native" understanding of the clinical mandate and possess credibility with students and faculty colleagues.

There is, however, a disadvantage. The seeds of change frequently may be found in the presence of 'strangers'. The very fact that the non-clinician anthropologist is not a native implies that new and different questions will be asked, research carried out to discover novel answers and novel suggestions made to improve practice. Implicit in this argument is the notion that it is not simply education in anthropology – or anthropology the discipline – that can contribute to health science education; it is also the presence of people whose basic commitment is different from that of clinicians. Yet they must also share concern for the clinicians' commitments.

There is also a disadvantage to anthropology. Applied anthropologists have long argued (Firth 1981) that anthropological theory benefits through testing those theories in real situations. The same is obviously true in clinically applied anthropology. Interdisciplinary projects such as those reported in this volume by Anderson and her colleagues and Weidman benefit anthropology while they enrich the health sciences. In addition, the literature in medical anthropology concerned with clinical problems from biomedicine has significantly increased over the last decade, in part because clinical problems have stimulated the interests of anthropologists in health science settings.

Another problematic area related to the culture of biomedicine facing the anthropologist is part of the set of expectations health practitioners have of anthropological teaching. "If anthropologists are interested in the 'cross-cultural', then they must be interested in *other* cultures." Thus, the teaching contributions might be expected only in the field of international health — significantly narrowing opportunities for anthropologists. Luckily, we have moved beyond that for the most part; but only to be caught in the next logical step. "Anthropologists must be interested in and knowledgeable about ethnic groups." Although it is certainly true that anthropologists are likely to be experts on one or a few ethnic groups, most of us desire to have a broader based set of contributions than just statements about ethnic cultural patterns and their relationships to health care. In this volume, both Weidman and Chrisman explicitly stress the importance of teaching a *perspective* in which cultural factors influencing all people's lives is the focus. And in fact the majority of chapters found here do not single out one ethnic group for consideration.

Clinically applied anthropologists should know a great deal about ethnic groups — racially or linguistically distinct and otherwise — especially those that are present in the local community and comprise the patient population. But our broader interests lie in the cultural characteristics of all kinds of groups: regional, age, religious, handicapped, chronically ill, immigrant, and the like. The difficulty our clinician colleagues have with this anthropological interest is perceptual. They frequently do not perceive that cultural patterns among these other kinds of groups make a difference in patient care. When confronted with a non-English speaking Southeast Asian refugee, the clinician is at a loss about what to do. And, to the credit of anthropological presence over the last few decades, clinicians now know that they need more than just linguistic knowledge to provide care. With patients whose cultural perspectives are not so obtrusive, however, health practitioners are likely to believe that the common sense that has served them so well in the past will do so in the future.

Another aspect of practitioner expectations about anthropological ethnic expertise is simultaneously problematic and the source of a solution. The problem is that clinicians view the ethnic knowledge they need as concrete and bounded — much like the biological knowledge with which they are more familiar. In other cases when such explicit knowledge is called for — e.g., ethics, pregnancy, diabetics, or the elderly — the teaching mechanism is a panel. Experts — including representatives of ethnic groups in some cases — deliver relevant knowledge in short bursts of verbiage.

A key to the solution is for anthropologists on panels to attempt to adopt the style of presentation — the short burst and high patient care relevance — and even some of the concreteness of ethnic or subcultural information. In addition, however, the anthropologist must also make a set of statements about perspective. Kleinman's chapter here suggests one way to accomplish this. That is, discrete concepts such as explanatory model, illness problem, or negotiation can be used in discussing the relationship of ethnic content — or other topics — to patient care. These concepts, with brief definitions, place the topical content in a broader social science framework and signal the existence of behavioral and social processes that must be known in addition to the trait list of ethnic characteristics.

At the University of Washington Health Sciences Center, the panel technique, combined with concrete concepts, has worked well in teaching family practice residents. Three faculty — anthropologist, psychiatrist/anthropologist, and family doctor — have for four years provided "Clinical Social Science Rounds" for the family medicine residency (Smilkstein et al. 1981). These rounds are monthly so there is the opportunity to build on past performances. However, the principle of providing data about various patient subcultures and ethnic heritage within the framework of a broader perspective has proven its value.

What these continuities, problems, and trends mean for anthropologists in health science schools is, in large measure, the persistence of challenge. In the presence of these challenges anthropologists must do more than just respond with tactical strategies to solve each problem on an ad hoc basis. The presence of anthropologists in health science schools for more than four decades indicates that we are capable of fathoming the needs and peculiarities of health science professionals. With this information and more importantly, with the increasing knowledge base in anthropology as it relates to understanding health needs and health care, anthropologists can act, not react, in clinical teaching and care settings. Of course, this means that we must be committed to collaborating with practitioners in pursuit of health care goals. Collaboration does not imply that we adopt their culture as it is — we do not need white coats. What we do need is specific information about cultural patterns related to health care, and specific — and communicable — concepts that aid in transmitting that information. In addition, clinically applied anthropologists must continue developing principles for our work that are generalizable as guides for those who follow us and that have been successful so that the clinical settings in which we work will be more receptive to anthropologists.

We hope that an advance toward those goals is reflected in the contributions to this volume. In designing the format and inviting authors we paid less attention to being representative and more to diversity. Although readers should find a great deal in the chapters that will help in day to day activities, answers will not be found. Instead, the reader should find role models for teaching and research in health science settings; contributions that experienced clinically applied anthropologists are making now that can be expanded upon for the future.

OVERVIEW OF CONTRIBUTIONS

The format for this book is based on the idea that most clinically applied anthropologists are involved in teaching in one way or another; ranging from formal teaching appointments to the sporadic desire (and need) to teach in the course of doing research. Thus, the first section is devoted to examples of what and how people teach. A second premise, and the basis for the second section, is that anthropologists in clinical settings need access to medical anthropological research that is clinically relevant.

Section I allows the reader a glimpse at the ways five anthropologists teach in health science schools. These include discussions based upon a number of settings in medical schools, one from a nursing school, and two more individualized contributions. We had hoped for a contribution from an anthropologist teaching in a school of public health, but a number of unavoidable personal difficulties prevented its completion. We begin with Robert Ness who teaches in the pre-clinical medical school curriculum. He demonstrates the need to become involved in team teaching efforts and the likelihood that an anthropologist will teach unfamiliar subjects. In his case, participation in the introductory clinical medicine course opens the door to two more specific and more anthropologically oriented teaching situations: teaching interviewing skills and cross-cultural seminars. Ness's chapter provides emphasis for the principle that an anthropologist be involved in the most clinically relevant course possible. Medical students usually complain about the irrelevancy of the Society and Medicine course in which social scientists typically teach. The Introduction to Clinical Medicine course has greater saliency and relevance.

Stein and Kleinman carry the theme of clinical relevancy still further, particularly since both work with residents who are delivering care. The setting for much of Howard Stein's teaching is the clinical conference. His chapter illustrates the need to be highly flexible in choices of discussion topic and to focus on the immediate concerns of the resident. As is true of so many other authors in this section, Stein's discussions are not narrowed to only the understandings of medical anthropology. This is particularly true in his emphasis on ethnography as a technique for clinical understanding. The chapter by Anderson and her colleagues and Gaines provide additional ethnographic insights into clinicians' perspectives.

Kleinman's chapter elucidates an extremely important method for teaching anthropology in a variety of clinical areas, based on the use of concepts that stimulate attention to discrepancies between patient and practitioner views. In addition, we are able to see the importance of consultation-liaison psychiatry as an avenue to a wide variety of clinical areas. Interviews to elicit patient and practitioner explanatory models, elaborated in Blumhagen's chapter, are central to Kleinman's clinical practice and teaching.

In his contribution on anthropology in a nursing school, Chrisman discusses the use of much the same information as used by those who teach in medical schools. Even though the thrust of nursing care varies from medical care, a biomedical perspective is still central in nursing and requires the same anthropological approach to expand horizons. However, the importance of patient life style to nursing practice accords greater legitimacy to topics such as family and community life. Among the many ways Chrisman's setting is different is the existence of Masters and Doctoral level graduate education. Thus, in addition to the need for clinical relevance of anthropology, there is also the opportunity to guide research in which graduate students themselves build the bridges between their clinical specialties and the behavioral science literature.

The last two chapters of Section I take a completely different tack. Ritenbaugh's chapter describes a single course — on nutrition and anthropology — that mixed anthropology and health science students. A systems approach and a culture and community focus are evident as core features. Her use of the case study method of teaching this important material to students is consistent with the similar teaching methods of other authors. Through her explication of obesity as an American cultural "illness", we gain insight into the kinds of cultural webs enmeshing both practitioners and patients. Irwin Press moves us to an even more microcosmic level in his extraction of principles for practitioner-patient relationships from his knowledge of folk healers. Usefully read with the Goods' contribution on patient requests, this chapter is not only important when one is working in a clinical setting, it also can form the basis for one or more lectures in the type of plenary sessions described by Ness.

Section II contains eight research contributions by authors who were asked to describe their research and findings as they relate to clinical problems. The assignment was phrased in this way to reduce the translation difficulties normally faced by anthropologists in clinical settings. That is, most research in medical anthropology is directed toward solving anthropological problems. To use the research in clinical settings, the clinically applied anthropologist frequently must use anecdotal material as a bridge. Of course, the clinical specificity of these chapters might cause the problem in reverse: the findings could be too narrow for the inherent flexibility and dynamism in clinical teaching. On the other hand, however, authors were also asked to discuss the anthropological issues surrounding clinical problems. This feature should allow readers to generalize to related clinical problems. We also could not provide a systematic sampling of relevant clinical or anthropological issues. Yet, the selections here do represent problems in mental and physical health, chronic and acute problems, various kinds of delivery settings, and issues in public health.

It is appropriate to begin Section II with Hazel Weidman's chapter. In essence, it is a second introduction to the book. She addresses both the substance and terminology involved in the debate about what anthropologists in health science settings should call themselves, explicitly distinguishing anthropologists as therapists from anthropologists in other roles in the health sciences. We (the editors) believe that this is the important distinction, regardless of terminology. However, anthropologists must be careful about our labels so we do not imply to clinicians that we are yet another competitor for their turf.

With the Miami Health Ecology project as the context, Weidman shows the significance of anthropological research on health for the wide range of activities in which clinically applied anthropologists engage. Her use of discrete concepts such as health culture, culture broker, and contextualization parallels Kleinman's experience with other concepts. Most significantly, the direct relevance of her research for patient care – and the mechanisms by which she involved students in research – promoted the integration of anthropological perspectives into a number of health science disciplines.

Gaines' chapter introduces us to the types of knowledge about popular culture needed by an anthropologist. His approach to each of the illustrative cases included a much wider net of data to be considered germane; data overlooked or misinterpreted by clinicians. An implication of his paper (and Weidman's) for other clinically applied anthropologists is that we would be well advised to conduct at least some of our research in the local setting (bucking anthropological tradition once again by studying at home). Gaines also provides insight into how anthropologists behave as members of health care teams, including the pitfalls of restricted understanding of hierarchical relationships among medical professionals.

One technique for aiding clinicians to probe further into their patients' illness meanings and illness problems is the use of patient requests, considered here by Mary-Jo DelVecchio Good and Byron Good. As a concept, patient request, with its supportive literature, is another concrete notion for potential use by the clinically applied anthropologist. The Goods' detailed research findings allow many avenues for further exploration in conferences with students. A second advantage of this paper is its demonstration of an important research tool. The approach contrasts with traditional ethnographic field methods, retaining open ended depth interviews only in initial stages. Subsequent development and use of more structured instruments, characteristic of health services research, is nonetheless directed toward solution of health problems from an anthropological perspective.

Dan Blumhagen's chapter on the meaning of hypertension expands our knowledge of the sociocultural factors linked to an illness commonly seen in ambulatory care settings. This contribution illustrates the use of explanatory model interviews as the basis for research in addition to their importance as a clinical tool. In clinical teaching, the data provided here are invaluable. Clinicians rarely recognize the variation in patient understanding that is hidden in the common sense terminologies of practitioner-patient encounters. Hypertension is a useful paradigmatic illustration of such variability. In addition, the case study illustrates the tenacity of popular culture beliefs in the face of (or in collusion with) consistent contact with providers who presumably maintain biomedical explanatory models. All of the illnesses discussed in other chapters are susceptible to similar analysis, suggesting a rich area for further and highly relevant anthropological research.

Explanatory models and negotiations about them were a key element in the planned change program documented here by Anderson, Toledo, and Hazam. Although this element was presented as clear teaching and sensitive listening, the reader can find good examples of explanatory model negotiation in the case vignettes. Of equal, or greater importance was recognition by health professionals that patients and their families had very different experiences in their interactions with clinicians and hospital settings than the practitioners knew about or thought. Careful anthropological research into patients' lives disclosed essential and compelling understandings that could be transmitted to caretakers. The Anderson

Toledo, and Hazam chapter can be read, along with Weidman's and Gaines', as an example of a type of collaborative relationship between anthropologists and health scientists.

Through the medium of two detailed case studies, Linda Alexander considers an issue with a great deal of potential in teaching and research for clinically applied anthropologists: the chronic sick role. An important feature of the chronic sick role is that it is simply not well known by clinicians, for whom it may be seen as "failure"; by social scientists, whose conceptual tools for explanation are poorly developed; and by the American populace, who do not as yet have cultural guide posts for understanding. In her analysis, Alexander explicates the conceptual difficulties facing clinicians and social scientists as they attempt to make sense out of a health care phenomenon that derives from the past successes of medical science in controlling many disease processes. The case studies provide ethnographic insight into the meanings of chronic illness on personal and societal levels.

Sue Estroff's chapter provides an understanding of the lives of those with chronic mental illness. Her sensitive ethnographic picture of the conflicts experienced by the mentally ill in community contexts corroborates many of Alexander's findings and complements Gaines' data from the acute psychiatric setting. Of great significance, however, are the health policy implications of this work: with steadily eroding state and federal funds for maintaining these people in hospitals or in the community, and given the problems now experienced, new health care alternatives must be developed. Anthropologists must move beyond simple ethnographic reporting and begin to also work on solutions. (And, as this goes to press, Dr. Estroff is working in an administrative position.)

The final chapter of this volume, by Byerly and Molgaard, shows the relevance of anthropological analysis for epidemiological issues in public health. Through their exploration of selected ethnographic understandings of a New Age healing commune, they demonstrate how cultural patterns act as risk factors for hepatitis and how the group responded to an outbreak. The eclectic approach to health care, "holistic health" in popular parlance, is nicely demonstrated in both the community response to threat and in the described healing gathering. This chapter is also an important reminder that clinically applied anthropologists must maintain the traditional anthropological focus on the community level of analysis, especially because most clinicians with whom we work conceive of health care on the one-to-one level.

We recognize that this volume can only scratch the surface of teaching and research activities in clinically applied anthropology. The teaching contributions are personal and idiosyncratic; research reports are highly specific. However, these contributions should be viewed as models of anthropology in novel territory; as a set of suggestions open to choice and modification depending on individual circumstance. With the advantage of having read all the papers, each of us has adopted a number of ideas for our teaching and has used the research material in various ways in clinical situations. We hope that others will do likewise.

REFERENCES

Alexander, Linda
   1977 The Double-Bind. Theory and Hemodialysis. Archives of General Psychiatry 33:
         1353–1356.
   1979 Clinical Anthropology: Morals and Methods. Medical Anthropology 3: 1: 61–
         107.
Bateson, Gregory
   1972 Toward a Theory of Schizophrenia. In G. Bateson (ed.), Steps to an Ecology of Mind.
         Los Angeles: Chandler Publishing Co.
Benedict, Ruth
   1934 Culture and the Abnormal. Journal of Genetic Psychology 1: 60–64.
Brink, Pamela (ed.)
   1976 Transcultural Nursing: A Book of Readings. Englewood Cliffs, New Jersey: Prentice-
         Hall, Inc.
Brink, Pamela
   1979 Medical Anthropologists in Schools of Nursing. Medical Anthropology 3: 3: 297–
         307.
Brown, G. W., et al.
   1975 Social Class and Psychiatric Disturbance Among Women in an Urban Population.
         Sociology 9: 225–254.
Caudill, William
   1953 Applied Anthropology in Medicine. In A. L. Kroeber (ed.), Anthropology Today: An
         Encyclopedic Inventory, Chicago: University of Chicago Press.
   1958 The Psychiatric Hospital as a Small Society. Cambridge: Harvard University Press.
Devereux, George
   1956 Normal and Abnormal. In Some Uses of Anthropology: Theoretical and Applied.
         Anthropological Society of Washington D.C.
Edgerton, R. B.
   1967 The Cloak of Competence. Berkeley: University of California Press.
Eisenberg, Leon
   1977 Disease and Illness. Culture, Medicine, and Psychiatry 1: 1: 9–23.
Engle, George L.
   1977 The Need for a New Medical Model: A Challenge for Biomedicine. Science 196:
         129–136.
Fabrega, Horacio
   1974 Disease and Social Behavior. Cambridge: Mass.: MIT Press.
Firth, Raymond
   1981 Engagement and Detachment: Reflections on Applying Social Anthropology to
         Social Affairs. Human Organization 40: 3: 193–201.
Fox, Renée
   1959 Experiment Perilous: Physicians and Patients Facing the Unknown. Glencoe: The
         Free Press.
   1979 Essays in Medical Sociology: Journeys into the Field. New York: Wiley.
Garrison, Vivian
   1978 Support Systems of Schizophrenic and Nonschizophrenic Puerto Rican Migrant
         Women in New York City. Schizophrenia Bulletin 4: 4: 561–596.
Goffman, Erving
   1961 Asylums. New York: Doubleday (Anchor Books).
Good, Byron and Good, Mary-Jo DelVecchio
   1981 The Meaning of Symptoms: A Cultural Hermaneutic Model for Clinical Practice. In
         Leon Eisenberg and Arthur Kleinman (eds.), The Relevance of Social Science for
         Medicine. Dordrecht, Holland: D. Reidel Publishing Co., pp. 165–197.

Henry, Jules
    1972 Pathways to Madness. New York: Random House.
Illich, Ivan
    1975 Medical Nemesis: The Expropriation of Health. London: Calder and Boyars, Ltd.
Kay, Margarita
    1978 Clinical Anthropology. In Eleanor E. Bauwens (ed.), The Anthropology of Health,
          St. Louis: C. V. Mosby Co., pp. 3–12.
Kleinman, Arthur
    1980 Patients and Healers in the Context of Culture. Berkeley: The University of Cali-
          fornia Press.
Kleinman, Arthur, Eisenberg L., and Good, B.
    1978 Culture, Illness and Care: Clinical Lessons from Anthropological and Cross-Cultural
          Research. Annals of Internal Medicine 88: 251–258.
Kleinman, Arthur, et al. (eds.)
    1975 Medicine in Chinese Cultures: Comparative Studies of Health Care in Chinese and
          other Societies. Washington, D.C. U.S. Government Printing Office for Fogarty
          International Center.
Langness, L. L.
    1967 Hysterical Psychosis: The Cross Cultural Evidence. American Journal of Psychiatry
          124: 143–152.
Leininger, Madeleine
    1978 Transcultural Nursing: Concepts, Theories, and Practices. New York: John Wiley.
Leslie, Charles (ed.)
    1976 Asian Medical Systems. Berkeley: University of California Press.
Linton, Ralph
    1956 Culture and Mental Disorder. In George Devereux (ed.). Springfield: Charles Thomas.
Logan, Michael H.
    1979 Directions of Research in Medical Anthropology. Implications Concerning Non-
          academic Employment. Medical Anthropology 3: 3: 353–364.
M. A. N.
    1980 Open Forum: Clinical Anthropology. Medical Anthropology Newsletter, 12: 1:
          14–25.
Maretzki, Thomas
    1981 The Culture Paradigm. In C. Eisdorfer, D. Cohen, A. Kleinman, and P. Maxim (eds.),
          Theoretical Bases for Psychopathology, New York: Spectrum Publications.
Mead, Margaret
    1939 From the South Seas. New York: Norton and Company.
Murphy, Jane
    1976 Psychiatric Labeling in Cross-Cultural Perspective. Science 191: 1019–1028.
Murphy, Jane and A. Leighton
    1965 Approaches to Cross-Cultural Psychiatry. Ithaca: Cornell University Press.
Opler, Marvin K.
    1967 Culture and Social Psychiatry. New York: Atherton Press.
Paul, Benjamin D.
    1955 Health, Culture and Community: Case Studies of Public Relations to Health Pro-
          grams. New York: Russel Sage Foundation.
Sapir, Edward
    1949a Cultural Anthropology and Psychiatry. In D. Mandelbaum (ed.), Selected Writing of
          Edward Sapir, Berkeley: University of California Press, pp. 509–522.
    1949b Why Cultural Anthropology Needs the Psychiatrist. In D. Mandelbaum (ed.), Selected
          Writings of Edward Sapir, Berkeley: University of California Press, pp. 569–577.
Schreiber, Janet M., and Scrimshaw, Susan C. M.
    1979 Anthropologists in Schools of Public Health. Medical Anthropology 3: 3: 309–338.

Smilkstein, Gabriel, et al.
    1981 The Clinical Social Science Conference in Biopsychosocial Teaching. Journal of Family Practice 12: 2: 347–353.

von Mering, Otto
    1970a Bibliography. Medical Anthropology Newsletter 2: 6: 59–64.
    1970b Medicine and Psychiatry. *In* O. von Mering and L. Kasdan (eds.), Anthropology and the Behavioral Sciences, Pittsburgh: University of Pittsburgh Press.

Wallace, Anthony
    1961 Culture and Personality. New York: Random House.

Young, Allen
    1976 Some Implications of Medical Beliefs and Practices for Social Anthropology. American Anthropologist 78: 1: 5–24.
    1981 Editorial Comment. Social Science and Medicine 15B: 1–3.

Zborowski, Mark
    1969 People in Pain. San Francisco: Jossey-Bass.

Zola, Irving K.
    1966 Culture and Symptoms. An Analysis of Patients Presenting Complaints. American Sociological Review 31: 615–630.
    1973 Pathways to the Doctor – from Person to Patient. Social Science and Medicine 7: 677–689.

SECTION I

CLINICALLY APPLIED ANTHROPOLOGICAL TEACHING

SECTION I

CLINICALLY APPLIED ANTHROPOLOGICAL TEACHING

ROBERT C. NESS

MEDICAL ANTHROPOLOGY IN A PRECLINICAL CURRICULUM

INTRODUCTION

The purpose of this chapter is to describe and analyze my teaching activities as a medical anthropologist working within a medical school setting.[1] My efforts to incorporate medical anthrpological theory and concepts within the first year curriculum at the University of Connecticut Medical School have involved four inter-related contexts: (1) plenary lectures within a required 100-hour course called the Social and Behavioral Sciences Teaching Committee; (2) a 22-hour elective seminar entitled Alternative Strategies of Healing: A Cross-Cultural Review; (3) a 24-hour elective seminar entitled Social Factors in Health and Mental Health; and (4) a year-long course called Introduction to Clinical Medicine I.

My discussion will be structured in terms of the scope and format of each of these teaching contexts. Although attention will be directed occasionally to course content, the emphasis will be on teaching strategies and their relevance to the concerns and backgrounds of first-year medical students. The paper includes my evaluation of these multiple teaching efforts and concludes with some reflections about generic issues in preclinical medical school teaching.

THE STUDENTS

It is important to understand the background and concerns of beginning students because the nature of this audience has a direct bearing on how medical anthropology is introduced and what is taught. This section will therefore briefly combine some descriptive statistics and my perceptions of these students in order to outline some major features of this group.

All my teaching activities, except Introduction to Clinical Medicine, involve medical and dental students in their preclinical years. Trying to generalize about their backgrounds and concerns, I am more impressed with their range of variation than with the commonalities. These students have, for example, a variety of opinions about the effectiveness of our health care system, the need for change, and their own anticipated role in the system. There is also considerable variability in their previous occupational experience within the health care system, ranging from physician's assistants to students with virtually *no* contact with the system as either a patient or a provider of care.

There is great heterogeneity as well in students' early career interests in medicine/ dental medicine. Some arrive with clearly defined career goals in geriatric medicine, laboratory research, or pediatrics, for example, while others have no specific plans. Subsequent postgraduate training, after four years of medical or dental school,

35

N. J. Chrisman and T. W. Maretzki (eds.), Clinically Applied Anthropology, 35–59.
Copyright © 1982 by D. Reidel Publishing Company.

indicates that a clear majority of students where I teach develop careers within primary care specialties. The table below summarizes this pattern by showing the residency placements of the 407 graduates from the University of Connecticut School of Medicine between 1972 and 1979.

TABLE I

Residency Placements from the University of Connecticut School of Medicine, 1972–1979

Specialty	Percent of Graduates
All Primary Care	68.3
Medicine	42.0
Family practice	7.1
Flexible	11.1
Pediatrics	8.1
Surgery	13.0
Obstetrics/Gynecology	5.4
Psychiatry	4.7
Pathology	3.9
Radiology/Anesthesiology	4.4

Data from Office of Student Affairs, University of Connecticut School of Medicine.

These figures are similar for the Class of 1980 as well, although there have been increases in this class in the proportion of graduates entering primary care (76%) and psychiatry (7%), and a slight decline in the proportion entering surgical training (10%). In general, then, the majority of students where I teach are attracted to careers in primary care. And it is precisely these graduates who may effectively incorporate medical anthropological theory/concepts within their practices.

I have summarized below in Table II selected characteristics of the in-coming medical and dental classes I have worked with since 1976.

TABLE II

Selected Matriculation Data from the Schools of Medicine and Dentistry at the University of Connecticut

Year of entry	Number of students[a]	Average age	Percent female	Number of self-described minority students[c]	Undergraduate major: social science or psychology
Medical School					
1976	80	22	28	4	9
1977	80	22	30	9	5
1978	80	23	30	8	2
1979	82	22	29	8	5
1980	80	23	32.5	8	6

Table II (continued)

Year of entry	Number of students[a]	Average age	Percent female	Number of self-described minority students[c]	Undergraduate major: social science or psychology
Dental School					
1976	52	23.5	15	1	b
1977	51	24	11	1	b
1978	50	25	14	0	b
1979	55	23	21	0	b
1980	51	b	23	b	b

Data from the Office of Student Affairs in the Schools of Medicine and Dentistry.
a First-time entering students.
b Data not available.
c Includes both economically disadvantaged and ethnic minorities.

Except for the sixth column indicating the small number of students with a social science or psychology major, the figures in this table would probably not change radically if they were describing students in a graduate anthropology program.[2] It is noteworthy, however, that most beginning medical students have very little formal background in the social or behavioral sciences. These sciences have not been a central interest of students who have concentrated primarily in the biophysical sciences in order to pursue careers dominated by a clinical service orientation. Consequently, the conceptual utility and research paradigms of the social and behavioral sciences are *not* familiar to medical/dental students. These backgrounds and career interests probably account for my repeated observation that theoretical issues, conceptual distinctions, and research findings that excite students in anthropology often fail to do so in a medical/dental school context. The question, therefore, of what materials from medical anthropology are "relevant" is a persistent question of considerable urgency for an anthropologist attempting to teach within a medical school setting.

What is thought to be educationally "relevant" is, of course, a value judgment reflecting an opinion about what kinds of skills physicians ought to have. From my perspective these skills should reflect three levels of expertise: (1) healing, (2) educating, and (3) planning. *Healing* includes the application of appropriate biomedical procedures/medicines as well as an effective response to the psychosocial concerns of patients. *Educating* involves the ability to effectively share relevant knowledge from the biomedical and sociobehavioral sciences with patients. Educating is closely related to healing, and re-establishes the meaning of the Latin term by which we address physicians (< L. *doctor*: teacher). *Planning* skills include the ability to assess and interpret epidemiological data, health care evaluation studies, and behavioral science information about the maintenance of preventive health care behavior. The promotion of these skills is relevant for the growing number of physicians who try to contribute effectively to the planning, implementation, and evaluation of health care services.

The preclinical curriculum is the proper context in which to introduce the basic science material relevant to these three skills. (The subsequent refinement of these skills will, of course, vary from one specialty to another.) Medical anthropology can be successfully integrated within this context because the field can contribute answers to (at least) seven questions that interest students and relate directly to the skills discussed above:

(1) How are diseases distributed in natural communities and what factors affect the distribution? (planning).
(2) How do people assess the meaning of symptoms and decide what to do when they feel sick? (healing, educating).
(3) What are the relationships between social stress, social support, and personality on the one hand and the onset, course, and outcome of disease processes on the other? (planning, educating).
(4) What factors affect a person's adherence to a treatment plan? (healing).
(5) What determines how a person will cope with a chronic disease? (healing, educating).
(6) How is effective communication with patients achieved and what kind of information should be exchanged with patients in order to provide quality care (healing).
(7) What is the value of the various treatment approaches *not* informed by bio-medical theory and research? (healing, educating).

The remainder of this chapter will describe how materials from medical anthropology are utilized in four related teaching settings to address these questions.

THE SOCIAL AND BEHAVIORAL SCIENCES SUBJECT COMMITTEE

My teaching responsibilities in plenary meetings of this committee have included the following topics: Alcoholism, Child Abuse, Stress and Illness, Cultural Forces Affecting Change in the Medical System, and Socio-cultural Definitions of Health and Illness. These materials are presented in 50 minute lectures to the first year class, accompanied by a syllabus which develops the material of the lecture in further detail.

Within this teaching context, one's style of presentation is important because the lecture is usually only one of a series that may span four consecutive hours. Intellectually sound material is easily "lost" in this environment where students commonly complain that they feel like they are trying to "get a drink from a fire hose". I have found that the best approach requires enthusiasm, avoidance of jargon or "buzz-words", the judicious use of audio-visual materials, and an explicit tie between the lecture and the written syllabus.

Although the topics of alcoholism and child abuse were not part of my academic training, I assumed responsibility for developing lectures and syllabus on these materials in order to help maintain the topical format designed by this teaching committee. In fact, any member of the committee may be occasionally asked :o develop lecture materials on topics outside his/her central interests. Medical anthropologists may be particularly vulnerable to these requests because the scope of our discipline is not well understood by other scientists in medical schools. As a result, there may be a tendency to view us as "jacks of all trades". This perspective has advantages and disadvantages: (1) it serves to open teaching opportunities and involve us in interdisciplinary teaching committees, and (2) it may place us in the awkward position of refusing teaching requests or undertaking a lecture for which we have no interest or prior training. The lesson here is twofold. First, one must be prepared to discuss and describe the boundaries of his/her interests and competence without being defensive or feeling threatened. Work within a medical school requires that one create, "advertise", and exchange "world views"; it cannot be assumed that one's colleagues share similar intellectual interests as, for example, may be appropriate in a department of anthropology. Second, medical anthropologists must be knowledgeable about specific diseases and public health problems confronting industrialized societies. Familiarity with the biological dimensions as well as the sociocultural aspects of these health problems is essential in order to maintain credible teaching (and research) activities within a medical school setting.

Two examples from my lecture experiences with alcholism and child abuse may make this point clearer. During my first lecture experience with alcoholism I drew from the ethnographic literature to emphasize the way in which sociocultural environments (cultural expectations) affect the behavior of people who are drinking. While this was interesting to me, the students complained that they learned little about the psychomotor affects of ethyl alcohol. During the second experience with this lecture, I reviewed the psychophysiological material first. Then, using illustrations from the ethnographic literature, I introduced the concept of "drunken comportment" (MacAndrew and Edgerton 1969) in order to examine the role of social learning and cultural context. The lecture ended with a discussion of the relative impact of ethyl alcohol per se and the sociocultural environment on the behavior of people who are drinking. This holistic approach is not only compatible with the major premise of our discipline, but also attractive to medical students.

The topic of Child Abuse is a second example of material about which I had little prior academic familiarity or research experience. In preparation for this two-hour lecture, my interests led me to consider two aspects of the topic: (1) The development and use of the term "child abuse" in historical perspective; and (2) the current models of explanation used to understand child abuse.

I spend about 25 minutes outlining the historical development of the concept of child abuse. In this effort it is necessary to describe the clinical phenomenon (especially radiological findings) which led investigators in the 1940s to formulate the concept of child abuse. I use these historical materials to emphasize two points:

(1) A major impetus to the development of this diagnostic term were radiological findings rather than signs and symptoms noted during a clinical examination. This point raises the issue of how discernible the "syndrome" of child abuse actually is and illustrates that a clinician, like any other observer, often "sees" only what he is prepared to see.

(2) Early theories of the etiology of child abuse, based on clinical experiences in hospital settings, emphasized the abuser's psychopathology. More recent work, based on community studies and parent-infant interactional studies, has greatly altered our earlier understanding of child abuse.

A major portion of the lecture then reviews the evidence supporting or refuting several models of explanation; viz., (a) psychological, (b) social ecological, and (c) interactional models of child abuse. An effort is made to integrate the models in an ecological framework, emphasizing the multiple interacting causes of several types of abuse (emotional, physical, and sexual). Anthropological perspectives on child abuse (Korbin 1977) are utilized in order to highlight the cross-cultural validity of an ecological interpretation, but are not given as much prominence as they might be in an anthropology seminar. Concluding the lecture, strategies of prevention and rehabilitation which flow from these models are assessed in terms of the data currently supporting each model.

My favorite lecture topic has been Cultural Forces Affecting Change in the Medical System, a presentation designed to discuss the limitations of medical interventions in the treatment of human illness. A 16-page syllabus, in conjunction with the lecture, is designed to achieve the following objectives:

(1) Understand the theoretical utility of distinguishing between *disease* and *illness*.
(2) Conceptualize the events and processes characteristic of The Natural History of Illness Episodes (in contrast to the Natural History of Disease).
(3) Outline the formal properties and functions of cultural beliefs about illness.
(4) Review the major classes of cultural beliefs which appear in urban North American communities.
(5) Formulate some general conclusions about the effectiveness of non-medical treatment approaches in order to understand their meaning and persistence within our society.
(6) Discuss the significance of the preceding five elements for improving clinical care.

Each of these objectives, except number four, is discussed during the lecture, drawing from recent publications by Kleinman (1978), Chrisman (1977). and Murdock (1978). Material relevant to objective four, in the form of ethnographic descriptions of *Rootwork, Curanderismo, Espiritismo*, and (Pentecostal) *Faith Healing*, are presented in a series of appendices to the syllabus. These materials draw from the work of Wintrob (1973), Alegria et al. (1977), Garrison (1977), Pattison (1973), and Ness (1980). Students are encouraged to study the syllabus in advance in order to become familiar with the major themes to be discussed in the lecture. It is made clear that ethnographic details of the belief systems presented in the appendices to the syllabus will not be potential examination material. This is an important caveat to these obsessive students who are, after all, not training to be anthropologists.

A central teaching device within this hour is a 10-minute film entitled *The Shaman of Northern Nepal* (International Films Bureau 1968). The students are asked to draw upon the ethnographic material in this film and their syllabus in order to compare the health care provided by a non-medical healing practice with the care provided by the western biomedical tradition. In order to make this comparison explicit and orderly, I ask the students to compare the following conceptual dimensions: (1) the kinds of data of interest to the practitioner and patient, (2) the amount of interest paid to internal bodily processes; and (3) the extent of attention paid to questions of (a) efficient cause (who?), (b) instrumental cause (what?) and (c) ultimate cause (why?). In collaboration with the class I construct a chart on the blackboard which enables the students to appreciate that the biomedical model of health care they are learning (and probably already ascribe to) focuses heavily on *disease* problems, while other forms of care focus on problems of human *illness*. This conclusion is acceptable and compelling because it is drawn *inductively* by comparing ethnographic materials from non-western *and* western traditions with their own understanding of biomedical care. This primary conclusion leads subsequently to discussions of (1) the role of indigenous healing traditions in urban communities and (2) the limitations and potentials of patient care structured by biomedicine.

I believe it is crucial in teaching contexts such as this (and in medical/dental schools generally) to present a *balanced* comparison of biomedicine and indigenous healing approaches. Overly forceful and unbalanced critiques of medical science or practice are not well accepted and only serve to alienate the audience. "The medical model" must not become a straw man which confuses important differences between medical theory and actual health care. Students, for example, are quick to argue that elements of the "medical model" described by Engel (1977), for example, only partially determine the delivery of health care, that concern for and attention to the whole illness *are* features of western health care. Accepting this point, it is easier to move to a discussion of the *relative* effectiveness of biomedical approaches and indigenous healing traditions in the care of human illnesses.

An effective way to "unpack" the medical model concept is to examine the idea that there are, in fact, different *types* of medical models. A very useful article by Lazare (1973) uses clinical vignettes to demonstrate how, in the practice of psychiatry, the "model" one uses determines (1) the kind of interview data selected for emphasis, (2) the nature of diagnosis, and (3) the form of treatment. Drawing on the article by Lazare and their own experiences as patients, students are encouraged to formulate the kinds of "models" which serve to structure clinical activities in pediatrics and surgery, for example. This model-building activity highlights the impact of one's training and "world view" on patient care. Extending this point to cover non-medical healing traditions, students appreciate more effectively that *all* patient care is affected by the beliefs and values of practitioner and client. This kind of discussion is most effective, however, in small groups, rather than plenary sessions for the whole class. The next section describes my experience with this teaching format.

THE SOCIAL AND BEHAVIORAL SCIENCES ELECTIVE SEMINAR

Concurrent with the SBS plenary sessions, students choose to participate in one of 15 seminars which provide the opportunity for in-depth exploration of one segment of the SBS plenary curriculum which is of particular interest to them. The seminar consists of eleven sessions; each session meets for two hours.

During the past four years I have offered an elective seminar entitled "Alternative Strategies for Coping with Illness: A Cross-cultural Review". The purpose of the seminar is to examine the process of diagnosis and therapy within a variety of treatment settings other than western biomedicine in order to accomplish the following objectives:

(1) Understand the beliefs, attitudes, and experiences which motivate people to utilize these types of healing strategies.
(2) Describe and understand the dynamics of diagnosis and therapy in these treatment settings.
(3) Formulate some general conclusions about the effectiveness of such treatments in order to understand their meaning and persistence within our society.
(4) Translate these conclusions into concepts which can be clinically applied to the process of biomedical diagnosis/treatment in order to make this approach more responsive to patients' needs and concerns.

The seminar readings cover three topical areas in order to achieve the objectives outlined above: (1) diagnosis and therapy in non-industrialized settings using case examples from the Kalahari Bushman and the Alaskan Eskimo; (2) the health cultures of selected minority groups (blacks, Hispanics), religious groups (Pentecostals, Christian Scientists) and treatment orientations (Chiropractic, Naturopathy) in our society; and (3) the nature of illness behavior within "mixed medical systems" which provide traditional/popular, folk, and biomedical modes of diagnosis and treatment. A central assumption of this seminar is that it makes good sense to study strategies of coping with illness from a cross-cultural, ethnographic perspective in order to arrive at an insightful view of what constitutes effective diagnosis and healing.

On the average, twelve students elect this seminar each year as their first choice. About one-quarter of these students have some academic background in the social sciences. More commonly, they share an interest in non-medical healing through personal experience or the experience of a close friend or relative. There has been no consistent pattern in terms of the sex distribution of students electing this seminar, although the clear majority have always been medical students rather than dental students.

One specific interest these first-year students share centers on the question: "How do these indigenous healing strategies work?" Many believe that such healing efforts can help people but are unclear about how this happens. Foreshadowing a difficulty I will discuss later, some students expect the answer to the question of effectiveness to be framed solely in terms of human physiology. Other students join the seminar rather convinced that such healing strategies cannot affect diseases and are curious about "why people believe things like that". It is worth noting also that students beginning this seminar often view the practice of biomedicine as qualitatively different from other forms of healing, a view not considerate of the idea that study of non-medical healing strategies might serve to eventually improve their own delivery of care. This attitude is one that I try to alter throughout the seminar.

A question that has concerned me involves the organization of the seminar syllabus; namely; whether to order the material inductively by beginning with a series of ethnographic materials, or to organize in a deductive fashion with some conceptual papers first, before the ethnographic descriptions are presented. Given the very limited anthropological background of these students, much can be said for both of these approaches. I have become convinced, however, that what matters most is how a seminar of this type *ends* rather than how it begins. This point will be discussed more fully later in this section.

I have, in practice, been most comfortable with a seminar which begins with two meetings devoted to conceptual issues. These discussions provide tools for ordering and analyzing the ethnographic accounts which the students examine in the remainder of the course. The conceptual materials that I have found most useful are introduced in the following order:

(1) The distinctions between illness, disease, and sickness developed by Cassell (1976) and Eisenberg (1977) form the basis for later discussions of illness behavior, the culture of biomedicine, and the functions of non-medical healing strategies.

(2) The structural and idiomatic similarities and differences between western science and traditional African thought discussed by Horton (1967) is an analysis applicable to health belief systems generally. This article is very useful for medical students who often assume scientific reasoning to be qualitatively different from other forms of belief. I have also found Young's (1978) discussion of the "mode of production of medical knowledge" a useful companion piece to Horton's work because Young's work more clearly focuses on the social and technical relations of production in western and non-western societies which both generate and constrain the development of medical knowledge.

(3) In order to help students develop cross-cultural comparisons and classifications when they read the ethnographic material, I assign articles by Glick (1967), Foster (1976), and Murdock (1978). These latter two authors provide classificatory schemes for ordering theories of etiology and Glick discusses the boundary problems associated with the application of the term "medicine" cross-culturally.

During the first two sessions which examine the readings outlined above, as well as in all subsequent sessions, specific students are asked to function as oral reporters. This role requires the following responsibilities: (1) a clear presentation of the author(s)' major contributions(s), and (2) the student's personal response to the article, including both positive and negative reactions to the author's work. As the seminar progresses, students are encouraged to compare authors' ideas during their personal assessments of an article. These reports help students sharpen their skills of oral presentation, provide me with one means of evaluating students, and lay the basis for class discussion of the assigned readings. I try to limit my own role to clarifying key conceptual distinctions or ideas that may have been neglected during students' presentations and class discussions.

Four films, shown in the following order, are presented during the seminar in order to increase the impact of the written ethnographic materials:

(1) *N/um Tchai*. (Marshall 1966) This film documents the Medicine Dance of the Kalahari Bushmen, showing the intense group effort and individual trance activity of the participants as they apply both preventive and curative techniques.

(2) *The Shaman of North and South Nepal*. (International Films Bureau 1968) The first film portrays a shaman applying his diagnostic and therapeutic skills for a family in distress. The second film follows a shaman who has undergone some medical acculturation, practicing with a mixture of traditional, Ayurvedic, and western perspectives on several different patients.

(3) *The Holy Ghost People*. (C.R.M./McGraw-Hill Film Division 1968) This film documents the multi-faceted nature of a fundamentalist church service in West Virginia. Trance and possession behavior, as well as a snake-handling ritual, are clearly portrayed.

(4) *Puerto Rican Espiritism and Santeria*. (WCVB-TV Boston, n.d.) This videotape documents the complex healing approaches of *Espiritismo* and *Santeria* as practiced in the Boston area. The use of possession as a diagnostic and therapeutic strategy is clearly shown.

I have found that these films help students to think *comparatively* about (1) the degree of healer specialization; (2) the role of *materia medica*; (3) the distinction between trance and possession and the functions of these behaviors in healing contexts; (4) the relationship between the healer's practice shown in the films and the broader health care system of which it is a part; and (5) the nature of "internalizing" and "externalizing" discourse (Young 1976) and "personalistic" and "naturalistic" medical systems (Foster 1976). Each of the films is discussed in terms of these five points. As the seminar proceeds, of course, a shared fund of cross-cultural knowledge develops which students can draw upon during discussion and class reports.

One of the most consistent themes to emerge in these films is the role of trance and possession in different healing strategies. These dramatic behaviors attract students' interest because most students are unfamiliar with their meaning or function. Exploiting this interest, I ask students to function as ethnographers in comparing *N/um Tchai* with *The Shaman from North Nepal*. My goal in structuring this comparison is to develop *inductively* the conceptual distinction between trance as an altered psychophysiological state and possession as behavior derived from a specific belief system (Bourguignon 1976). The cross-cultural variability in possession behavior (and its diagnostic/therapeutic utility) is subsequently demonstrated by the shaman films, the film on *Espiritismo*, and *The Holy Ghost People*.

This latter film introduces the phenomenon of glossolalia which often absorbs students' interest. The review article by Pattison (1968) is an excellent way to cover questions about temporal distribution, induction techniques, and psychopathology related to "speaking in tongues". The reports by Kane (1975) and Tellegen et al. (1969) enable seminar participants to explore questions about the presumed psychopathological nature of glossolalia. The research by these authors is particularly appropriate because it was conducted in the region of the United States where *The Holy Ghost People* was filmed.

These issues concerning the nature of trance and possession must be examined because the students are intensely curious and often poorly informed about this type of behavior. The danger, I have found, is that the seminar may become preoccupied with psychological issues related to possession so that too little time remains for the structural analysis of healing strategies. The most effective way to handle this dilemma has been to: (1) defer extended discussion of trance/possession until after *The Holy Ghost People* has been viewed, and (2) limit the discussion and class reports on this topic to one seminar period.

At the beginning of this section I noted that a major student interest in this seminar is the question of the effectiveness of indigenous healing strategies. Students often have their own answers to this question before the seminar begins, and it is useful to be aware of these perspectives. My experience has been that students usually embrace one of three positions. Some students presume that the direct physiological impact of *materia medica*, in the form of herbal preparations, accounts for the reported beneficial effects. Other students feel the impact is strictly psychological, with no effect on human physiology; and, finally, some students are convinced there are few or no beneficial effects attributable to most indigenous healing strategies. Given these views, one of the main outcomes of this seminar has been to demonstrate the wide variation in the "clinical impact" of indigenous healing strategies.

I have found it useful to begin by analyzing the connotation of the verbs "to heal", and "to cure", as well as the term "symptom" in order to establish the idea that these words usually convey a focus on disvalued *physical* sensations or conditions (diseases). Students perceive more clearly, then, that the meaning of these terms is linked with the selective attention of biomedicine in our society generally and in their training specifically. Sources of *physician* satisfaction, therefore, involve primarily the amelioration, elimination or control of a set of physical signs and symptoms.

In order to build an appreciation for the fact that an individual's satisfaction with treatment may be based on criteria other than the reduction of physical distress, I assign readings which document the improvement of social relationships (Turner 1964), the reduction of psychological distress (Ness 1980), the strengthening of cultural beliefs (Pattison 1973), and improvements in daily functioning (Kleinman and Sung 1979; Cay 1973) as alternative bases for treatment satisfaction in a variety of cultural settings. These readings serve to broaden the students' understanding of "healing"' as a multidimensional phenomenon and lead to discussions about the sources of patient dissatisfaction with biomedical treatments in our society.

Turning now to a different issue, it has been difficult to adequately respond to students' interest in herbal preparations and other *materia medica*. Until recently, the literature in medical anthropology has been dominated by sociocultural analyses of indigenous treatment practices, making it difficult to describe for students the potential physiological impact of *materia medica* utilized in indigenous treatments. After viewing the film entitled *N/um Tchai*, for example, the students raise questions about the possible efficacy of plant substances carried in a tortoise shell by one of the male curers. In addition, *The Study Guide* by Marshall and Biesele (1974) accompanying the film claims the !Kung recognize and use 17 medicinal plants, but nothing further is said about their use or effectiveness. Other studies addressing this issue have been hard to find, generating frustration for me and the students.

Recently, however, a series of papers has been published on the biomedical evaluation of indigenous medical practices in several different cultural settings (Etkind 1979). These papers will greatly improve the scope of the students' reading and add balance to a syllabus which, admittedly, has emphasized sociocultural analyses of indigenous healing practices. But still to be done is a *biocultural* analysis of a single indigenous healing practice, integrating both biomedical and sociocultural assessments of the healing practice.

Since this seminar is an elective, students approach the material with interest, but they rarely expect that the seminar material will contain concepts which are applicable to their future clinical practice. The last two sessions of the seminar are organized, therefore, to examine the clinical relevance of the ethnographic materials that have been discussed earlier.

Building on the distinction between disease and illness, I have found Chrisman's discussion of "The Natural History of an Illness" (1977) a useful model that helps students conceptualize the particularistic ethnographic accounts they have read. First, the model highlights the interlocking effects of (1) symptom perception/ evaluation by the ill person and (2) the advice he/she derives from "lay consultation" on the *range* of treatment actions that might be attempted before, after, or concurrent with a visit to a physician. Second, Chrisman's model forms an important contrast with the idea from public health that diseases have a "natural history". The juxtaposition of these models clarifies the fact that an understanding of the "natural history of a disease" cannot effectively explain the behavior and cognition of individuals who feel dis-ease. Most importantly, the model discussed by Chrisman (see also Fabrega 1974) emphasizes that *adherence* to a therapeutic regimen has *multiple* determinants, many of which are located outside of the healer-patient relationship. It is sobering, I think, for students to consider the idea that their lengthy and expensive training will be of *no* value clinically if patients fail to adhere to their treatment plan. Learning, then, about the multiple factors affecting adherence is clinically relevant.

The basic point I try to develop here is that during a patient interview it is just as important to elicit information about the history of the illness as it is to record information about the history of the symptoms. In a real sense, this information helps the physician understand "where the patient is coming from" as well as where the patient is likely to go(!).

In order to establish the idea that as an illness episode unfolds the sick individual may be confronted with a number of problems which generate as much suffering as the disease itself (or even more), I ask the students to list the kinds of problems that could arise at each point in Chrisman's model of the Natural History of an

Illness Episode. Many of the problems formulated by the students are discussed in Kleinman's (1977) essay which is read to reinforce the multidimensional nature of illness. In Kleinman's terms these dimensions are:

(1) Problems related to patient and family beliefs and values about the cause, nature, and significance of the symptoms.
(2) Problems related to family malfunctioning that either has preceded or has resulted from the sickness episode.
(3) Problems related to a change from the patient's pre-morbid social status and social role.
(4) Problems related to financial pressures created by the sickness and its treatment.
(5) Problems related to the choice of and interaction with different health care providers as part of the health-seeking process.
  (a) Conflicts in the labeling of the sickness and in the sanctioning of a particular type of sick role (e.g., acute, chronic, disabled, psychiatric, etc.).
  (b) Misconceptions between patient and care-givers.
  (c) Divergent patient and healer evaluations of therapeutic outcome and the quality of care.

A discussion of these materials inevitably generates questions about how to most effectively elicit this information during a patient interview. Besides encouraging students to develop their own answers to these issues, I assign the article by Kleinman et al. (1978) because it serves as a clear summary of the clinical relevance of the seminar. In this essay students are introduced to the concept of culturally constructed "explanatory models" about illness which are utilized by both patients and physicians to "make sense" of a specific illness. The authors enumerate eight questions which will elicit features of the patient's explanatory model as well as the scope and intensity of illness problems which the patient may be experiencing. (Although Kleinman provides clinical vignettes in much of his work to demonstrate the operation of explanatory models, the only comprehensive analysis of a clash between professional and patient's explanatory models I have found is by Redlener and Scott (1979). This article is well received by students because of its clinical-case structure and clear demonstration of the cultural construction of clinical realities.)

Students are eager to read about these kinds of specific interviewing suggestions because at this point in the medical school curriculum (early fall) the medical students begin a two-year experience called Introduction to Clinical Medicine (ICM) where they will develop their interviewing skills. The latter half of this chapter is devoted to a description of this teaching context and my role within it as a medical anthropologist.

SOCIAL FACTORS IN HEALTH AND
MENTAL HEALTH: AN ELECTIVE SEMINAR

The third context within which I teach is a multidisciplinary, elective seminar which is part of the Medical Sciences electives program that all medical and dental students are required to complete during each of their first two years. The major goal of this electives program is to permit the student to select an area of concentration related to, and derived from, the Medical Sciences core curriculum. An additional goal of the elective seminar is to make the student aware of how information in a given discipline is acquired and interpreted, and how current data relate to the existing body of knowledge in that discipline.

During the past four years I have collaborated with a cultural psychiatrist and a medical sociologist to present a Medical Science elective seminar that surveys selected materials from cultural psychiatry, epidemiology, medical sociology, and medical anthropology. The primary goal is to critically examine theory and data which develop links between sociocultural factors in urbanized societies and the health/mental health of people living in those societies. Although the required readings are primarily basic research reports, three themes in this seminar reflect issues inherent in clinical care: (1) the interrelationships between physical and emotional health; (2) the structure and function of treatment settings, including psychiatric facilities as well as indigenous, community-based approaches to health care; and (3) the identification, interpretation, and evaluation of symptoms as a sociocultural process. While the clinical relevance of these materials is discussed, the primary emphasis in this seminar is developing skills which will enable students to assess the research which has generated our current knowledge base. Graduates from this seminar will be, we hope, interested and competent evaluators of the social and behavioral sciences as they relate to issues in health and mental health.

Two additional themes in this elective seminar are developed from epidemiological studies: (1) the distribution of types of emotional distress as a function of community organization, and (2) the relationships between sociocultural change and emotional distress. These materials are particularly challenging to examine with preclinical students because the research highlights the relevance of concepts such as "poverty", work roles, sex roles, social class, ethnic identity and social mobility for understanding the distribution of various types types of physical and emotional illnesses in urban societies. These are new concepts to most students: their operationalization and associated measurement techniques are not familiar and therefore require some introduction and explanation. In addition, their status as "causal variables" often raises challenges for students accustomed to thinking (solely) of biophysical organisms as causal factors in human illnesses. In a real sense, then, the epidemiological material expands the concept of "patient" from the individual through the familial, communal, and societal levels of analysis. In this context there is often very lively debate about the most appropriate level for intervention and prevention projects.

While this elective seminar, held during May each year, draws some students who have previously taken my *SBS* seminar in the fall (see pages 41–47 above), the majority are students who become interested in the area during the Social and Behavioral Sciences Committee earlier in the year. During the past three years this elective seminar has attracted about 12 students each year. The sequencing of this seminar appears, therefore, to be effective in providing students an opportunity to follow-up interests developed earlier in the year.

It is important to emphasize that the material in this seminar is designed specifically to introduce levels of anlaysis which are clearly different from clinically-related concerns. The enthusiastic interest of students selecting this seminar indicates to me that there is an important "market" for aspects of medical anthropology, medical sociology, and cultural psychiatry which are often neglected in discussions stressing the clinical relevance of our teaching material.

INTRODUCTION TO CLINICAL MEDICINE (ICM)

ICM is a course which extends throughout the first two years of medical school, occupying one-half day a week. This course has three inter-related goals which provide: (1) an early and continuing contact with patients and faculty so that students can develop the perspectives and attitudes requisite to functioning as physicians; (2) a clinical setting where the relevance of what is being taught in medical science subject committees can be observed and practiced; and (3) the clinical skills necessary to assume the clinical responsibilities of the third and fourth years as a clinical clerk.

The first year of ICM includes four inter-related objectives and is the context within which I have worked:

(1) Introduce the concept of a patient-centered data base and provide opportunities to elicit clinical information through patient interviews.
(2) Develop the skills of eliciting, recording and presenting data through:
    (a) a working familiarity with the format of the medical history and the functions served by each portion of the history.
    (b) experience in recording data, including an appreciation for the problems of reliability, completeness and reproducibility.
    (c) experience in oral presentations before a group.
    (d) continuing practice in interviewing patients.
    (e) initial experience with a physical examination of the head and neck.
(3) Provide specific clinical problems as the focus for an expanded understanding of the clinical relevance of the basic biological, behavioral and social sciences.
(4) Gain experience with patient-physician relationships and small group interactions through (a) observing and participating in patient interviewing, and (b) the continuing experience of small group preceptor sessions.

In order to accomplish these objectives, the first year medical student class is divided into eight groups with approximately twelve students in each group. Each of these groups meets one-half day a week at a participating hospital with at least two preceptors. These preceptor teams include at least one physician and may involve social or behavioral scientists as well.

I have served as a preceptor in ICM I for the past five years. Since 1978 I have also functioned as co-chairperson of ICM I, working with a family physician to organize and administer the activities of all preceptor groups in ICM I.

The preceptor I work with is a pediatrician who is able to arrange regular access to pediatric patients as well as patients from a general medical/surgical ward. In addition to these patients we have utilized patients at a medical care facility for the elderly near the general hospital where our preceptor group meets. These patients form the clinical base for all of the ICM I activity in our group.

The history of participation by social/behavioral scientists in ICM I has been variable. In fact, since the early 70s there has been an overall decline in the number of participating social/behavioral science preceptors. This erosion has been due, I believe, to the inability (in some cases, unwillingness) of some clinical and social science preceptors to appreciate each other's expertise and meld these effectively in a preceptor group setting. Given the clinical orientation of ICM I, it has been particularly difficult for some social/behavioral scientists to demonstrate in a sustained way the clinical relevance of their knowledge/skill base. In addition, the knowledge base of some social/behavioral scientists has oriented them primarily as critics of current medical care delivery. The clinical relevance, then, of their perspectives has often become so divisive that on-going cooperation between preceptors is eroded.

This is not to say that first year medical students, or clinical preceptors, are not interested in critically examining the structure of medical care and their roles in the system of health care. These preceptor groups are an excellent context for discussing issues of this kind. The problem, rather, is one of balance. First year medical students are very eager to try-out their career roles in a concrete way, and ICM I provides that context. Compared to the vast amount of academic/theoretical material they must learn, the skills developed in ICM seem "more real" and directly "relevant" to their emerging self-image. One student summed up her feelings this way:

If it weren't for ICM, I think I'd drop out. It's the only part of the week when I feel I've made the right decision [to go to medical school]. It's what I thought it would be like, and I'm gaining confidence talking with patients.

If preceptors do not contribute to the development of student feelings such as those expressed above, by helping them acquire effective basic interviewing and history-taking skills, students perceive them as marginal members of the preceptor team no matter how astute or useful their analyses of medical care delivery may be. It is important, therefore, for social/behavioral science preceptors to offer knowledge which is applicable to the task of patient interviewing.

My contribution to the ICM I preceptor group includes seven topical areas: (1) helping students understand the structure and function of each section of a medical history; (2) helping students learn how to elicit a medical history; (3) introducing the concept of the mental status exam and its role in the patient interview; (4) explaining the clinical relevance of patients' and doctors' "explanatory models" and helping students learn how to elicit these models; (5) sharing sociological and anthropological perspectives about health issues such as child abuse and substance abuse; (6) sensitizing students to the psychosocial adjustments required by chronic illness; and (7) helping students assess relationships between patients' life-styles, current health status, and illness behavior.

These activities do not appear in any specific chronological sequence during ICM I; they arise primarily in response to issues raised by students' interview experiences. For example, after an interview on the pediatric ward a student felt that parental neglect, perhaps even abuse, was responsible for a child's physical condition. During our preceptor group discussion (held regularly after the patient interviews) the pediatrician outlined the importance of differential diagnoses and I helped students evaluate the quality of the psychosocial history in order to expose the difficult judgments required in cases of suspected abuse. During another group meeting, the impact of a young woman's chronic illness (multiple sclerosis) on her family and her own coping strategies prompted a lengthy discussion about adjustments to chronic illness and the associated role of the physician and other health care providers.

Each week, then, the range of interview-related problems varies so that it is not possible, or effective, to prepare a block of material in advance. Developing confidence with the topics enumerated above is therefore an on-going process. During my first years of ICM I teaching, I felt most comfortable with those areas numbered four through seven above. Skill in topical areas one through three has been acquired gradually through my continuing participation in ICM I.[3]

It is not my intention to describe all of these activities in detail, but I would like to discuss a few approaches that have proven useful. When I first joined the ICM teaching committee, I took the position that a medical history could be conceptualized as a specialized sub-species of a key-informant interview (an activity all cultural anthropologists should be able to perform). Through ICM I have come to appreciate, in fact, the large overlap between the contents of a "medical history" and my interests as a medical anthropologist. Emic data obviously relevant to the medical history include the patient's physical/psychological complaints, a history of those complaints (including efforts to cope with them), a social/family history, and a history of past illnesses, their treatment and resolution. The patient (informant) thus constitutes a case-study about the popular and professional health culture within which his/her illness has unfolded.

There is, of course, a body of information relevant to internal disease processes which the beginning student would like to elicit from the patient. Specialized questions about the presenting complaint and the "review of systems" are the major places in a medical history where this information may be sought. In ICM I, however, where the students' knowledge of pathophysiology is not well-developed, these questions cannot be pursued in depth. My clinical co-preceptor may discuss the pathophysiology of particular patients in our group case discussions, but a systematic effort to relate disease processes to symptom data is set aside until the second year.

First-year medical students are very cognizant of this dilemma, but find, in general, that mastering the overall structure of the patient interview (in conjunction with a head-neck examination) is a large enough task for ICM I. This first year is, in fact, a time when preceptors can *exploit* the students' lack of knowledge about pathophysiology, highlighting instead the *patient's* view of the illness and his/her efforts to cope with it.

The basic text for the course is *Interviewing the Patient* by Engel and Morgan (1973). The senior author is a well-known physician who emphasizes a holistic assessment of patients by integrating biological, psychological, and sociological levels of information. The structure and function of each part of a medical history is discussed in this text, which serves as a basic reference throughout the course.

My co-preceptor and I have found that students benefit from seeing a complete medical history performed for them early in the course. One of us may be video-taped conducting a patient interview or we may interview a patient before the group during one of our first meetings. No attempt is made to standardize our interviewing methods or approaches to data collection and the differences between our interviews, in terms of what data we choose to explore or neglect, is an important subject of discussion.

A major distraction for students during their first interviews is a fear that they will forget the basic elements of a comprehensive interview. We have found it useful, therefore, to spend at least one session with role-playing, allowing each student an opportunity to act as the patient as well as the physician. This helps students fix the sequence of interview topics more firmly in mind. In addition, during the first month of interviews we ask students to slowly add to the length of their interviews by beginning, for example, with only the Chief Complaint and History of the Chief Complaint and adding additional parts until they have completed the Review of Systems (ROS).

There has been some debate within the ICM committee about the utility of the ROS, given the fact that these beginning students have completed none of their basic science subject committees related to pathophysiology. Our feeling is that a minimal set of questions, simply committed to memory, is a useful exercise because (1) the review of systems intensifies the contact with the patient, and (2) quite often students elicit information related to the Chief Complaint which they had not uncovered earlier in the interview. In addition, the clinical preceptors can utilize specific patient problems to demonstrate the clinical relevance of specific questions within the ROS.

I have found that the ICM I small group format is an excellent opportunity to teach and illustrate the clinical relevance of patients' and physicians' "explanatory models" and the conceptual distinction between disease and illness. Students are introduced to the empirical bases for these concepts through a discussion of Kleinman et al. (1978) which I time to coincide with my plenary lecture on "Cultural Forces" (see pp. 40–41 above).

Throughout the year students practice eliciting the patient's explanatory model (EM) in addition to the traditional components of a medical history. Students utilize a set of questions derived from Kleinman et al. (1978: 256), take notes during their interviews, and formulate a report on their patient which they deliver to the group. I have tabulated the results of interviewing during one month in order to illustrate the range of information about the patients' explanatory models derived by first-year students during their interviews.

TABLE III

Questions about Illness: A Survey of 57 Patients[a]

I. *Chief complaint*
Excess fat (3); hernia (4); dizziness (1); a growth on or under the skin (3); gastro-intestinal distress, including diarrhea, constipation, gas, and/or pain (9); rectal bleeding (3); muscle cramps (3); Localized pain, including arm, back, foot, or chest (13); weight loss (2); bruises related to an accident (4); loss of sight (1); unable to urinate (1); yellow skin (1); depression (1); other miscellaneous complaints (8).

	Number	Percent
II. *Perceived cause*		
Don't know	18	31
Patient's behavior[b]	7	
Patient's personality[c]	3	21
Family history	2	
Accident	7	12
Biomedical cause	20	35
III. *Reason for timing of symptoms*		
Don't know	30	52
Current or past accident	11	19
Biomedical term concepts[d]	16	29
IV. *Understanding of internal processes*		
Don't know	27	46
Biomedical terms	28	49
Other	2	4
V. *Adjective used to describe illness*		
Serious	9	
Long-term	10	33
Not serious	6	
Short-term	29	61
Not sure	3	5

	Percent of problems
VI. *Illness problems*	
Pain/tiredness	16
Decreased mobility	45
Interpersonal relations[e]	8
Psychological or behavioral change[f]	20
Financial stress	11
No problems	26

a   There were 22 males and 35 females interviewed. Mean age was 57 years.
b   "Over-work", eat poor food, "held my water", over-eat.
c   Loneliness, frustration, nervousness.
d   Previous injury/surgery/illness; at risk due to age; heavy lifting; incorrect diet.
e   Marital difficulty, family functioning.
f   Feel ugly, sexual functioning declining, requires special diet, cannot use alcohol.

The figures in Table III indicate a wide variety of Chief Complaints: the most frequent complaint, localized pain, constitutes just 23% of all the complaints. This variety reflects the fact that the interviewing usually occurred on the general medical and surgery floor of a large public hospital.

Thirty-one percent of the patients were not able to identify the cause of their health problem, while an additional 21% felt that the cause of their problem was related to their own behavior (seven patients), their psychological status (three patients), or an illness vulnerability related to family history (two patients). Excluding those seven patients reporting "accidents", the remaining 35% conceptualized the cause of their problems in biomedical terms.

Students are surprised at the number of patients who cannot identify a cause for their illness. Although a portion of these patients may have ideas about causality which might be elicited with more effective interviewing skills, I think these figures support Kleinman's observation that explanatory models are often incomplete and fragmented (Kleinman et al. 1978: 256). It is intriguing that so many patients are unable to give an answer in (at least) biomedical terms, and several students during group discussions have suggested the hypothesis that patients with no sense of causality seem at higher risk for emotional distress.

Turning to the question about the timing of symptoms, 52% of the patients had no idea why their symptoms appeared at the time they did. Excluding the 19% who blamed a current or past accident for timing of their symptoms, the remaining 29% of the patients accounted for the timing of their symptoms primarily in biomedical terms. Thus, the figures in Table III indicate that patients fail to understand the timing of their symptoms more frequently than they fail to understand the cause of their symptoms.

The following question was asked to elicit patients' perceptions of internal body processes: "What do you feel is happening inside you to make the symptoms you have?" Almost half of the patients interviewed (i.e., 47%) had no idea what might be occurring internally to account for their symptoms. An equal percentage answered the question using terms, phrases, and concepts derived from biomedicine. Some of the patients, however, described ideas related to body imagery or internal processes which were clearly at variance with a biomedical perspective. For example, one student discovered that a middle-aged woman would not consent to surgery for stomach cancer because she believed that cancer is spread by airborne particles that would infect other parts of her body if it were opened during surgery. In group discussion, it was decided that the attending physician should be informed of this woman's views and encouraged to talk with the woman (as, in fact, the student interviewer had already tried). Follow-up by the student indicated that the woman had finally consented to surgery.

The number of patients with no answer to the question about internal processes is surprising, and I agree with one student who suggested that no answer to this question may reflect, in part, the nature of doctor-patient communication. In fact, the students often recorded that these patients were eager for information about their internal bodily processes but were often not able to obtain understandable explanations from their doctor or the nurses. Group discussions about this finding have concluded that physicians may know how to elicit information from patients but frequently do not know how to effectively *exchange* information with patients. Beginning students are very challenged by this idea, but also frustrated with their inability to fully address patients' questions. The formulation of such answers is an important part of group discussion.

Patients' evaluations of the consequences of their illnesses were assessed using two questions. First, the following questions were asked: "How serious do you feel your illness is? Will it be short-term or long-term? All the patients except for three were able to give a specific answer to these questions: Sixty-one percent felt their illness would be either "short-term" or "not serious", while 33% responded that their illness would be "long-term" or "serious". In spite of the fact that a large majority claimed their illness was short-term or not serious, only 26% responded that they had "no problems" when asked to describe the chief problems their sickness had caused for themselves. Analyzing the remaining responses in terms of the numbers of problems listed (since patients could mention more than one problem), the figures in Table III indicate that: (1) sixteen percent of the problems were described in terms of pain or tiredness; (2) forty-five percent of the problems were related to decreased general mobility; (3) eight percent of the problems were described as interpersonal difficulties; (4) twenty percent of the problems were psychological or specific behavioral changes caused by the illness; (5) eleven percent of the problems described involved financial stresses related to the patient's illness.

These figures clearly illustrate the array of difficulties associated with illness and I have found this kind of data useful in group discussions to supplement the clinical vignettes used by Kleinman et al. (1978). As students collect this kind of information, I provide monthly tallies which constitute an "epidemiology of illness problems" within the students' patient base. The data patterns stimulate discussion about the causes for the variation in the data and highlight the fact that "illness" is a generic phenomenon applicable to every clinical situation. In addition, the kind of data presented here suggests that patients' explanatory models are often quite fragmentary and incomplete. This apparent vagueness may be a function of three interacting influences (excluding the students' level of interview skills): (1) the modified and attenuated assimilation of biomedical knowledge within our popular health culture, (2) the erosion of alternative explanatory models of illness within our popular health culture, and (3) ineffective communication of biomedical knowledge between doctors and patients. Explanatory models of this fragmented kind are often evaluated during students' discussions as dysfunctional, constituting part of the patient's illness rather than providing meaning and order during a time of stress and disorder.

Finally, the range of information derived from questions about explanatory models and illness dimensions highlights for students ways in which the "Problem-Oriented Record" format can be improved when they write out their interview data. This recording format (Weed 1970; Voytovich 1974) recognizes the importance of "patient problems", particularly *behavioral* dysfunctions secondary to disease, but does not identify key questions that can be used to uncover the *cognitive* and *psychological* dimensions of a patient's *illness*. For example, the section entitled "Patient Profile" within this recording format requires only a cursory description of selected sociological features of the patient, but does not require students to record the patient's conceptualization of his/her health problem. Thus students learn to critically evaluate and improve the recording instrument they will be required to use during the clinical clerkships in their third and fourth years of training.

In conclusion, I have found that the *Introduction to Clinical Medicine* in the first year is a very effective context for demonstrating the utility of several key concepts. The organizing power and clinical relevance of "illness", "illness behavior", and "explanatory model", for example, become especially evident to students as their interviewing skills improve. This improvement, in turn, serves the important function of confirming their nascent clinical abilities and dispelling doubts about the appropriateness of their career plans. Perhaps most significant, from my view, is that these interview activities continually demonstrate how patients, families, and physicians draw from their cultural and personal milieux in order to construct, modify, and reconstruct explanations for suffering and misfortune. The role of cultural constructions in the practice of medicine is therefore more firmly understood than it ever could be from simply hearing a series of lectures.

REFLECTIONS

Teaching within the preclinical curriculum described above has been a very rewarding experience, both personally and professionally. The experience has convinced me that medical anthropology can contribute significantly to the preclinical training of medical students.

I have tried to identify the rationale for the teaching strategies and materials I have found useful as I have moved through a description of the contexts within which I work, so a lengthy summary here is not necessary. There are, however, several persistent issues which, I suspect, are generic to preclinical teaching efforts undertaken by medical anthropologists.

First, I recognize a continuing need to develop material which attracts the attention of dental students as well as medical students. Case materials and field data, for example, need to be developed which clearly illustrate the clinical relevance of medical anthropology for dental students. Beyond the traditional contributions of physical anthropologists, very little help can be identified in the current discussions about clinically applied anthropology. Yet this is a persistent problem for a medical anthropologist whose preclinical lectures may be directed to a class with about 35% dental students. (This may not be an issue, of course, in other schools where the preclinical education of medical and dental students is separated.)

Second, the tight schedule of the preclinical years makes it very difficult to devise extra-classroom teaching experiences which, by comparison, are accomplished very easily in graduate anthropology programs. Moving groups of preclinical students in and out of field settings effectively is a difficult task logistically and academically. Students often view these visits as simply "fun and games" unless there is good preparation prior to the trip, a clear task during the field visit, and planned discussion after the trip. I have found, in general, that bringing visitors from local communities and treatment programs *to* the class is just as effective and less time consuming (but I keep hoping to put together that "perfect" field experience).

Third, I believe that effective teaching in a preclinical curriculum is significantly influenced by one's own research activities. Research materials that clearly promote the development of healing, educating, or planning skills usually attract student interest, regardless of whether the research was done in a remote, small-scale society or in urban North America. I believe, however, that the development of research focusing on *local* patient populations or community samples is an important tactic: information about illness/disease and the health care system in the United States is viewed by students as especially relevant. One potential difficulty is that biocultural research efforts are often by necessity collaborative and take time to develop. A medical anthropologist may therefore face a year of preclinical teaching before he/she can draw from on-going localized research to strengthen and embellish lecture material. There is no easy answer to this dilemma and each "solution" will have to derive from a combined use of one's previous research, the general literature, and the earliest possible development of research within the region or community where the school is located.

Finally, the question about what aspects of medical anthropology are relevant for a preclinical curriculum will persist. The answer will, of course, be formed in part by the teaching opportunities available within the preclinical curriculum. My role, for example, in *ICM* has provided a clear opportunity to introduce materials from medical anthropology which are clearly relevant for the skill of *healing*. But I have argued above that there are other substantive materials within medical anthropology which can contribute to the development of preclinical students' skills in *educating* patients and *planning/evaluating* services. Working toward an optimum balance of material from medical anthropology which promotes all three of these skills constitutes the essential excitement of teaching in a preclinical curriculum.

NOTES

1. I have been a member of the department of psychiatry within the medical school at the University of Connecticut Health Center since 1976, supported in part by an NIMH grant for undergraduate medical education. This sustained support is gratefully acknowledged. I have also maintained a joint appointment with the department of anthropology at the university, contributing specifically to the doctoral training program in medical anthropology.
2. It is probably true, however, that the proportion of women in graduate anthropology is higher than the proportions shown in Table II for medical/dental students.
3. My graduate training in anthropology also helped me cope with my role in ICM. Specifically, a graduate seminar on stress and interviewing in fieldwork and the field interviews about illness completed for my dissertation proved to be two very relevant experiences for teaching in *ICM*.

REFERENCES

Alegira, D. et al.
  1977 El Hospital Invisible. Archives of General Psychiatry 34: 1354–1357.
Bourguignon, E.
  1976 Possession. San Francisco: Chandler and Sharp Publishers, Inc.
Cassell, E. J.
  1976 Illness and Disease. Hastings Center Report 6: 27–37.
Cay, E. L. et al.
  1975 Patient's Assessment of the Result of Surgery for Peptic Ulcer. Lancet 1: 29–31.
Chrisman, N. J.
  1977 The Health Seeking Process: An Approach to the Natural History of Illness. Culture,
       Medicine and Psychiatry 1: 351–377.
C.R.M./McGraw Hill Film Division
  1968 The Holy Ghost People.
Eisenberg, L.
  1977 Disease and Illness. Culture, Medicine and Psychiatry 1: 9–23.
Engel, G. L.
  1977 The Need for a New Medical Model: A Challenge for Biomedicine. Science 196:
       129–136.
Engel, G. L. and W. L. Morgan
  1973 Interviewing the Patient. London: W. B. Saunders Co., Ltd.
Etkind, N. L.
  1979 Biomedical Evaluation of Indigenous Medical Practices. Medical Anthropology 3:
       393–400.
Fabrega, H., Jr.
  1974 Disease and Social Behavior: An Interdisciplinary Perspective. Cambridge, Mass.: The
       MIT Press.
Foster, G. M.
  1976 Disease Etiologies in Non-Western Medical Systems. American Anthropologist 78:
       773–782.
Garrison, V.
  1977 Doctor, Espiritista or Psychiatrist?: Health Seeking Behavior in a Puerto Rican Neigh-
       borhood of New York City. Medical Anthropology 1: 65–180.
Glick, L. B.
  1967 Medicine as an Ethnographic Category: The Gimi of the New Guinea Highlands.
       Ethnology 6: 31–56.
Horton, R.
  1967 African Traditional Thought and Western Science. Africa 37: 50–71, 155–187.
International Films Bureau
  1968 The Shaman of North and South Nepal.
Kane, S. M.
  1975 Ritual Possession in a Southern Appalachian Religious Sect. Journal of American
       Folklore 87: 293–302.
Kleinman, A.
  1977 Recognition and Management of Illness Problems: Therapeutic Recommendations
       from Clinical Social Science. Massachusetts General Hospital Series on Psychiatric
       Medicine.
Kleinman, A., L. Eisenberg, and B. Good
  1978 Culture, Illness and Care: Clinical Lessons from Anthropologic and Cross-Cultural
       Research. Annals of Internal Medicine 88: 251–258.
Kleinman, A. and L. H. Sung
  1979 Why Do Indigenous Practitioners Successfully Heal? Social Science and Medicine
       13B: 7–26.

Korbin, J.
   1977   Anthropological Contributions to the Study of Child Abuse. Child Abuse and Neglect
          1: 7–24.
Lazare, A.
   1973   Hidden Conceptual Models in Clinical Psychiatry. New England Journal of Medicine
          288: 345–350.
MacAndrew, C. and R. B. Edgerton
   1969   Drunken Comportment: A Social Explanation. Chicago: Aldine.
Marshall, L.
   1966   N/um Tchai.
Marshall, L. and M. Biesele
   1974   N/um Tchai: The Ceremonial Dance of the Kung Bushmen. A Study Guide. Docu-
          mentary Educational Resources, Inc.
Murdock, G. P. et al.
   1978   World Distribution of Theories of Illness. Ethnology 17: 449–470.
Ness, R. C.
   1980   The Impact of Indigenous Healing Activity: An Empirical Study of Two Fundamen-
          talist Churches. Social Science and Medicine 148: 167–180.
Pattison, E. M.
   1968   Behavioral Science Research on the Nature of Glossolalia. Journal of the American
          Scientific Affiliation 20: 73–86.
Pattison, E. M., N. A. Lapins, and H. A. Doerr
   1973   Faith Healing. Journal of Nervous and Mental Disease 157: 397–409.
Redlener, I. and C. Scott
   1979   Incompatibilities of Professional and Religious Ideology: Problems of Medical
          Management and Outcome in a Case of Pediatric Meningitis. Social Science and
          Medicine 13B: 89–93.
Tellegen, A. et al.
   1969   Personality Characteristics of Members of a Serpent-handling Religious Cult. In J. N.
          Butcher (ed.) MMPI: Research Developments and Clinical Applications. New York:
          McGraw-Hill.
Turner, V. W.
   1964   An Ndembu Doctor in Practice. In A. Kiev (ed.), Magic, Faith and Healing. New
          York: Macmillan.
Voytovich, A. E.
   1974   Understanding the Problem Oriented Medical Record. The University of Connecticut
          Health Center, Farmington, Connecticut.
WCVB-TV, Boston
   n.d.   Espiritismo and Santeria (videotapes).
Weed, L. L.
   1970   Medical Records, Medical Education and Patient Care. The Press of Case Western
          Reserve University.
Wintrob, R. M.
   1973   The Influence of Others: Witchcraft and Rootwork as Explanations of Behavior
          Disturbances. Journal of Nervous and Mental Disease 156: 318–326.
Young, A. A.
   1976   Internalizing and Externalizing Medical Belief Systems: An Ethiopian Example.
          Social Science and Medicine, 10: 147–156.
   1978   Mode of Production of Medical Knowledge. Medical Anthropology 2: 97–121.

HOWARD F. STEIN

THE ETHNOGRAPHIC MODE OF TEACHING CLINICAL BEHAVIORAL SCIENCE

INTRODUCTION

In recent years the salience of behavioral sciences in medical education in general has become increasingly recognized (Montagu 1963; von Mering 1970; Spiegel 1971; Mauksch 1974; Fabrega 1975; Egnew 1977; Eisenberg 1977; Residency Review Committee 1977; Mauksch et al. 1978). This can be readily adduced from the presence of a behavioral science component of the National Board Examinations; from the proliferation of courses on family dynamics, human sexuality, death and dying, aging, human development, and ethnomedicine; emphasis on the transactional process of communication in medical interviewing; from the widespread interest in such self-awareness-oriented programs as Human Dimensions in Medical Education (affiliated with the Center for Studies of the Person, La Jolla, California); and from the development and institutionalization of two new primary care professions, Family Medicine and the Physician's Assistant, as specialists in the comprehensive and continuous treatment of the whole person and family.

If behavioral aspects of health and illness are indeed becoming accepted as integral rather than peripheral to medical education throughout the future practitioner's training, the question of how such learning best takes place then becomes paramount. Throughout education, not merely medical education, there has raged for over a decade the controversy between those who advocate programmed-modular learning (as exemplified by the "behavioral objectives" approach) and those who prefer a more open-ended approach to the learning-teaching experience (Green 1975; Gardner 1977). The present argument, not a particularly new one, is that in order to teach future health care personnel an openness to human complexity, the structure of the learning experience must itself be open-ended rather than finalistic or reductionistic. It is not that skills, techniques, and goals are unimportant. Rather, the *context* in which they are acquired determines whether they will become creative tools or restrictive prisons. The ethnographic approach to teaching suggested in this paper attempts to ensure a congruence between open-ended outcome and open-ended process.

THE ETHNOGRAPHIC PARADIGM

My thesis is that a holistic medical care that conceptualizes and treats a whole person and a whole family can come about only if the personal wholeness of the student or apprentice clinician is fostered. An ethnographic teaching-learning methodology emphasizing what might be called experience-based clinical behavioral science is offered as a means of achieving this desired end. According to this method,

N. J. Chrisman and T. W. Maretzki (eds.), Clinically Applied Anthropology, 61–82.
Copyright © 1982 by D. Reidel Publishing Company.

students at all levels in health care fields in which the writer teaches are encouraged
to utilize and discipline their own subjectivity rather than avoid or deny it. Several
principles of this approach are outlined, and clinical vignettes are offered to illustrate their operation: (a) the self as medical instrument, and the clinician-client
relationship as the most important "medicine" (Balint 1957); (b) serendipity; (c)
leading by following, (d) timeliness of interpretation and insight; (e) the value of
emotionally-charged learning situations; (f) teaching basic concepts by eliciting and
examining the students' own definitions, values, beliefs, premises, expectations, and
stereotypes. This mode of knowledge acquisition about oneself and about patients
is not designed to supplant existing rigorous scientific methods of determining
etiology, diagnosis, treatment plan, and prognosis. Instead, it is advanced as a complementary instrument for investigating psychodynamic, psychosomatic, psychosocial, and sociocultural aspects of the illness process, part of the "spectrum" that
is frequently overlooked. The diverse cultural settings in which this model is discussed are family practice residency training; psychiatry residency training; medical
student, physician's assistant, public health and medical anthropology classes,
seminars, and workshops.

Specifically, the classroom, seminar, and clinic setting are utilized as opportunities for *self-ethnography*, which leads to an ability to be a *clinical ethnographer* in
the service of patient care. It is the writer's assumption that the successful clinician
(as measured, say, in terms of patient compliance and satisfaction, [Korsch and
Negrete 1972]) must *prima facie* be *an astute ethnographer of his or her patients*.
A patient-encounter is every bit as legitimate a focus of study as is the traditional
"ethnic" or "national" unit-of-culture with a cast of hundreds or thousands. The
quality of the ethnography has nothing whatever to do with "sample size". Rather,
it has everything to do with the quality of the relationship and with the ability of
the clinical ethnographer to utilize his or her sensorium with the sensitivity of
electrophoresis. The method of *ethnographic teaching* discussed in this paper
emphasizes that not only are patients the "natives" whose personal and shared
worlds of symbol, relationship, and meaning need to be understood, but that the
students themselves and likewise their instructors are "natives" who, in becoming
"informants" on their own experiences (with identified patients, in assigned field
sites, *and* beyond the officially compartmentalized "professional" domain of their
lives), are able better to inform themselves about the experiential context of their
patients' lives (Balint 1957; Bion 1959; Devereux 1967; Bowen 1978; La Barre
1978).

The "field" is not separate from oneself — this, not limited to the ethnographer's
role, but co-extensive with teaching, learning, therapy — in fact, life. The personal
experience of classroom and clinic are *part of the "field"*. By extension, for one
who indeed is a good participant observer in the human condition, life itself is a
continuous ethnographic experience! One should not have to be among the Bonga-
Bonga to conduct *bona fide* fieldwork. Any rigid compartmentalization distorts
one's ability to perceive holistically, and hence makes it impossible to treat holistically. If one must travel a thousand miles to discover some acceptable form of

mankind, one wonders what part of himself the ethnographer is so eager to leave behind.

According to the model offered here, the educational experience is intrinsically a therapeutic experience — this because ultimately the ethnographic "subject" is the relationship between self and subject. I have used such settings as the clinic office, hospital grand rounds, consultations, home visits, case conferences, seminars, and even lectures as a means of learning the "culture" of the group by participant observation, in order to provide timely feedback of my observations to the members of that culture. It is possible that in the future the clinician-patient relationship will be based on this ethnographic clinical method. What Erikson writes of the relationship between analyst and analysand surely ought to be no different than that between the teacher of a future clinician and the student, and finally between practitioner and patient. "The 'classical arrangement' [of the patient on the analytic couch, and the therapist seated on a chair beyond the head of the couch, out of the patient's view] was only a means to an end — namely, a human relationship in which the observer who has learned to observe himself teaches the observed to become self-observant" (Erikson 1963: 422). What La Barre says of the psychiatrist holds equally for any clinician, scientific observer, or teacher: one "will not be able to see in his patients what he cannot afford to see in terms of his own defenses" (La Barre 1978: 269). Continuous self-ethnography, not unlike psychoanalysis, is a means of testing and transcending one's out-of-awareness assumptions (Hall 1977). Such self-discipline is necessary to the delivery of clinical care if the practitioner is to be emotionally and cognitively capable of distinguishing his or her own needs and perceptual organization of the world from those of the patient. There is all the difference in the world between therapy and acting-out.

In this chapter I argue that holism as an analytic framework and an organizing principle of therapy ought not only be applied *by* the practitioner to the patient population, but must first be applied *to* the student, in order that the future practitioner be able to treat the patient holistically. As a part of the therapeutic process, the practitioner must be able to locate himself or herself in that process — and not simply take for granted that the role of detached, objective, observer (which is the ideal according to the biomedical model) is actually possible, let alone preferable (Devereux 1967). According to the traditional medical model, one must determine a diagnosis before therapy proper can be initiated. However, the student and apprentice clinician discover that the communication itself in the good interview and history are inherently "therapeutic," precisely because patients appreciate being taken seriously as persons. Students, moreover, need this "ethnographic" framework in order to discover that information-gathering of a highly specialized type is only one aspect of the communication between patient and clinician, and that the communication process itself — if the clinician permits it — can be therapeutic: part of an end, rather than simply an instrumental means to the therapeutic goal that, according to medical semantic punctuation, commences at some later point. Here, self-knowledge is essential, since the patient's transference and the practitioner's own counter-transference constitute a considerable part of the communication process. Indeed, they function as meta-communications that can easily nullify the most expertly performed "skills".

Throughout all varieties of medical education — and, this writer would add, anthropological education — we have tended to devote so much time and effort to "packaging" and transmitting often highly abstracted information to students about prospective patients' cultures, that we have neglected the psycho-cultural realities of those whom we are training. (In anthropological training, it should be noted in passing, students are told of the professional perdition that awaits them should they "go native" in the field, and are admonished by their advisors not to take personal or cultural preconceptions to the field — as though a word to the psychodynamically naive should be sufficient!) We expect them to be humanely concerned about the subjective worlds which their clientele inhabit (or, more correctly, project), yet our educational methods, congruent with those of Western physicalistic medicine, have tended to neglect the fact that those whom we train are persons whose worlds of meaning — not unlike that of the practitioners — unconsciously influence clinical perception and decisions. The holism and integration we expect *of* them toward their patients we ought to provide *for* them in their training.

A word must be said for the use of psychoanalytic concepts and techniques in the clinical teaching of medical holism. Holism is an orientation which explores the patterned network of intra-personal (including somatic function) and inter-personal relationships and meanings among humans. As such, to ignore intrapsychic process and its representation in social action is to omit one potent avenue to decoding the meaning of meanings and relationships — for purposes of this paper, the experience of illness and clinician-patient encounters.

Holism, shall we say, must begin at home. This is not a matter of ideology, but of practical clinical ethnography. One must be able to distinguish between oneself and another before one can accurately perceive that other. Otherwise, the ethnography one writes will be little more than a species of disguised autobiography. Moreover, simply to know one's own cognitive categories is not enough (though our culture certainly supports the splitting of cognition from affect). One must come to know which taxonomies are more a matter of convenience or indifference, those which are more deeply invested in, those to which one is committed — and why (De Vos 1975). It is at this point that one begins to recognize the pervasiveness and fundamentality of transference phenomena not only in the clinical setting, but throughout cultural life. The discovery of one's own data (at many levels) becomes the key to understanding the patient unencumbered by one's unaware preoccupations and preconceptions. If all this sounds like an epistemology that is "too Freudian," the writer can offer no apology. One must go to where the data lead, else one will distort social reality in accordance with personal ideology-rationalized and culturally supported resistances: demonstrating in act what is denied in word.

THE SELF AS INSTRUMENT

It has been my observation that for the most part we instruct future clinicians as though they, as persons, were not really present. We hope that their years in professional training have effectively socialized *out* of them any and all subjectivity — the bane of scientific, objective medicine. We might hold an ideological commitment to the treatment of a vaguely conceptualized "whole person", but in practice approach the patient as a machine, an assemblage of parts "out of tune", heir to the tradition of John Colt and Henry Ford. Whether our model derives exclusively from the mechanical-assembly line image or metaphor of the Age of Industrialization, or is also influenced by the language of the Computer Age (feedback, biofeedback), it is important to recognize that not only does the practitioner perceive and treat the patient in this mode, but often shares this worldview and accepts its premises about human nature. The Newtonian-linear-Industrial model has bequeathed to us the legacy of the germ theory, organ systems, transplants, and behavioral objectives for specific goal-oriented programmed learning or treatment. The cybernetic-circular-systems model has more recently given us new approaches to understanding psychosomatic illness, the role of family conflict in pathogenesis, and the like. But both approaches avoid subjective experience, seeing it as not genuinely empirical or objective, as contaminating "hard" scientific data. In the process, *both* clinician and patient become depersonalized (Weizenbaum 1976; Stein and Kayzakian-Rowe 1978). What is worse, because at least in mainstream American culture the lay cultural model and the professional medical model overlap considerably, the selective *in*attention to illness experience is a matter of shared definition of the situation, and not an imposed "medical nemesis".

In my ethnographic teaching of clinical behavioral science, I have attempted to reintroduce subjectivity as a valid and necessary clinical tool. The concern here is how a *holistically* conceptualized health care training can foster in the student a finely calibrated "instrument" for dealing with the inner and inter-personal experiential worlds that span organ-system, personality-system, family-system, and culture-system. This approach does not discard biomedical science which the practitioner must master; rather, it demonstrates to be scientific what was heretofore discarded.

Human beings, we learned long ago from Freud, often perceive and treat other human beings not as they actually are, but in terms of previous, often very early, relationships. What is more, because this process is unconscious, one does not realize the inappropriateness of what is taking place. The distinction between transference and countertransference refers simply to whether patient or practitioner is the one who is "transferring" the emotion, perception, etc. Because all health restoring relationships are built on the dialectic of taking care of/taken care of, they are especially vulnerable to parent-child transferences (Simmel 1927). How can we best teach about this aspect of clinical relationships that is so conspicuously present, yet which students and residents with whom I have worked either take for granted or deny? By themselves, behavioral science textbooks, including works of

Freud himself, fail to convince residents of the clinical, practical value of their contents. What does gradually convince them is a clinical or interpersonal experience, which, upon interpretation, vividly illustrates the process *in them*. Life illuminates, indeed animates, the text. But life must first be illuminated: which is precisely why the ethnographic method shares so much dynamically with the psychoanalytic method.

One technique I use to teach about the importance of culture — including values, attitudes, beliefs, expectations, and especially how these are reflected in illness and health-seeking behavior — is to discuss his or her own culture with each resident in an open-ended fashion. One resident had remarked that his father had come from a wealthy family, had lost everything due to political and economic circumstances, and had taken a service job. With urgent speech, the resident related how his father had placed great pressure and expectations on him to succeed in school — perhaps to vindicate his father's life, to reestablish his father's past through his son's future. Later the same day, during a conference with all Family Practice residents, he was worriedly concerned about understanding the assignment the writer had just made. He wanted to be sure he knew exactly what his instructor wanted so that he could do his work as "perfectly" as possible. After the other residents had left the room, he remained behind in his chair, pressing me to clarify the assignment. An exactingly conscientious man, he wanted to do what was right — the first time. He persisted with tense posture and anxious voice. I felt that no amount of specification could satisfy him *in his wish to satisfy me*.

Suddenly our earlier discussion came to mind. Perhaps he had not heard my voice and message: namely, that process was more important than next week's product. Perhaps he was responding to his instructor's "demands" with the same urgency and vocabulary with which he described his earlier family life, education, and most specifically, his father. I paused, and quietly said: "Dr. X, relax. I am not your father. I think that you're hearing me as though I were him." He did indeed relax: his full broad smile and eased posture confirmed the hypothesis. I then briefly interpreted what I felt to be taking place: that the resident acted as though his teacher expected from him the same as had his father; that he did not hear his teacher's voice, but that of his father in its stead. Perhaps for this reason he could not quite understand the assignment as precisely as he wished, even though he repeated the assignment "perfectly". This seemed to me the *timely* opportunity to reintroduce the concept of "transference", which we had on a previous occasion discussed cognitively, intellectually. Again, he beamed: he had been ready now to comprehend *experientially* with conviction the meaning of this abstract concept. (Interestingly, this student subsequently said that he wished to get to know me better as a person.)

I do not wish to imply that the transference was miraculously "cured". Nor is my teaching style self-consciously designed to be "therapeutic". Nonetheless, I long ago discarded the spurious distinction between teaching and therapy. So long as the personhood of teacher and student is permitted to be present, the educational process must, by consequence if not intent, involve the emotions as well as the cognitive apparatus. In fact, to permit the presence of affect is to modify that very cognitive apparatus. Over subsequent weeks, this resident's exactitude and intensity returned, though not quite with his earlier desperation. Resistance and transference should be expected in the future: a single breakthrough from gentle confrontation and insight does not eliminate the influence of his thirty years. Now this resident proudly proclaims that he is beginning to take notice of many "psychological" aspects of his patients that he had heretofore overlooked; that what was initially an incomprehensible behavioral science has now become "second nature". Over time the less resistance he has to insights about himself, the more superb a clinician he will become.

On another occasion, two residents presented a case conference. Here, I used the group-process both to illustrate certain concepts about group-process (and family dynamics), and to demonstrate the necessity of understanding and working through their feelings about the patient before they could formulate a treatment plan in the best interest of the patient.

Briefly, the patient was a middle-aged "hippie" from a large eastern city, a regular smoker of "grass", spoiled by a wealthy family, a man who left his children to join a commune and indulge in all varieties of group-sex, and whose personal God would give him everything he wanted. He had been seen by each of the residents, each time wanting a pain killer for his lower G. I. pain which continued to hurt him despite the fact that no pathology could be found. (His father, however, had died of cancer of the colon — which identification we later pursued.) As the residents presented the case, a group consensus about this patient was quickly reached: he was an addict, lazy, manipulative, overindulged, and so on. These words, it must be noted, were those used by the residents to describe *the patient*. Only much later did the group come to recognize that these "loaded" words equally described how the residents *felt toward* the patient.

The residents delegated to their instructor the task of finding some quick way of ridding them of this bad patient, or at least telling them how to manage him. During the case presentation, they alternated between laughter and ridicule toward the patient. His life-style was obviously "crazy" — an affront to those values the residents cherish and represent. I declined the role they wished to assign: the "expert" in behavioral science who would make a magical recommendation that would solve (expunge) their problem. That is, I refused to join in their group-fantasy, their wish to exculpate the "bad" or "problem" patient (Stierlin 1973a; Stierlin 1973b). I returned the responsibility for the patient to the group — a group of which I was a member, but not the Savior. This proved no easy task, for a thinly disguised hostility was directed at me when I refused to give them the answer.

After the formal case was presented, my goal was to help the residents recognize their own disdain for this patient, a task that was exhausting, but ultimately rewarding. The "conference" was structurally a group (proto-culture) who could not begin *rationally* to attempt to solve the patient's problem until they solved their own. When asked if they disliked the patient, they vehemently denied any such feelings, becoming hostile toward me for even suggesting the notion. I then reflected to them what feeling-tone (not merely content) I had heard during the presentation. I temporarily added "fuel" to their fire (joining, rather than challenging, the defense) by vividly describing a common picture of "addicts": their manipulation, their seductiveness, their seemingly bottomless neediness, their need to frustrate attempts to help or cure them, and the like. I attempted to see this patient through the residents' eyes: physicians are not supposed to dislike any patient, but are called upon to treat everyone, to *care* for everyone. What do you do with "negative" feelings when you're not even supposed to have them?

Gradually, the residents began to concur with this portrait of the patient and of themselves. Their words became less defensive, and their feelings came out. They acknowledged and accepted their frustration and anger, and began to perceive how this influenced the type of therapy they wanted to give the patient: immediate detoxification, bluntly confronting him and exposing his lies. Together we recognized that the initial "treatment plan" was a disguised form of punishment, one designed to meet their needs rather than genuinely help the patient. This patient, in fact, highlighted their needs through his threat to them: omniscience, omnipotence, omnibenevolence. This patient had made them feel totally inadequate, helpless, and impotent.

We gradually worked from an initial group-transference to the patient (as evil) and to their clinical teacher (as redeemer) to the possibility of *identifying with* the patient and trying to understand why he was so voraciously needy, manipulative, deceptive. Looking at the family history, we considered the possibility that, having never received enough from his mother, he was determined to re-create inadequate mothers everywhere he went, to "set up", so to speak, the early frustrating relationship and prove how terrible people are. How easily the Family Physicians could adopt and be enveloped in this role, and devoured by the patient's needs! After all, Family Physicians are supposed to care about people, not merely organs; and these Family Physicians were being delegated the role of mother-who-can-never-be-good-enough. Yet a physician is also expected to Know — with almost God-like perfection and prescience and availability. Was it possible, we briefly explored, to be a professional and be vulnerably human, to realize the limitations of one's knowledge, and admit it even to a patient? Or, to revise one's medical-cultural rules of benevolence, and help the patient to set limits without becoming sadistic in order to have vengeance on the patient? After fully exploring both the residents' group-transference onto the patient, and the patient's transference to the Family Physicians, we *then* (and only then) could explore the task of how best rationally to help the patient (Bion 1959).

During yet another case conference in which the identified patient was a chronically ill man in his seventies, the presenting resident felt strangely confused and paralyzed, unable to evaluate how best to care for his patient. Then he came out with a "Freudian" slip: "I just couldn't see putting my father in a nursing home". He suddenly realized that his transference to the patient was the decisive obstacle to a clinical decision. He had been unable to separate the patient's needs in the context of the family, from what he had not until that moment realized were his own needs. The resident's breakthrough was the point at which the patient existed separate from the resident's needs and guilts: the resident's resistance had first to be overcome.

None of these illustrations has a magical, "fairy tale" ending. Indeed, to force a conclusion compromises the process that is the core not only of this learning-teaching method, *but of patient care itself.* These vignettes illustrate the need for *serendipity* in medical education. Had I rigidly adhered to a pre-planned agenda, or to formalized objectives, or to the classical arrangement of the case conference in which only the patient is discussed, these emotionally-charged learning experiences would not have been *permitted* to arise. These vignettes also illustrate the pervasiveness of what is too often compartmentalized as "psychiatric" in day-to-day primary care medicine. Likewise, they illustrate the need to take the residents' subjective worlds seriously, when the pay-off (if we think in terms of cost-efficiency) in the long run is greater and there is more subtle attentiveness to the interplay between human biology, psychology, and socio-cultural factors. What the residents are able to notice and accept in themselves they will be more skilled in observing, accepting, and treating in their patients.

Although students and residents are asked to read a plethora of material on family dynamics and psychodynamics and cultural ethos, it is their emotionally-charged personal experience of what is initially the remote printed word that makes for their conviction that these behavioral, subjective domains are every much as "tangible" facts as are blood-sugar and urine-sugar counts. The only thing that changes is the "instrument". The instrument they add to their already formidable array is themselves, which offers a field of vision, a parallax, they would otherwise lack. Indeed, in one complex case we discovered that it was our own field of vision — and the likewise too biomedically focused perspective of physicians who treated this patient for over twenty years — that prevented us from looking beyond the patient's out-of-control diabetes to discover that his psychopathic personality; his seductive, overprotective, and over-indulgent mother; and now his wife (who would furtively bring hamburgers, soft drinks, and cakes into the hospital — all medically contraindicated) were together part of an *out-of-control system.*

LEADING BY FOLLOWING

For several years I taught behavioral science to first year medical students, Family Practice residents, and Psychiatry residents at Meharry Medical College and became convinced of the value of "serendipity" as a tool for the development of clinical insight by the resident. The less their instructor needed to prove that he was in "control" of the class, the freer students and residents became with their hypotheses, inferences, and observations. One fourth year medical student who had earlier participated in my Community Psychiatry seminar, decided to take a psychiatry externship in Cleveland. Upon his return, he remarked with surprise and the pleasure of discovery:

You know, Dr. Stein, all those different ethnic groups you were always talking about – Poles, Italians, Jews, Irish. I never gave too much thought about them. I'm not saying what you taught wasn't true, but I'd never seen it, so it didn't have anything to do with me. I just couldn't believe that Whites could be at each other's throats like Blacks and Whites are in the South. I grew up in rural Alabama, and we just didn't have much to do with Whites. There'd be some troubles now and then, but we each kept to ourselves. When you talk about racism, I think Black and White. Then I did that externship in Cleveland, at a child guidance clinic associated with the Department of Psychiatry. I couldn't believe what I saw. There was this one Polish lady absolutely irate over the fact that her daughter was planning to marry an Italian fellow. I don't know if they ended up disowning her or not, but it was like the end of the world. Down here in the South, I guess we're so used to thinking only Black and White, we can't imagine anybody else being like that.

During an eight-week rotation of Family Practice residents, I brought up the issue of ethnic factors in individual and family responses to illness, but issued a warning about over-generalizing, even stereotyping, about an individual based on assumptions about that patient's ethnicity. A Family Practice resident born and reared in New Orleans gave a more cogent illustration of intra-ethnic diversity than any textbook (or "cookbook") could provide.

When I first talked with residents and students from New York, I couldn't believe them! (He smiled, continuing:) They'd tell me that up in Harlem you locked your door as soon as you got home; you kept your door locked at night; and you'd better be careful if you go out. I said to myself, 'Are these the same people I know?'. Down in New Orleans when I was growing up, Black folk were out on the streets at all hours of the night. Everybody was always visiting somebody. You never locked your doors. That would have been unfriendly. Besides, nobody was going to try to break in, even in the middle of the night. People would stay up till all hours on their porches. They weren't afraid of getting mugged or murdered or anything.

It was at *experientially* opportune times such as this that I could introduce, say, the issue of regional variation in family structure, or the community social support system. What I was doing is foreign neither to the anthropological fieldworker nor to the psychoanalyst: a paradoxical method of *leading by following*, and interpreting only as the student or resident is ready. Eventually, during the various courses, all the formal topics had been covered, all the readings assigned. Rather than to program courses from start to finish, I tried to use the group-process as a means of eliciting and analyzing cultural material.

SEIZING THE MOMENT

On one occasion, all but one of the residents had arrived in the seminar room and had joined the "circle" of chairs. The last resident was evidently still in another building on the wards. The class would begin obviously late. The Family Practice residents began looking hither and yon, at one another, fidgeting about, and the like. Finally, I broke the silence, and causally introduced the issue of "time", "waiting", criteria underlying "who waits for whom", and the like. How, through the manipulation of "time" is it communicated that the "subject" is more important than the "person", or that one status-person merits a longer wait than another?

As a group, we then explored how the use of time reflects status, expectation, authority, power, money, and so forth. The residents, to a person, said that they had never thought of it before, that time is something we all take for granted. Yet, they began to realize that this is an assumption that must be examined. We discussed the American cultural meaning of "being on time", punctuality, tardiness, how these are bound up with ideas about efficiency, a sense of place, and moral judgments about who is a good and who is a bad person — or patient. We then discussed many of the value and economic assumptions underlying the issue of time-scarcity in medicine, and how time is crucially linked to patient compliance and satisfaction.

What, for instance would we make of a Latin patient, whose sense of time is much more fluid, much less urgent, than "Anglo" time; a person for whom a two o'clock medical appointment might mean two thirty or two forty-five? Or, how would we think of a Black patient who expresses her resentment toward the White world (which largely also includes those from all groups who have "made it" in medicine) by passive-aggressive lateness? Are these irrelevant questions, or are they central to the type of physician-patient relationship that forms? Such topics as cultural relativism, the unconscious, and transference emerge readily as the class and the intructors together learn to lead by following — by listening, and by introducing novel ideas or perspectives when they are *timely*, embedded within a suddenly familiar context. We could then delve into an ostensibly "academic" topic such as the fact that culture is largely *internalized*. Perhaps in the past we had missed many subtle cues which expressed the patient's cultural orientation, and also had interpreted these cues in terms of *our* cultural meanings. In this particular discussion, we had discovered that *we* had taken "time" as a fixed "given", while it "exists" only as part of a larger cultural ethos or pattern whose rules are mostly out-of-awareness (Hall 1977).

The residents quickly realized that this was not some intellectual game or exercise. Rather, it was a way of communicating types of information through using ourselves, and the relationships in the group, as sources of information. Types of "facts" which initially seemed only peripheral to the practice of Family Medicine emerged as focal. But those categories of "facts" became relevant to medicine only after they became salient to the residents themselves. The Family Medicine residents could lead their patients by following them only after they had learned how to "follow" themselves — how to listen to themselves.

ESTABLISHING BASIC CONCEPTS

At Meharry, in attempting to convey varieties of family structures, division of labor, roles, statuses, and how these are related to health care, I often avoided the lecture or formal case format. Instead, I began by asking each resident his or her understanding or definition of what a "family" is. Since Family Medicine distinguishes itself as being a specialty for the treatment of the entire family, I felt that we ought to cover the concept of family. I did so by inquiring, rather than telling – at least at first. Some residents were from India, some from New York, some from New Orleans, some from the rural South, and so forth. Each had a different concept of family. I expanded the discussion to include the "extended family", with similar results. Finally, I pursued the concept of family to its limits in anthropology, to subsume "fictive kinship" (e.g., a godfather) and the "personal network" of reciprocity that may extend far beyond relation by blood and marriage. The residents spoke of their own families, often coming to recognize that they assumed that all "normal" families should be like their own. Some suggested that perhaps the Black church could be regarded as an extended family, not only in the past as the singular institution controlled by Blacks, but in the present as well. *The group* took the idea further: perhaps, when we work with a Black patient who has "no" family in the American culture-bound sense, we might look into the social supports offered by his or her church.

On another occasion, I raised the question of the relationship between diet, nutrition, and culture – even culture change. Three residents from India shared their experiences, which turned out to be far more diverse than this American writer would expect! One resident laughingly said that he had been introduced to beef hamburgers by a fellow Indian, but that his wife, also from India, refuses to this day to eat meat from the cow. We talked about disgust, not merely the somatic dis-gust, but the system of meanings that elicits the gastric response. No one needed to forcibly make the obvious point that food is never mere nutrient, but is always bound up with some symbolic or ritual meaning.

I related an incident my parents had told me, in which the pediatrician had recommended to them, Orthodox Jews, that bacon would be a good supplement to my early diet, since at that time I was apparently undernourished! They said they politely told him that we were Jewish; and, would a substitute be possible? I further recounted one of my father's stories. During the years his parents and siblings were living in the squalid Jewish ghetto of Chicago, he was often sent to the Jewish butcher shop to get the "leavings" of what the others did not want: lungs, liver, intestines, etc. He laughed, saying that today these are considered expensive luxuries. No sooner had I finished than a Black Family Practice resident from the Deep South added that what Blacks were, out of poverty, compelled to eat in the past, has now become "Soul Food": chitterlings (chitlins), greens, and fried chicken. Having begun to think about the meanings which food can have, the residents quite naturally gravitated toward the issue of attempting to work within a patient's frame of reference when prescribing a diet, and making certain that they understood the patient's and patient's family's diet in particular, rather than assuming that conventionally held stereotypes corresponded to reality (e.g., "Italians only eat starchy and greasy foods", versus the reality of an individual family's diet).

During an individual consultation, one resident reported that he had just read on the sports page of a local newspaper that potato chips, cookies, candy, soft drinks, and bread were all considered to be "junk food". He asked: "Why is bread a junk food?" I took that opportunity to explore with him the specific, yet conceptually broader, issue of how and why people classify foods in particular ways. I inquired into the resident's taxonomy of foods, and the assumptions that lay behind them (e.g., nutrition, balanced diet, etc.), and then broached the issue of the importance of affect in cognitive classifications (Stierlin 1973b). We explored more closely the significance of the idea of "junk foods" within the "natural health food movement" (Brisset and Lewis 1978), and discovered a strict dualism between natural or organic, and artificial or synthetic. Furthermore, we discovered that attitudes toward food were related closely to other attitudes toward the social and natural world, that what began innocently as a food classification belongs to the wider issues of identity, conversion, ideology, worldview and the Manichean dualism between "good" and "evil" that characterizes the current "holistic health" movement.

The resident had brought up the subject of "junk food" independently. We had discussed the symbolic significance of foods on previous occasions, but now he was taking the initiative, making new connections, raising the issue of food classification *himself*. What is more, his source for the question was not a journal of *scientific* medicine, but a local newspaper, a rich source of insight into *popular folk medicine*, a distinction we had dealt with formally (academically) earlier, but which now made *experiential* sense. A further outcome of this incident was his greater attentiveness to the varieties of American "folk medicine" such as are presented in newspapers, magazines, radio, television, and the like. In order better to know his patients, he was discovering that he must not only keep up with the medical journals, but with popular-folk culture(s) as well.

A later incident with this same resident facilitated the illustration of a number of basic concepts: taboo, culture change, acculturation, values, to mention only four. The resident was an experienced Vietnamese physician who was undergoing residency training in the U.S. to qualify him for board certification and practice. Though neither taciturn nor loquacious, during one case conference in which pastoral counselors and family practice physicians collaborated on a case, he seemed to be unusually quiet, offering no comments but listening attentively behind arms tightly crossed in front of him.

The minister summarizing the case stated that the identified patient, a woman in her thirties, married, and with two children, seemed unconsciously to use her overprotectiveness and solicitousness toward her multiply handicapped three year old son as a means of avoiding and rejecting her husband, sexually and otherwise. Thus the mother's worry over her child was later seen by most members attending the case conference as a symptom of a disturbance in the family system as a whole.

Later that afternoon, during my regular private consultation with the resident, I opened with the question: "What did you think of the case this morning?" During the conference, I had not wished to press the resident, but recognized that "something" was different about today, and did not want to make a *public* confrontation out of it. (I utilized a "face-saving" approach, waiting until a private occasion was available to bring it up. The resident already felt quite "different" and "foreign"; hence to make an issue of it in the group, even in the guise of discussing case *content*, would be to heighten the sense of cultural-personal difference even within a group of professionals.) He replied very candidly:

In this conference I just wanted to observe. You know I want to learn a great deal about
American culture — very fascinating. Since I am over here I need to learn how people think and
do things. In there this morning I would not know what to say. You do things very different
here in America than we do in my country, Vietnam. And since my patients will be Americans
I learn as much as I can about American culture — I read the newspaper, every page (broad
smile). About the case, I can tell you this: In my country you would never hear of a case like
this. A person would never go to the doctor or to the priest about family problems, especially
sexual problems. Here (laughs briefly), everyone talks openly about everything, even sex. You
can even have conferences about it. But in Vietnam the patient would be ashamed to talk about
it. Sex is, how do you say, very personal. A patient would be embarrassed to talk about it to
anyone. You just don't talk about it. Here, people talk with their friends about very intimate
things. In Vietnam, nobody will know. But now I am here, and I listen and watch closely how
people think and what they talk about, so that I can learn to counsel them.

At this point it was easy to discuss the interpersonal dynamics and consequences of
taboos, culture change, acculturation, and value orientations, in relation to a "case"
which is only fictitiously separate from himself, but which in fact engages his own
personality.

Values and taboos are not readily discardable, violable, and instantly substitut-
able. It is necessary, over time, to nurture the resident's own personal integration,
which requires something of a meta-cultural adaptability. The resident will be
better able to *understand* his patient, his patient's culture(s), and culture changes
the patient undergoes, when he understands these concerning himself — which is
in turn facilitated by a process in which he comes to feel that *he is understood by
another who is interested in him*. Another way of putting it is to say that basic
clinical-ethnographic concepts are truly established when they become a matter
of *conviction*; that is, when affect-laden insight is fused with cognitive skill. The
clinical-ethnographic task can be summed up as a process of overcoming cultural
(which is to say, shared-defensive) resistance to insight (Devereux 1967; Hall 1977;
La Barre 1978). Paradoxically, this may prove easier for one who is originally
"alien" to the culture than for the student or clinician who takes the culture for
granted, shares in its defenses, and ethnocentrically assumes that all mankind lives
by the same rules as does he!

TOOLS FOR ELICITING DATA

One tool I recently introduced to Family Practice residents is an adaptation from the
"kinship diagram" (genealogy) that is standard fare in anthropological field research
(Schusky 1965; Pendagast and Sherman 1977; Rakel 1977; Medalie 1978). However,
it is used for much different ends. Although I ultimately suggest to the residents
that a kinship diagram can be effective in interviewing patients, eliciting medical,
family, and social histories, I initially use it with the residents. Since we are all
"natives", if we can learn about ourselves in a particular way, then we may be
better disposed to use that way in learning about our patients. The kinship chart
functions simultaneously as (1) a means of building rapport between instructor
and residents; (2) as a means of obtaining information from them not only about

individuals but about relationships; (3) and as a device analogous to "projective tests" in psychology (e.g., the Rorschach inkblot) in which associations or connections are made that are not written onto the chart, which in turn lead to questions based on those associations. Soon the portrait is no longer (primarily) a one-way question-and-answer. The residents begin to add to the expanding diagram, relating stories about relationships, feelings, illnesses, and the like. This further suggests questions I could not have known to ask. Moreover, it convincingly (over time) suggests that a "family" consists, even medically, of more than discrete individuals who share only a genetic history: the emotional and relationship history and structure come to play a direct part in the no-longer-compartmentalizable "medical history". In short, what began as a rigid, virtually closed exercise, ends as an open-ended free association in which the ethnographer interjects questions about facts or relationships to which the residents have led him. While initially it may be time consuming to do this, in the long run it is not only more "efficient", but more *valid*. This is so because the physician is able to learn about the patient's network of relationships, meanings, and feelings that most likely would be missed in the exclusively questionnaire-like directed medical interview. This approach promises much return on the physician's investment of time, since it encourages the patient literally to draw a picture of his or her life. The physician only needs be attentive to where the patient is leading, and ask relevant medical (e.g., diagnostic) questions as they are timely.

Participant observation, another familiar anthropological technique, should also be adaptable by the Family Physician. In field research, the anthropologist often becomes a part of (a participant in) what is being observed, not merely standing on the sidelines as a pure observer. The *clinical* participant observer simply takes this one step further: the clinician communicates or interprets to the patient what he or she observed the patient saying or doing. My activities as a clinical behavioral scientist with Family Practice residents is no different from what I hope they would do with their patients. The familiar X-ray viewer, for example may have additional surprisingly novel and unlikely uses: (a) as a marvelous potential "Rorschach" of what the patient is thinking about, (b) for the physician to compare what he or she sees with what the patient sees (in both instances: what each pays attention to), and (c) as a medium for enhancing the physician-patient relationship. Viewing the X-ray negative with the patient offers the opportunity for the Family Physician to lead by following. The physician, however, must be prepared to *recognize* the opportunity.

I discovered these things about the X-ray box by accident. I had been consulting with one Family Practice resident in his office, when a nurse came to the door and brought an X-ray negative. The resident told me that we would have to interrupt briefly our conference, so that he could talk with the patient — or, he asked, "Would you be interested in seeing us together?" I welcomed the opportunity. The resident began walking toward the door to the examination room to bring in the patient. I suggested that he first ask the patient's permission. He concurred. Returning momentarily from the examination room (the door was closed when he discussed the matter with the patient) he briefly introduced us, and placed the negative in the X-ray box on the wall. The patient stood slightly to the left of the box, the resident directly in front, and I stood slightly to the right.

The resident directed the patient's attention to a fuzzy spot on the left lung, telling him that the pneumonia was gradually clearing up, but that he wanted to be sure there was not a small tumor obscured by the pneumonia. The physician's plan was to keep him on antibiotics until the lung completely cleared.

From the beginning of this interaction, however, the patient had not been looking at his left lung. He had been examining his heart. Quavering, he said: "Is the heart the way it should be? It looked different the last time". He had previously had angina, and was concerned about the size of his heart. Was he about to have another attack? was the unasked question. The physician, still thinking about clearing the lung, replied that his heart was fine. He then gently instructed him to continue taking his antibiotics, and to make an appointment for two weeks, at which time another X-ray would be taken.

After the patient left, I suggested to the resident that we postpone continuing our earlier discussion, and that we examine the interaction that took place in front of the X-ray box. What had seized my attention was the fact that while the physician and the patient were looking at the same "stimulus", the X-ray negative, they were noticing, directing their attention to, entirely different parts of it. I wanted to share this discovery with the resident and see where it might go. First, I emphasized that neither physician nor patient was "right" or "wrong" in observing what he did. Then I began to speculate about how the seemingly unambiguous X-ray negative might serve as a marvelous tool to compare what is on the physician's mind with what is on that of the patient. The resident became enthusiastic. He remarked that in the previous X-ray, which he had viewed with the patient, the heart seemed to be slightly distended in one place, and that he wanted this X-ray to evaluate the condition of the patient's heart, in addition to wanting to follow the pneumonia. Having viewed the X-ray before the patient's arrival, he remarked that he was convinced that what he had seen in the earlier X-ray was only a shadow, caused simply by how the patient was standing. He saw no need to talk about the heart, because for *him*, there was no pathology to discuss. But he began to see where I had been leading: what for the physician was of no concern remained paramount with the patient; and the "medium" for discovering what was on the patient's mind was the "Rorschach" that might easily go unnoticed because it is merely (in the medical eye) a conventional X-ray negative (this point, incidentally, is equally salient for the radiologist, cardiologist, or pulmonary specialist).

Both the resident and the writer were excited about this serendipitous discovery. There was no need to assign him to use the X-ray as a formal "psychological test". Through this experience, he made the connection, and it is inexpugnable. He was *ready* to admit a new perspective to his clinical repertory, and not pre-select admissable data on criteria of professional compartmentalization. The point is not the specific discovery of the X-ray box as a potentially important interpersonal tool in the physician-patient relationship. Rather, by viewing the physician-patient relationship as one involving clinical participant observation by the clinician, an enormous realm of *unanticipatable* possibilities opened up. It is an *attitude* that admits, or excludes, the type of data discussed in this paper. (This casts an entirely new light on the issue of evaluation; for if one seriously uses the method of clinical ethnography, any assessment of specific predetermined academic, cognitive and behavioral skills must be supplemented with a willingness to recognize the residents' own creative inferences — no less real because they cannot be predicted.)

This experience raises a more generic conceptual issue, which in turn will be illustrated by a final vignette. In recent years, medical anthropologists have been emphasizing the importance of being aware of differing "Explanatory Models" (Kleinman et al. 1976) as sources of problems in communication, compliance, and patient satisfaction (Korsch and Negrete 1972; Mumford 1977). Foster (1976) distinguishes between "naturalistic" and "personalistic" etiological models; von Mering (1961) identifies at least seven distinct disease models and treatment pathways; Eisenberg (1977) distinguishes between "illness" as a subjective and intersubjective experience, and "disease" as a diagnostic category for classifying entities identified by Western medical science; Fabrega (1974) and Kleinman (1978a) contrast the "biomedical" and the "ethnomedical" model; and Weidman and Egeland (1973) note that a "health culture" as a social institution is a central organizing concept for understanding patient (and, by extension, practitioner) attitudes, beliefs, expectations and the like. This list is by no means exhaustive. While these different explanatory models *of* "explanatory models" (Foulks 1978; Kleinman 1978b) have been the subject of my classroom lectures, seminar presentations, and case conferences, the question remains as to how or whether they make a difference in students' and residents' clinical work.

One example must suffice to demonstrate the process by which the necessity for considering these models became a matter of clinical conviction *to the practitioner*. I had been asked to serve as both observer and "coach" by one Family Practice resident who was working with a chronically depressed, immature, very little girlish woman whose twenty-six years chronicled a series of traumatic recurrent losses: early abandonment by an alcoholic mother; orphaned by a father who had no time for children; a first marriage ending in divorce; several miscarriages; two previous live births, both children having been taken from her under questionable legal and family circumstances; remarriage and rejection by her present in-laws; and constant pain during intercourse, which made her afraid that her "very understanding" husband may also eventually leave her.

Two years ago she gave birth to twins who are quite healthy according to her evaluation. Recently she became unintentionally pregnant, and she and her husband agreed that she should seek an abortion. Following the abortion, the gynecologist suggested that she have a vaginal hysterectomy, which medically "promised" both to relieve her painful menstruations and eliminate pain during intercourse. During an office visit, in which the resident, the patient, and the anthropologist were present in the examining room, the resident sought to alleviate her anxiety about the forthcoming surgery by explaining thoroughly the exact procedure which would be used and its outcome. As the resident spoke, she became increasingly anxious, as was evident by increased fidgeting with a large wad of facial tissue in her hands. The more the physician explained, the more she twisted and tore at the paper, the more frequently she averted eye contact, and the more she withdrew by bringing her arms and legs together leaning forward, and lowering her head. Her voice was silent, but her body spoke — a different language from that of anatomy, physiology, or endocrinology.

The resident explained that a vaginal hysterectomy would leave no scars, since the surgeon would not have to enter "through the belly". And within a few weeks she would be fully recovered, and would be able to have sex without any pain. The careful, complete explanation lasted perhaps ten minutes. When the physician had finished, the patient very briefly lifted her head, looked up, still rolling the paper into a ball, pulling at it, and asked worriedly: "When everything is over — I know this sounds ridiculous — but how do I know that I will still be a woman? And I'm afraid that after going through all of this that my husband won't want me anymore . . . " The resident leaned forward to reassure her, but began to repeat his previous *anatomical* explanation, only this time more urgently. The patient responded by avoiding eye contact, and attacking her wad of facial tissue with renewed anxiety. When the resident paused, I said to the patient in a very quiet voice, speaking slowly: "You are afraid of losing even more: your insides, your husband. And you'll be an orphan again". Whereupon the wringing anxiety ceased, and the patient broke into heavy sobs. As she cautiously began making eye contact, and gesturing with her hands, she literally poured out her dread of loss — body parts, body image, sexual identity, marriage. The patient now had the opportunity to give vent to her "Explanatory Model" of what might happen to her, even though she — ambivalently — sought the surgery.

Later I discussed this session with the resident. The resident recognized that I simply had observed the patient closely and listened to the present circumstance through the "third ear" of her experiential past and anticipated future. Not that the *instrumental* aspect of the surgery was unimportant; but rather that it needed to be contained within the patient's *expressive* concerns, however irrational or unwarranted they may appear to the observer. Here was a situation structurally identical with that of the X-ray episode: Physician and patient looking at the same "stimulus," but experiencing and explaining it differently. In these cases, the physician will stand a greater chance of having the patient pay attention to his view if he attentively inquires into what the patient "sees". It is from clinically vivid episodes such as have been described in this paper that I have discovered the process by which such conceptual and abstract issues as "Explanatory Models" become salient to the student and practitioner. The issue for a truly ethnographic pedagogy is, ironically, the same as in psychoanalytic psychiatry: "how" to teach is bound up with "when" to teach. One must be observant enough to learn that from one's students and residents.

CONCLUSION

I have argued in this chapter that if health care givers are to practice medicine holistically, then their medical education must itself be holistic. If we accept the fact that content is inseparable from context, then we must include the student or resident as a person in the experiential context of his or her medical training. Although the health care giver as "person" and as "professional" can be radically compartmentalized, its result is the impoverishment of medical care — rationalized, to be sure, by the invocation of "scientific objectivity". Yet, as this paper has suggested, the "choice" to exclude the subjective domain is itself subjectively (defensively) motivated. We can either deceive ourselves and our residents (and bolster their defensive self-deception) by naively pretending that only a certain type of data, and only certain instruments and tests that observe and analyze such data, are genuinely medical. Or we can enlarge the scope of medicine and welcome those phenomenological, personalistic aspects of the practitioner and the patient we have traditionally berated and suppressed. Improved medical care towards a whole person and a whole family can come about only when the personal wholeness of the practitioner is fostered. Far from being unscientific mysticism, we are discovering this to be empirically verifiable — and to be good medicine.

If holistic medicine — which is to say comprehensive, systemic care — is not to be merely an elusive ideological shibboleth, then we must develop a means to convey the holistic approach that has simultaneously personal and clinical immediacy for the student and resident in all clinical sciences. In this paper a number of vignettes have illustrated the promise of experience-based learning not only as a tool for the learning of clinical behavioral science, but more widely, as a tool for integrating those overdetermining and multidetermining variables present in every case (Stephens 1978; Stein 1979a, b). This perspective insures that the determination of etiology, diagnosis, treatment plan, and prognosis will be comprehensively thought through.

If this approach places a greater burden on the student or resident in dealing with the subtleties and complexities of human behavior, it equally places a greater burden on the teacher of clinical behavioral science whether to medical anthropologists, physician's assistants, or family practice physicians. For if the practitioner is to be "on call" in the full human sense discussed here, the clinical behavioral scientist must likewise be prepared to be "on call" *with* his or her colleague, both in the literal sense and in the figurative sense of genuine clinical collaboration: reciprocity, or better, mutuality. Didactic instruction, case consultation, and the like are only the beginning. In many ways, they confer on the behavioral scientist the "safety" of remoteness and freedom from responsibility; luxuries the physician cannot share. We should not expect of a resident what we are ourselves unable or unwilling to do. Thus the onus of experience-based learning in clinical behavioral science rests *not* with the student as an "isolate", but with the *relationship* built between behavioral scientists and apprentice practitioner. This paper has offered one model by which this relationship can be fostered and built both between clinical behavioral scientist and student, and between clinician of any type and patients.

ACKNOWLEDGEMENTS

The author wishes to express his gratitude to Arthur Hippler, Ph.D., Weston La Barre, Ph.D., and David Werman, M.D., for their generous criticism and encouragement; and to Margaret A. Stein, M.A., for her editorial assistance.

REFERENCE

Balint, Michael
   1957 The Doctor, His Patient and the Illness. New York: International Universities Press.
Bion, Wilfred R.
   1959 Experiences in Groups. New York: Basic Books.
Bowen, Murray
   1978 Family Therapy in Clinical Practice. New York: Jason Aronson.
Brissett, Dennis and Lionel S. Lewis
   1978 The Natural Health Food Movement: A Study of Revitalization and Conversion. Journal of American Culture 1: 1: 61–76.
Devereux, George
   1967 From Anxiety to Method in the Behavioral Sciences. The Hague: Mouton.
De Vos, George A.
   1975 The Dangers of Pure Theory in Social Anthropology. Ethos 3: 1: 77–91.
Egnew, Thomas R.
   1977 Behavioral Training for Family Physicians. Journal of Family Practice 5: 779–781, November.
Eisenberg, Leon
   1977 Disease and Illness: Distinctions Between Professional and Popular Ideas of Sickness. Culture, Medicine and Psychiatry 1: 1: 9–23.
Erikson, Erik H.
   1963 Childhood and Society, revised edition. New York: Norton.
Fabrega, Horacio Jr.
   1974 Disease and Social Behavior. Cambridge: MIT Press.
   1975 The Need for an Ethnomedical Science. Science 189: 969–975.
Foster, George M.
   1976 Disease Etiologies in Nonwestern Medical Systems. American Anthropologist 78: 773–782.
Foulks, Edward F.
   1978 Comment on Foster's 'Disease Etiologies in Nonwestern Medical Systems'. American Anthropologist 80: 660–661.
Gardner, Leonard
   1977 Humanistic Education and Behavioral Objectives: Opposing Theories of Educational Science. University of Chicago School Review 85: 3: 376–394.
Green, Maxine
   1975 Curriculum and Cultural Transformation: A Humanistic View. Cross Currents 25: 2: 175–186.
Hall, Edward
   1977 Beyond Culture. Garden City, New York: Doubleday, Anchor.

Kleinman, Arthur
1978a International Health Care Planning from an Ethnomedical Perspective: Critique and Recommendations for Change. Medical Anthropology 2: 2: 71–96.
1978b What Kind of Model for the Anthropology of Medical Systems? American Anthropologist 80: 661–665.
Kleinman, Arthur et al.
1976 Medicine in Chinese Cultures. Bethesda, Maryland: NIH, pp. 645–658.
Korsch, Barbara and Vida Negrete
1972 Doctor-Patient Communication. Scientific American 227: 66–74.
La Barre, Weston
1978 The Clinic and the Field. In George D. Spindler (ed.), The Making of Psychological Anthropology, Berkeley: University of California Press, pp. 258–299.
Mauksch, Hans O.
1974 A Social Science Basis for Conceptualizing Family Health. Social Science and Medicine 8: 521–528.
Mauksch, Hans O., Edward Brent, J. Timothy Diamond, and Susan Elder
1978 Going Through Medical School and Considering the Choice of Family Medicine: Prescription or Antidote? Manuscript.
Medalie, Jack H. (ed.)
1978 Family Medicine: Principles and Applications. Baltimore: Williams and Wilkins.
Montagu, Ashley
1963 Anthropology and Medical Education. Journal of the American Medical Association 183: 7: 577–583.
Mumford, Emily
1977 Culture: Life Perspectives and the Social Meanings of Illness. In Richard C. Simons and Herbert Pardes (eds.), Understanding Human Behavior in Health and Illness, Baltimore: Williams and Wilkins, pp. 173–183.
Pendagast, Eileen G. and Charles O. Sherman
1977 A Guide to the Genogram Family Systems Training. The Family 5: 1: 3–14.
Rakel, Robert E.
1977 Principles of Family Medicine. Philadelphia: W. B. Saunders.
Residency Review Committee for Family Practice
1977 Residency Review Committee for Family Practice, official definitions of "Family Practice" and "Family Physicians", Denver, Colorado.
Schusky, Ernest L.
1965 Manual for Kinship Analysis. New York: Holt, Rinehart and Winston.
Simmel, Ernst
1927 The 'Doctor Game', Illness and the Profession of Medicine. International Journal of Psychoanalysis 7: 470–483.
Spiegel, John
1971 Transactions: The Interplay Between Individual, Family and Society. New York: Science House.
Stein, Howard F.
1979a Rehabilitation and Chronic Illness in American Culture: The Cultural Psychodynamics of a Medical and Social Problem. The Journal of Psychologial Anthropology 2: 2: 153–176.
1979b The Salience of Ethno-Psychology for Medical Education and Practice. Social Science and Medicine 13B: 199–210.
Stein, Howard F. and Soughik Kayzakian-Rowe
1978 Hypertension, Biofeedback, and the Myth of the Machine: A Psychoanalytic-Cultural Exploration. Psychoanalysis and Contemporary Thought 1: 1: 119–156.
Stephens, G. Gayle
1978 The Integration of Family Practice into Today's Medical Education (abridged). Rural Health Communications 3: 4: 2–11.

Stierlin, Helm
   1973a Group Fantasies and Family Myths: Some Theoretical and Practical Aspects. Family
      Process 12: 111–125.
   1973b Interpersonal Aspects of Internalizations. International Journal of Psychoanalysis
      54: 203–213.
von Mering, Otto
   1961 Healing Experience and Disease Causation. *In* Family-Centered Social Work in Illness
      and Disability: A Preventive Approach. Monograph VI in the Series, 'Social Work
      Practice in Medical Care and Rehabilitation Settings'', Medical Social Work Section,
      National Associations of Social Workers.
   1970 Medicine and Psychiatry. *In* Leonard Kasdan and Otto von Mering (eds.), Anthro-
      pology and the Behavioral Sciences, Pittsburgh: University of Pittsburgh Press, pp.
      272–306.
Weidman, Hazel Hitson and Janice A. Egeland
   1973 A Behavioral Science Perspective in the Comparative Approach to the Delivery of
      Health Care. Social Science and Medicine 7: 845–860.
Weizenbaum, Joseph
   1976 Computer Power and Human Reason: From Judgment to Calculation. San Francisco:
      W. H. Freeman and Company.

ARTHUR KLEINMAN

THE TEACHING OF CLINICALLY APPLIED MEDICAL ANTHROPOLOGY ON A PSYCHIATRIC CONSULTATION-LIAISON SERVICE

PROLOGUE

Most Wednesday afternoons for the past five years I have conducted teaching rounds with a group of four or five medical students, two or three psychiatry residents, a postdoctoral fellow, and in the spring semester when I teach a course in medical anthropology, several anthropology students, graduates and under-graduates. We visit two or three patients whom the residents and medical students have already interviewed and whose case histories have been briefly presented. I interview each of the patients in the presence of the entire teaching group, some of whose members contribute to the interview. After we leave the patient's room, we return to my office or a seminar room and puzzle over what we have seen and heard. We try to make sense, both clinical and anthropological, of distinctive individuals and families struggling with difficult illness problems in complex life situations. We bring to bear psychiatric knowledge and anthropological knowledge, and a great deal of shared common sense. Our focus is patient care, but in illuminating illness problems and searching for therapeutic solutions we also deal with knotty conceptual and methodological concerns in the borderland between anthropology and medicine.

By the end of the afternoon, I am often very tired. I find the constant effort to make anthropology clinically applicable and psychiatry anthropologically informed exhausting. Coming up with a therapeutic synthesis that helps a patient can be difficult. Occassionally, I feel frustrated and am unhappy with my work both as a clinician and a medical anthropologist. But most of the time I find myself engaged in a richly rewarding intellectual and practical experience that confirms my conviction that there is a unique relationship between consultation-liaison psychiatry and medical anthropology that makes this setting a specially powerful one for the clinical application of anthropology and for the anthropologizing of medicine.

In this paper I will review my personal experience with teaching clinically applied medical anthropology on a psychiatric consultation-liaison service in a general teaching hospital. I will outline the many advantages and a few of the difficulties of fostering close working relationships between medical anthropologists and consultation-liaison psychiatrists. I will argue that this type of engagement in practical medical work illustrates well the significant role that medical anthropologists can play as *consultants* in clinical settings. I also will discuss barriers to such work, some erected by physicians, others by anthropologists, yet others by the institutional setting. Finally, I will generalize to meet the editors' charge that I cover the wider situation of anthropological teaching of any kind in departments of psychiatry.

83

N. J. Chrisman and T. W. Maretzki (eds.), Clinically Applied Anthropology, 83–115.
Copyright © 1982 by D. Reidel Publishing Company.

CONSULTATION-LIAISON PSYCHIATRY

To set the stage, I will first introduce consultation-liaison psychiatry. This relatively recent and rapidly growing clinical subspecialty of psychiatry consists of psychiatrists working with patients and health professionals in general hospital and primary care settings (cf. Hackett and Cassem 1978; Lipowski 1974). The *consultation psychiatrist* is called by physicians and nurses on internal medicine, surgery, obstetrics and gynecology, pediatrics, and family medicine wards and clinics to assess patient care problems. These problems may result from psychopathology, the psychosocial burden of medical disorders, staff-patient conflicts, or the stresses associated with special treatment settings (e.g., coronary care unit, respiratory care unit, hemodialysis unit, burn center, rehabilitation ward, etc.). The consulation psychiatrist like other medical consultants renders a diagnostic opinion and offers suggestions for treatment, but does not provide care to the patient. The *liaison psychiatrist*, in contrast, participates as a regular member of these treatment units, and consequently performs in many other roles besides that of a consultant. For example, he may routinely attend ward rounds, hold special teaching sessions with staff and trainees, participate in clinical case conferences, lead support groups for staff, patients or family, provide cotherapy for patients and family with a staff member or trainee, participate in the administration of a unit, engage in collaborative research, and so forth. Unlike his consultation colleague, the liaison psychiatrist often delivers direct care to patients. The consultant "treasts" the staff.

In a family medicine or primary care internal medicine clinic, the liaison psychiatrist may supervise residents' treatment of patients with psychiatric disorders or psychosocial problems; contribute to the diagnostic workup of complex cases; participate in weekly clinical and teaching conferences; organize special training sessions, such as sensitivity groups for residents; and offer lectures on such topics as depression, dementia, supportive psychotherapy, family therapy, psychopharmacologic agents, hypnosis, biofeedback, etc. The liaison psychiatrist, then, spends considerable time in one unit where he becomes part of the treatment and teaching team. The consultation psychiatrist is most often asked to very briefly consult on a wide variety of units, which he visits as an outsider and with which he maintains contact only with respect to specific patient problems. In a recent study of our consultation service, Ries et al. (1980) found that out of 260 consecutive consultations, 30% had to do with the management of what we have termed illness-related problems (i.e., psychosocial concomitants of serious disease and treatment), including financial and other social loss and gain, family breakdown, marital discord, maladaptive coping styles, etc. Another 17% of consultations were deemed to be the result of staff/patient conflicts. Hence a substantial amount of consultation psychiatry is concerned with the social causes, processes, and consequences of sickness and care. Inasmuch as many staff/patient conflicts reflect the different (and often conflicting) ways each construe and construct the clinical world as a social reality, consultation psychiatry can be thought of as providing a window on cultural problems in care that result at least as much from the culture of biomedicine as from the culture of patients. Liaison psychiatry is focused even more on sociocultural issues, and might even be thought of as a special form of clinical ethnography.

These fields, then, can be seen to be especially relevant to anthropologists because the work approximates participant-observation in an applied mode. They offer access to the fundamentally sociocultural basis of sickness and health, yet at the same time disclose that it is inseparable from the microclinical, biological and psychological realities that constitute much of care. Consultation-liaison psychiatry, therefore, places the anthropologist in a clinical stance, the same exigent state of discourse and action that patients and care-givers assume, and yet at the same time allows him, like his psychiatric colleagues, to travel back and forth between microclinical and macrosocial levels in the search for help. Anthropology, as we shall review below, also has much to offer the consultation-liaison psychiatrist with respect to how best to understand and change this dialectic between sociocultural structure, sickness, and care.

PERSONAL EXPERIENCE

In 1976 I came to the University of Washington with the expressed interest of integrating anthropological teaching and research into a Department of Psychiatry and Behavioral Sciences. I moved to Seattle as Head, Division of Social and Cross-Cultural Psychiatry, the usual venue for relating social science to psychiatry. But in 1977 I also became Head, Division of Consultation-Liaison Psychiatry, a major clinical service that is my chief clinical interest. I had trained in this subfield of psychiatry at the Massachusetts General Hospital, where I had also gained substantial personal experience developing teaching and research methods for relating anthropology to clinical work that could be applied specifically in psychiatric consultation and liaison (see Kleinman 1977). It was in this setting, for example, that I had developed the "explanatory model" approach to analyze and change doctor-patient communication, systematically recorded "illness problems" as a means of assessing and treating the psychosocial and cultural issues associated with major sickness, conducted clinical ethnographies of the influences of cultural meanings on popular and professional care, and first taught students and residents how to utilize these and other clinically applied anthropological methods in doctor-patient negotiations (see Kleinman, Eisenberg and Good 1978). At the Massachusetts General Hospital, I had also cut my teeth on the predictable but surmountable difficulties of working as an anthropologist on clinical services and teaching clinicians how to think anthropologically about their work in the midst of the exigent press of the therapeutic mandate.

When I arrived in Seattle, therefore, I had a fair idea of what I wanted to accomplish and how I wanted to go about doing it. My task was made easier (though by no means easy) by my position as the director of the Consultation-Liaison Service at University Hospital. This post meant that I was in charge of the day-to-day teaching, research, and clinical work on the service, and therefore could establish the policy of integrating medical anthropology at each of these levels. And that is what I set out to do. Of course, I had to demonstrate to the service's clinical attendings, residents, medical students, and, not least of all, the physicians we consulted to on other services (family medicine, internal medicine, surgery, etc.) that this was an effective direction to travel; and this meant most of all that our approach had to have clearly demonstrated benefits for patient care and clinical teaching. Since, as I have noted, roughly one-third of the clinical problems we encountered on the service related not to psychopathology *per se*, but to such things as the psychosocial burden of physical illness, staff-patient conflicts, and difficulties associated with the institutional structure of the hospital and the ecology of special treatment settings, it was not too difficult to win the confidence of colleagues and the interest of trainees. But we had to show them that medical anthropology and other medical social sciences provided concepts that offered a better understanding of these problems than common sense or traditional bio-medical notions, and that these concepts could be practically applied to successfully guide patient care. It was more difficult, however, to gain the same support for similar efforts by trainees or anthropologist teachers who were not themselves clinicians. This has remained a source of tension and a major challenge up to the present. Meeting it has taken a great deal of time; time spent making each clinical attending on the service familiar with the use of relevant anthropological ap-proaches; time spent helping anthropologist trainees and instructors learn how to work in a clinical milieu; and therefore time spent in removing stereotypes each held of the other and in negotiating a pluralistic service with distinctive and legitimated roles. The end result is that we have a program in which psychiatry and anthropology are very closely interrelated, and in which there is general sensitivity to the strengths and limitations of both and willingness to relate both orientations as complementary within an integrated clinical framework.

This model reproduces my own very special experience, and therefore may not be generalizable: not only because of the unusual administrative control I can exert, but also because I feel personally comfortable crossing the border back and forth between anthropology and clinical medicine in clinical practice as much as in teaching and research. To be sure, there have been certain difficulties in maintaining this integration in the everyday workings of the service. At times psychiatric and anthropological orientations are in open conflict with respect to the determinants of problems and the focus of intervention. Not infrequently I find myself rejecting one approach or the other as nonilluminating or unhelpful. At times even both together do not suffice to clarify a complex patient-care question and provide a successful therapeutic intervention. But most often the very tension that results from examining a problem from these two distinctive viewpoints proves to be a creative source of clinical judgment and stimulating teaching.

Doubtless, the "fit" between clinically applied anthropology and clinical psy-chiatry is facilitated by the current theoretical pluralism in psychiatry. Lacking a single framework of analysis, psychiatrists learn to bring distinctive biomedical, psychodynamic, behavioral, and social perspectives to the same problem (see

Lazare 1973; Manschreck and Kleinman 1977; Kleinman 1980). Medical anthropology, along with medical sociology and psychology, contributes a scientific basis to the "social" perspective of psychiatry. In turn, the ethnographer's skill in working with plural beliefs and values in particular contexts of action and his interest in assessing how cultural construals of the social world help construct behavior contribute to the insertion of anthropology in consultation-liaison psychiatry. My colleagues and I have built on these complementary strengths in developing a model of consultation and clinical communication generally as *interpretation* and *negotiation* that I will review in another section of this paper (see Katon and Kleinman 1980, 1981).

Among the problems I encountered in developing this interdisciplinary program, one of the easiest to resolve is the unfamiliarity of anthropologists (teachers and students) with medical settings and activities. Anthropologists approach biomedicine often with the erroneous view that it is homogeneous and unchanging. Some are deeply hostile to physicians whom they view as patients' jailers, and also maintain naively romantic caricatures of patients as victims. Others so overidentify with either healers or patients that they view care as either a conspiracy or a heroic drama. Still others approach first-year medical students with an almost missionary zeal to convert them to other fields. Ethnographic immersion may not change their ideological orientation, but does offer the needed understanding of clinical categories, interests, norms, and practices as related elements in a cultural system: the medical school and physicians' training program. Such an immersion, particularly if it requires the anthropologist to become a teacher and consultant on patient care, elicits the empathy for the physician's task that leavens critical analysis with insight into the press of uncertainty and the structural contradictions of bureaucratic practice; it also nurtures the sensitive appreciation of the dynamics of therapeutic communication that can awaken physicians to the central reality and powerful subtleties of patients' life problems. Clinical ethnography teaches the anthropologist relevant aspects of medicine, sensitizes him to the stresses the physician faces, and widens his analytic framework so that he appreciates not just the typical burdens clinical settings place on patients but also the active control patients can exercise over the therapeutic process. It makes concrete and grounded his understanding of the limitations of a traditional biomedical approach and his ability to integrate social science into a more comprehensive biopsychosocial framework (Engel 1977). All in all, it clarifies the essentials of clinical work: diagnosis, triage, consultation, therapy. Such participant-observation offers the ethnographic insight that the anthropologist requires to be an effective clinical teacher and researcher by demonstrating massively and in-depth in a large number of particular instances how clinical reality is differentially culturally construed and thereby constructed; how social reality is clinically transformed in the dialectical interplay of professional and lay clinical categories; and, as a result, how clinical praxis is constituted and expressed as a meaningful product of clinical relations. Not the least of this insight is recognition of the influence of personal and professional values, shared cultural biases and stereotypes, and conventional metaphors of self, others, the body, and emotions on clinical assessment and decision making.

Such an experience makes unacceptable a superficial view of medicine as a monolithic structure; it compels an understanding of the plural beliefs, value orientations, structures of relevance, behavioral paradigms, relationships, and life worlds that coexist in biomedicine. It also makes much more complex and real the patient's perspective on and experience of help seeking, illness behavior, popular therapy, clinical communication, compliance, satisfaction, and therapeutic outcome. Following such an exposure, the anthropologist and the anthropologically oriented clinician will find it much more difficult to maintain a tendentious, unidimensional view that caricatures patients or health professionals as black or white. The ethnographic immersion I believe liberates them from their own professional and personal biases, and in turn enables them to liberate physicians from their professional, cultural, and idiosyncratic biases. Effective clinical teaching benefits enormously from an ability to apply distinctive perspectives, social science and biomedical, physician's and patient's.

The anthropologist as clinical teacher faces the creative but very difficult challenge of enabling clinicians (and increasingly patients and families also) to see *in particular instances* how their categories socially construct illness, how these constructs compare and contrast with patient constructs, and how both constrain therapeutic action and yield predictable outcomes, including problems for patients and practitioners. By treating biomedical understanding as emic, not etic, and comparing it with patient understanding, similarly viewed, the clinically applied medical anthropologist, as I shall outline below, can negotiate between these usually distinctive (and often conflicting) views and help resolve problems that emerge from them. This focus also offers obvious and powerful directions for clinical research and teaching.

The great challenge for the anthropologist is to be able to persuasively offer an anthropology of specific cases of illness and treatment that can stand side by side with biomedical and lay perspectives as a rich source of alternative theoretical and practical options that potentially can be applied to the healers and the healing process at least as much to those who seek healing. To accomplish this, the anthropologist must be so well trained and experienced, and have so balanced immersion (and acceptance) in the practical realities of particular clinical settings with *professional* alienation from the taken-for-granted meanings, norms, and differential relations of power in medicine, that he can confidently promote an anthropology of clinical care. If this strikes the reader as utopian, I assert that I have often witnessed the possibility for it in my own work, and occasionally have had the good fortune to see it realized.

Consultation-liaison psychiatry offers an especially suitable vantage for anthropologists to accomplish this goal, because it legitimates concern for the psychosocial and cultural aspects of illness, and because it focuses on how the treatment setting and the therapeutic relationship contribute to clinical problems. It also forces the anthropologist to act as a consultant and therefore to apply ethnographic insight and social science concepts to the practical solution of patient-care problems.

It provides a balance between acceptance in the biomedical domain and alienation from it (psychiatry is always marginal to medicine since meanings and social relations are not legitimated in the biomedical model), analogous to the actual experience of the ethnographer. This makes professional medical cooptation less likely and yet demands that clinical anthropology, like psychiatry, relate effectively to the practical realities of care. Furthermore, the consultant anthropologist, like the consultant psychiatrist, must assert his autonomy and that of his perspective, and at the same time translate it into a language that his clinician colleagues can understand and use within their framework. Despite the repeated frustrations of not getting his message across, of not being listened to or of not seeing how his views can be made relevant to medical work, the clinical situation that he shares prevents him from escaping into purist abstraction devoid of all practical utility or antimedical propagandizing to provide solace for a bruised ego. And to my mind it is precisely this applied orientation, the necessity of sticking with the situation and the mandate to effect change in it, that forces the anthropologist, sometimes even against his professed ideology, to be clinically effective in the same way that the physician must be and therefore is effective. That is to say, the clinically applied anthropologist in psychiatric consultation-liaison cannot stop with an analysis of the cultural construction of the clinical reality he faces, but must go on to clinically construct and thereby alter this reality. This makes for neither paradox nor ambivalence, but the very stuff of a clinical contribution. That contribution, in turn, offers marvelous opportunities for analyzing the inner workings of clinical practice and successfully teaching how they are influenced by cultural norms and social structure.

CLINICAL EXAMPLES

A few case illustrations drawn from my own experience in consultation-liaison psychiatry highlight both the kinds of problems this window on medicine offers the clinically applied anthropologist and anthropologically informed clinician, and the types of anthropological strategies that can be applied to help resolve them.

Case 1

Consultation was requested from the Orthopedic Surgery Ward to assess whether one of their patients could be certified as insane in order to permit them to amputate his infected leg in spite of his refusal. The orthopedic residents regarded the patient as insane because he would not take their advice that the infected leg was a serious threat to his life and must be amputated if he were to recover. On consultation the patient was found to be a 60-year-old Caucasian veteran who had been living alone in a downtown apartment in Seattle on a disability pension. The patient had had adult onset diabetes for more than 20 years, and had suffered many of the complications of this chronic metabolic disorder including most notably severe peripheral vascular disease. Five years before, one of his legs was amputated at another hospital for sequelae of this problem: stasis ulcers and osteomyelitis. In the interim the patient had adjusted well to his disability. Though living alone and possessing neither family nor close friends, he had managed to maintain a highly valued autonomous life style. He would drive his car to visit acquaintances, frequented several taverns where he was regarded as a valuable patron, would go fishing, and as he put it in a characteristically crusty way: "do whatever I damn well please whenever I want to!"

The patient was not at that time psychotic and had no history of mental illness, though he admitted he had periodically had a serious alcohol abuse problem, presently under control. He reported that he became infuriated and "threw those damn young doctors" out of his room after they told him that his remaining leg's stasis ulcer had become infected and had in turn produced osteomyelitis in the underlying bone necessitating amputation. He broke down in tears when he told me this, adding that he could not conceive of being able to live his independent life style without legs. He preferred death to dependence on others and loss of autonomy. As we talked, he claimed that if his life were truly in jeopardy from his infected leg, he knew he would feel a great deal worse than he presently did. Hence he could not believe that the doctors were correct in their assessment of the problem. If he were seriously ill or dying, he went on to state with some passion, "of course I would let them take off the leg. What choice would I have? But damn it all, I just don't know why they want to take it off now, all of a sudden. Why they have never really sat down and made a good case for it. They don't even let you decide yourself. These bastards just tell you what you got to do. Well, the hell with them! I don't plan to be forced into anything against my will".

After speaking separately to the residents on the case, it became apparent that the evidence for osteomyelitis was in fact marginal — a mere X-ray shadow about which the radiologist was uncertain. They were afraid he would quickly develop gangrene and sepsis that would jeopardize his life as had happened before when his other leg was amputated. They believed the situation was too dangerous because of his impaired metabolic state to warrant a two-week course of very high dose intravenous antibiotics, which the infectious disease consultant had recommended. They perceived the patient's stubborness "in the face of the evidence" as irrational, and wondered whether his prior alcoholism had made him demented and therefore incompetent to make this crucial medical decision.

Of note, the senior resident was about to finish his training and was aggressively searching out major surgical procedures to complete the requirements of his training program. (This information came from the intern who was less inclined to force the surgical procedure on such an unwilling patient.) The junior resident pointed out that the patient fit the orthopedic indications for amputation, and that the attending orthopedist had agreed, though he had left it to them to persuade the patient to undergo the procedure in view of the serious threat he faced. These surgeons had been extremely busy with other cases and had not had time to sit down with the patient and review the problem in detail. Instead they had very hurriedly informed him during morning work rounds on Monday of the fact they planned to schedule him for surgery at the end of the week. They viewed the psychiatrist's role not so much as "commiting the patient to surgery" against his will, but to "talk the patient into consenting".

Instead, I informed them of my belief that the patient's explanation seemed perfectly reasonable. I attempted to negotiate a different treatment plan with them that would have begun with the more conservative intervention of intravenous antibiotics, followed by surgery only if it failed and the disease progressed to a point at which it would be stated to the patient there was no other treatment short of amputation that could save his life. This plan the orthopedists would not accept, since they felt it contravened the best surgical care and therefore was both "technically and ethically unacceptable". As a result, the psychiatric consultation-liaison service arranged for the patient to be transfered to another hospital. There he received, as he so strongly desired, intravenous antibiotics. His progress was slow, and his diabetes worsened, but after six weeks his X-ray revealed no indication of osteomyelitis and he did not develop sepsis. His stasis ulcer took longer to heal, and never fully resolved, but eventually after several months it improved sufficiently that he was discharged without amputation.

It would be easy to blame this dismaying and nearly disastrous situation on the orthopedic surgeons' poor training in providing a caring relationship, their failure to communicate with the patient as a person, and their not-so-well disguised self-interest. If the anthropologist's or psychiatrist's primary interest were to indict the doctors for their treatment, here was a case that would generate enough shock and anger to be blown up into a full-scale atrocity used to attack American surgery and postgraduate surgical training. By others' lights, I suppose these orthopedic surgeons might be viewed as deviant, an aberration of the ideal of medical care due to personal failings — a situation that has more to say about bad individual physicians than about physicians and their training generally. But from the orientation sketched in the preceding section, this case came to represent for my colleagues and me an extreme instance of an otherwise common problem in medicine: breakdown in clinical communication caused by conflicting cultural constructions of clinical reality. We were able to help the patient, and, though the particular orthopedists involved remained resistant to our perspective, we came to effectively use this case with other surgical and medical residents in teaching a patient-centered approach to clinical care. Indeed, this became one of our paradigmatic exemplars for the model of doctor-patient negotiation we developed (see below) and now routinely teach to students and house officers.

Though the personalities and backgrounds of the physicians doubtless contributed to the dangerous impasse they created for this patient, my colleagues and I view their behavior as the result in large measure of their indoctrination into a professional surgical explanatory and normative system that made their cultural construal, however insensitive and tendentiously ideological it may strike the reader, compelling to them as the best way technically (and morally) to proceed. From their perspective this case could be understood in terms of a culturally constituted discourse based on probability assessment that results from biomedical research on the course and outcome of large numbers of patients with similar disease. In the very narrow terms of this discourse, sanctioned by the authority structure of statistics, it is not only reasonable but necessary to amputate the patient's leg. That decision is buttressed by the way this clinical discourse shapes the evidence, socially creating the biomedical "facts" as a surgical reality for which appropriate reality tests are available to demonstrate the validity of surgical judgement. Like almost all biomedical discourses, this orthopedic one does not legitimate psychological and social information as part of the scientific data base. As the note from the infectious disease consultant and the intravenous antibiotic treatment approach of the internal medicine physicians at the second hospital suggest, the discourse of internal medicine constructed the clinical reality of this case differently enough to support the patient's treatment choice. As the anthropologist working in clinic and ward soon learns, the cultural discourse of biomedicine is plural and not infrequently conflicting. Usually, however, trust and shared common sense, along with a modicum of interpersonal sensitivity and communication skills, enable patients and physicians to overcome professional and lay solipsism in the negotiation of medical uncertainty (cf. Holzner and Marx 1978: 259–277). When such culturally constituted conflicts arise, and they arise routinely in health care, medical anthropology provides a means for analyzing and potentially resolving them that is an essential complement of biomedical methods in the provision of effective patient care. A forceful cultural critique of biomedical categories and norms, one aimed at reforming them to protect patient interests, to reduce their frequently dehumanizing effects on patients *and* practitioners, and to provide more psychosocially and culturally appropriate treatment, is a desideratum for clinically applied medical anthropological research that could form the basis for systematically detoxifying iatrogenic effects of the culture of biomedicine such as those depicted in this case. The reader is also cautioned to be wary of potential side effects of medical anthropological intervention — no clinically efficacious intervention lacks side effects. In this instance, a negotiation approach actually alienated the surgeons who pulled out of the case. Fortunately, a suitable referral was obtained, but if there had not been one, the patient's situation would have been even more desperate.

Case 2

The patient was a 42-year-old woman in whom an intestinal bypass surgical operation had been performed 16 months earlier. She was brought to the Harborview Medical Center, Seattle, after taking an overdose of a sedative hypnotic drug. She had a history of obesity since early childhood, as well as a strong family history of extreme obesity, with her mother weighing 400 pounds, her sister 400 pounds and her father 700 pounds. The patient stated that she had been happy at her previous weight of 350 pounds, but due to constant pressure by her doctors, friends and peer group, she had decided to undergo the intestinal bypass operation. The only physical problem she had secondary to obesity was mild hypertension (in the range of 140/90 mm of mercury).

The patient stated she had devoted much of her life to proving that obese people could do most of the things that thin people could do, such as swim, water ski and hike. She had been exceedingly active, raised three children on her own after a divorce and worked regularly as a vocational nurse. Before the operation she had lived with a man for two years. She said that there were no significant problems in their relationship. Finally, 16 months before admission, at age 40 she decided to have the intestinal bypass operation.

The technical results of the bypass were good. The patient lost 100 pounds; her surgical wound healed well; and her blood pressure decreased. However, the side effects of the procedure and resulting illness problems were considerable.

She began having 10 to 12 bowel movements per day, had occasional fecal incontinence and problems with flatulence. She was admitted to the hospital four times due to syncope and orthostatic hypotension. Before the operation she had described herself as jovial, often the center of attention, hardworking and enjoying her primary relationship with her boyfriend. After the operation and resulting symptoms, she had problems with her body image. She felt that the doctors had taken away a third of her body and that she was no longer a complete person.

The patient said that she had insomnia and decreased energy, and had been experiencing suicidal ideas for many months before taking the overdose. She had begun to miss work frequently because of the side effects of the operation, had financial problems due to the recurrent hospital stays, and her depression and irritability had started to cause problems with the man she was living with.

She visited at least five surgeons before taking the overdose. She was gradually more insistent that they reanastomose her bowel. All refused, however, stating that the operation was successful — that is, she had lost 100 pounds and her blood pressure had decreased. They offered to try to control her side effects with medication. Finally, in desperation, the patient decided that she no longer wished to live with her physical problems and her perception of a substantial decrease in the quality of her life. Thus, she took an overdose of sedative medication (Katon and Kleinman 1981).

In the narrow discourse of the surgical variant of the biomedical model, the operation appeared successful. The orthostatic hypotension, fecal incontinence, diarrhea, and flatulence were undesirable but understandable side effects of a procedure that could significantly benefit the patient's future health status. Yet from the patient's perspective, which was not elicited by her surgeons, the outcome was constituted as negative. Elsewhere Katon and Kleinman (1981) have described this case to illustrate a model of clinical negotiation which we actually employed here. The clinically applied anthropology and psychiatry consultants elicited the patient perspective, compared it openly with the contrasting surgical perspective in the presence of both parties so as to call attention to the tacit conflict, and helped patient and surgeons agree to a compromise plan which initially employed conservative management that proved unsuccessful, and thereafter went on to reoperation to return the patient to her original status. This resulted in a marked improvement in the patient's condition and in her relations with her surgeons. Both parties were in agreement that it was a mutually satisfactory settlement to this difficult problem. Subsequently the patient worked closely with the surgeons to better assess candidates for the same surgical procedure, and the surgeons became more receptive to psychosocial consultations and teaching.

Case 3

The patient was a 49-year-old Caucasian female who is the wife of a minister of a small fundamentalist church in rural Washington. For ten years she had suffered from chronic headaches that were so debilitating that every few months the patient took to bed for several weeks. The patient had visited many doctors for her headaches, and was addicted to narcotic pain medications. Her local physcans felt frustrated and no longer able to care for her, and therefore had referred her to the Pain Clinic at the University of Washington. The patient stated that if the Clinic failed to help her she would seek out neurosurgical treatment to "deaden the nerves in my head".

The liaison psychiatrist in the Pain Clinic was the first psychiatrist she had been asked to consult. She was ashamed to see a psychiatrist, denied any emotional problems, and stated that she and her husband and their church are "against psychiatry". Psychiatric assessment, however, disclosed a chronic major depressive disorder and long standing somatization as a chronic coping device to deal with stress. The MMPI supported this assessment. Anthropological interviewing and observation with the patient and her husband revealed substantial hostility in their relationship combined with a strong need for them to present an impeccable image to others. Both husband and wife were socialized in families where the expression of strong affects (especially negative ones) was discouraged, and where religious and somatic idoms were the chief channels for expressing distress. They had maintained this pattern in their marriage. The wife's pain was viewed by both as a test by God of her strength and character. After several interviews, however, it became apparent to the liaison team that the patient's pain elicited care and attention from her husband, allowed her to indirectly express her frustration with their relationship which she could not address openly, and helped her to distance him sexually. After treatment with antidepressants and biofeedback the patient's headaches greatly improved. She and her husband refused psychotherapy and marital counseling, and denied they had significant problems in their relationship. Follow-up at one year revealed the patient occasionally suffered exacerbation of her headaches at times of stress, and that she and her husband were considering divorce.

This case is an instance of the extremely common finding of somatization of psychological and social problems in primary care. The psychiatrist tends to think of somatization as the result of an underlying psychiatric disorder which when effectively treated will lead to loss of physical complaints. But from an anthropological perspective, chronic pain and other forms of somatization are more comprehensively understood in terms of personal, social, and cultural meanings. The care-giver needs to *interpret* what specific significances particular somatic complaints hold for the patient, family, network, employers, coworkers, and practitioners. Chronic pain may be (and often is) an idiom to symbolize unhappiness, indirectly express anger, sanction failure, manipulate a martial partner, change work, obtain financial compensation, and so forth. When undiagnosed by primary care-givers, and this routinely happens, somatization leads to unnecessary and costly medical and surgical interventions, iatrogenesis, and support for illness as a life career. Anthropological assessment of the context of meanings and social relationships within which somatization occurs is as important for the management of this common problem as are biomedical and psychiatric evaluations. In a later section of this paper, I will outline a clinically applied strategy we have developed (the explanatory model approach) to teach clinicians how to elicit and interpret their patients' emic meanings of their illnesses.

Case 4

Mrs. S. was a 27-year-old Native American female with a six-year history of systemic lupus erythematosis and treatment with steroids, who was referred to the University Hospital in Seattle at 30-weeks gestation with symptoms of preeclampsia. The patient had had four previous miscarriages in the last six years at early stages of gestation. She had one daughter, age 8, and strongly desired another child.

Due to severe preeclampsia, labor was induced during her second hospital day and a nonviable premature infant was delivered. Psychiatric consultation was obtained three days later due to "psychotic depression with hallucinations".

The following history was obtained from the patient. She was mourning the death of her baby and had "heard the baby cry" two days after the death. She stated that it was normal in her American Indian culture for loved ones to talk with close family members after death to try to bring relatives with them into the hereafter. Although she had no prior experience with this custom, many of her friends had spoken of their experiences with loved ones after death. The staff reacted with anxiety and alarm on hearing that Mrs. S. had heard her baby cry after it had been dead for two days and never bothered to elicit her cultural explanation. Thus, a psychiatric consultation was requested.

After talking with the patient and the staff, we recommended that the staff help the patient ventilate her feelings about the death of the baby and also enable her to perform any cultural ceremony that she and her husband would normally go through at home. During the next seven days of the hospitalization the patient "heard her baby cry" daily but with the help of the staff and her husband this became less alarming to the patient. She and her husband went through their indigenous rite of destroying all traces of the baby's existence, including blankets, baby clothes, and an echogram picture. The patient made an uneventful recovery both physically and emotionally (Katon and Kleinman 1981: 259–260). Reports of similar culturally constituted acute grief reactions can be found in the ethnographic literature on Native Americans.

This case illustrates a clinical problem brought about by cultural differences between patient and staff. Clinically applied medical anthropologists should be particularly skilled in the identification and analysis of such problems. Anthropologist contributors to Harwood's (1981a) recent volume on *Ethnicity and Medical Care* review how the illness beliefs and behavior of seven distinctive American ethnic groups (urban Blacks, Chinese Americans, Haitian Americans, Italian Americans, Mexican Americans, Navajos, and Puerto Ricans) influence clinical care and how knowledge of such influences can be applied to resolve problems in patient care that present obstacles to effective treatment. Our own training program has developed expertise in dealing with similar culturally constituted problems among Asian Americans in particular.

Harwood (no date) divides cultural differences in beliefs between patients and doctors that frequently yield problems that may undermine therapeutic relationships and interfere with clinical communications into five groups (cf. Katon and Kleinman 1981: 268–269).

(1) The patient and doctor use the same term but actually mean different things. This commonly occurs when the doctor and patient use the same biomedical term with the physician thus assuming that the patient understands it the same way he does. A common example occurs in the doctor's history taking when he asks the patient about allergies to medications. Many patients claim they are allergic to a certain type of drug but if the physician asks them about the reaction in detail, it is often only a minor side effect, not an allergy as the doctor understands that term.

(2) The patient and doctor use the same term, apply it to the same phenomena but have different etiologic concepts. The implication here is that the patient who views the cause of his or her illness differently than the physician may have differing expectations of treatment. An example is the folk model of hypertension (Blumhagen 1980). Hypertensive patients often view their illness as caused by acute stresses in their lives. The physician may view chronic stress as a component in the complex etiology of hypertension but usually views genetic predisposition and physiologic abnormalities as being primary. Acute stress is not regarded as etiologically important. The physician prescribes diuretics and perhaps occasionally counsels patients about decreasing the long-term stress in their lives; but he does not focus his recommendations or therapies on any particular acute stress. Many patients believe, however, that stress, especially acute stress, is primary, indeed that hypertension means too much tension not high blood pressure. They may try to reduce particularly bothersome acute stresses, but not alter habitual patterns of stress and their long-term coping responses nor take their medications.

(3) A similar problem is one in which the physician and patient share the same terms and referents but these terms are embedded in different nosologies. Harwood (1981b) gives an example from his study from Puerto Rican culture in which 23 of 28 adults interviewed stated that ulcers led to cancer. Obviously, the physician's diagnosis of peptic ulcer disease to many Puerto Rican patients may have far more serious connotations to the patient than to the physician. Moreover, these cultural meanings are hidden to the physician.

(4) Patients may stigmatize certain diseases so that physicians and patients

share the same term and the same referent for the term but may have very different emotive meanings attached to it. An example here is the stigmatization of mental disease. This often adversely affects the psychiatrist's history-taking. Patients frequently will not give an adequate family history during an interview due to the stigma of having mental disease in their family. Feeling ashamed of the "weakness" and other negative attributions associated in their network with emotional problems, depressed patients will tell their family doctors about physical complaints but not depressed affect, and as a result their depressive disorder will be misdiagnosed.

(5) The last communication difficulty (Harwood labels it a "lexicon" level problem) is where the doctor and patient simply do not use the same terms. Here the patient may speak a foreign language or dialect of the standard language or the physician may use medical jargon. Sometimes this problem is resolved by asking for clarification of one another's unknown terms. At times, however, the same word may have totally different meanings in the two cultures or there may be no equivalent of a term in the other language. Although such problems may be resolved by use of interpreters, interpreters may unwittingly amplify these problems. Few interpreters are trained in biomedical terminology, few may have systematic knowledge of their own culture's folk medical concepts and terms, and some may be so acculturated or otherwise alienated from indigenous concepts and norms that they fail to adequately interpret the native perspective. Indeed it is our experience that clinicians can anticipate frequent misunderstandings when using clinically inexperienced or untrained interpreters and need to monitor work-ups carefully to make sure such misunderstandings do not distort diagnostic assessment and undermine therapeutic plans.

In addition to clinical problems caused by differences in cultural conceptualization, distinctive value orientations and behavioral norms associated with ethnicity (as well as with different religions and social class backgrounds) may interfere with doctor-patient relationships. For example, cultural expectations about modesty among young Hispanic American females may make physical examinations by male physicians even when carried out in the presence of female staff embarrassing and difficult. Gypsy expectations that the polluted portion of the body below the waist should not contaminate the pure portion above it may mean that the physical examination is expected to be conducted literally downward from head to toe. Elderly Chinese and other Asian American patients may find the informality and egalitarianism of middle-class American doctor-patient relationships an unacceptable substitute for an expected Confucian-style authoritarian relationship. Numerous other ethnically based value and behavioral differences have been reported. The clinically applied medical anthropologist should be an expert in handling such problems and in teaching clinicians how to deal with them.

Many other clinical examples could be described to illustrate other issues relevant for clinically applied medical anthropology consulting and teaching. Included would be examples of clinical problems associated with structural constraints on the delivery of care such as the bureaucratic organization of time and space in the hospital, professional expectations of patient comportment, life problems created for patients and families by the unusual requirements of special therapies (e.g., hemodialysis, intravenous hyperalimentation, particular exercise and diet protocols, etc.), the psychosocial burden of highly stigmatized disorders (e.g., leprosy, tuberculosis, venereal disease, mental retardation), difficulties in clinical communication and relationships in the practice of foreign medical graduates, the maladaptive effects on doctor-patient relationships of the sleep deprivation and dehumanizing work schedules of residents and interns, among many others.

Case 5

The patient was a 23-year-old white female admitted to the hospital because of severe asthma. Psychiatric consultation was requested immediately prior to discharge because of the patient's history of chronic polydrug abuse, alcoholism, criminal behavior, and chaotic life style. She had moved fifteen times in two years, and had lived in four different states during that time. Her four children, all fathered by different men, were in foster homes. She had no close friends or relatives, and had more than a dozen sexual partners in the previous few months. The patient worked as a prostitute, and recently sold street drugs. She had a long history of violent behavior. She had been uncooperative on the ward, and would not allow the medical team or social workers to set up after-care plans for her so as to provide more effective care for her asthma, which she had failed to manage appropriately and for which she had utilized emergency room and inpatient services that she refused to pay for.

Psychiatric assessment disclosed that the patient's parents were alcoholics, and that she and her eight siblings were raised in foster homes. She experienced childhood sexual and physical abuse, including incest and rape. Her drug use began at age twelve and her adolescence was spent either on the street or in correctional facilities. At present she had no place to live, no job, no money, and no natural support networks in Seattle. The patient refused placement in a drug detoxification facility or contact with relevant self-help groups and social agencies.

Traditional psychiatric diagnosis would determine that the patient had a chronic personality disorder with sociopathic, narcissistic and borderline features along with chronic substance abuse. The clinically applied anthropologist involved with this case was no more successful than the psychiatrists, medical housestaff or social workers in establishing a therapeutic alliance and negotiating a mutually agreeable discharge plan for futher care and rehabilitation. But the combination of psychiatric and anthropological assessment was much appreciated by the house officers and students who had cared for this patient. This integrated approach to clinical teaching emphasized the dialectic between macrosocial determinants and microclinical behavior. While discussing the dynamic interrelationship between social and personal pathology, and even considering a possible genetic contribution as well, the anthropologist-clinician highlighted the intractable nature of the problems for the clinician and the feeling of impotence this produces — a feeling that leads care-givers to act with hostility to the patient who may then be further abused or rejected.

Recognition of the social structural and cultural foundations of the patient's situation led to a forthright and heated discussion of the limits of clinical work and of clinical social science intervention. This, in turn, led to an extended and (for the clinicians at least) insightful comparative analysis of social pathology and social interventions. Here the anthropologist had the marvelous opportunity to teach basic social science in a setting that riveted the attention of clinical trainees and that legitimated a forceful social critique of our health care system, family structure, and agencies of social welfare and control. I quickly reviewed the distinction between deviance and psychopathology, described labeling theory, and related each of these ideas to the tragic and deeply frustrating ethnographic situation posed by this case. Even if the theoretical niceties and technical language of the discussion were not fully appreciated by the clinical students, there was obvious recognition of the central importance of social and cultural analysis for understanding the problem and for coming to grips with the terribly difficult question of remedying it.

This particular case review also enabled me to demonstrate how shared cultural assumptions *and* professional "interests" can bias the formulation of a case and its treatment. But this rich educational opportunity was possible not because it offered an occasion for cynical hectoring or facile revolutionary crusading, but precisely because the social scientist joined his clinical colleagues in their painful practical predicament. Clinicians were enabled to widen their biomedical perspective. Anthropologist and clinicians were liberated from the tacit bias of the treatment setting and wider culture. And all were able to consider the powerful cultural meanings attached to social deviance, norm breaking, therapeutic impotence and inefficacy, and their effects personally on clinicians and their work. It is through intimate participation in the frustrating evaluation of very difficult cases that are not neatly dissected by analytic strategies and that do not respond to therapeutic intervention, as much as through contributing to the successful resolution of corrigible clinical problems, that the clinically applied anthropologist establishes his collegial role and ultimately wins the respectful (even if sometimes grudging) interest of his clinical audience. Thus, the anthropologist can situate himself strategically to effectively teach how clinical reality is socially constructed and how assessing different social constructions of clinical reality contribute to patient care and clinical practice.

Constraints on space prevent me from presenting other relevant case vignettes. Instead in the section that follows I will describe clinical anthropological techniques that my colleagues and I have developed that can be readily applied on a psychiatric consultation-liaison service. These should be of use to medical anthropologists starting up clinically applied teaching and consultation activities both in this particular clinical setting as well as in other clinical contexts.

CLINICALLY APPLIED ANTHROPOLOGICAL STRATEGIES

1. *Explanatory Models*

We teach medical students and residents to systematically elicit the *patient's explanatory model* (Kleinman 1975; Kleinman, Eisenberg and Good 1978; Kleinman 1980: 104—118). This consists of the patient's understanding of the cause, reason for onset at a specific time, pathophysiology, expected course and prognosis of his illness, and the treatment that he believes will be or should be administered. It is elicited by open-ended questions in lay terms, so that the model is not contaminated by the physician's assumptions. Independent of the important information it provides, this approach requires that the physician demonstrate warmth, empathy, and active interest in the patient's perspective. This action in itself moves the center of gravity of a doctor-patient relationship a bit closer to the patient's side and usually improves rapport. It also makes it more difficult for the physician to regard himself as the locus of responsibility for care. Most patients will tend not to answer questions about their explanatory model unless they sense some genuine interest on the physician's part in them and their concerns. Indeed, physicians need to overcome patients' reserve and fear of being intimidated by emphasizing that the information elicited may be crucial to the tailoring of a more appropriate treatment plan.

From an ethnographic perspective, the explanatory model approach may appear superficial, a quick and dirty elicitation that does not fit into an indepth assessment of personal and contextual meanings. For this reason it may offend the ethnographer as a less than adequate methodology. But in the exigent, time-limited setting of care, it is not feasible to expect more from students and fully qualified doctors. Trust and the importunate quest for therapy help overcome reticence and suspicion. I am continually amazed at how much can be expeditiously learned about the patient and his illness through this relatively simple technique. Teaching clinicians how to solicit and interpret meaning through the use of the explanatory model approach allows the anthropologist to introduce ethnography into the clinic, and the thin edge of this wedge thereby opens the door to understanding illness and its context of meaning more generally. One can effectively explore explanatory models to gain relevant information about many different cultural and psychosocial themes in patients' lives. By eliciting family models, the clinician can be taught to search for tacit family conflicts, assess support, and increase communication with key members of the patient's network. Though not as rigorous or exhaustive as ethnographic interviewing, the explanatory model approach is "good enough" for the purpose of improving patient care.

The consulting psychiatrist and anthropologist can use the explanatory model framework, moreover, to stand outside the doctor-patient relationship and compare physician and patient models in the hope of uncovering potentially important conflicts that may undermine effective care. Monitoring changes in explanatory models can help determine the effectiveness of clinical communication and prevent clinical misunderstandings. Recent research by Lazare et al. (1978) not only demonstrates that the patient's perspective can be effectively and briefly assessed in the clinical situation, but also that such assessment can positively influence clinical outcomes (cf. Blumhagen in this volume; Inui et al. 1976; Starfield et al. 1980).

The explanatory model approach also contributes to an understanding of the patient's perception and experience of stress, sense of support, coping strategies, relative degree of ethnic and religious commitment, and past experience with and current view of particular health care providers and therapies. Illness behavior, help seeking, compliance, and satisfaction all can be evaluated as "natural" extensions of explanatory models. Moreover, once oriented to patients' cognitive worlds the clinician rapidly comes to realize the inseparability of affects, psychodynamics and interpersonal communication from the illness, and, most importantly, gains confidence and skill in exploring these non-biological and often (for the clinican) threatening domains.

2. *Illness Problems*

While it may raise some philosophical problems for social science theory, a distinction between *disease* and *illness* remains an extremely valuable clinical heuristic. In our current formulation of this analytic distinction, we teach that sickness is initially perceived and experienced by patients and families in ethnomedical terms as *illness*; i.e., the life concerns and problems that it presents for common sense understanding as part of the everyday world of the sick person (Robert Hahn personal communication). When first brought to the attention of health professionals, sickness is discussed within a shared cultural common sense frame of reference. And over time clinicians repeatedly find this shared cultural idiom available for communicating with patients, and clearly many, and perhaps most, use it. But at the same time, clinicians refract illness through biomedical (or psychiatric, or alternative health professional) lenses so as to construct *disease*. In the instance of biomedicine, this means sickness understood in terms of a fundamentalist, biologistic Cartesianism as mechanical breakdown or disruption in biological structures and functions. The psychoanalyst, chiropractor, osteopath, Chinese-style doctor, Ayurvedic physician, all construct their own distinctive professional disease models.

The disease/illness distinction has the value of being able to drive home to health professionals the limitations of the biomedical model. At the same time it forces them to be aware of illness as a lay category and psychosocial reality. Recent work supports the view that most problems health professionals deal with can be thought of as relating to illness experience. Yet this group of problems is inadequately conceptualized and treated. In an attempt to draw on psychological and social science concepts to better define this domain, we have developed the notion of *illness problems*, the problematic effects of sickness on everyday life. The clinically applied anthropologist and the psychiatric consultant should formulate illness problems as specifically as possible so that specific strategies can be recommended to manage them. For example, the onset of chronic back pain in a construction worker may require him to curtail his work activities or even change careers, lead to significant economic problems, decrease his sexual relations, interfere with his life style and recreation, and perhaps result in marital discord, in disruption of his social network, in disability-related law suits, and in serious personal distress which may lead to seeking care from many physicians simultaneously. Each of these can be considered an illness problem. Just as biomedical physicians are taught to diagnose disease problems (e.g., metabolic abnormalities, infection, immunological dysfunction), record them in the medical record, provide disease interventions to treat them, and assess their cost/effectiveness, so too can they be trained to diagnose, record, treat, and assess the outcome of illness problems (Kleinman 1978; Kleinman and Smilkstein 1979; Katon and Kleinman 1981). Table I lists typical illness problems encountered on a consultation-liaison psychiatric service that we believe are applicable to any clinical setting.

TABLE I
Illness Problems*

1. Family problems created or worsened by sickness.
2. Financial problems created or worsened by sickness.
3. Major changes in a patient's personal identity and social role in the context of a terminal sickness or a permanent disability.
4. Lack of adherence with therapeutic regimen due to the unusual nature of a procedure or its expected outcome.
5. Maladaptive coping responses that patients and families use to manage sickness, such as denial, passive-hostile behavior, etc.
6. Conflict in personal beliefs between patients (and family) and practitioners concerning cause or nature of sickness and expected course and objectives for treatment.
7. Inappropriate resort to sick role and illness behavior owing to psychological or social gain.
8. Conflict in cultural values concerning treatment style and interpersonal etiquette between patients and practitioners due to substantial differences in social class, life style and ethnic norms.
9. Inappropriate use of alternative or indigenous health care agents and agencies.
10. Breakdown in communication between patient (and family) and practitioners.
11. Transference and countertransference problems in the doctor-patient or doctor-family relationship.
12. Life problems stemming from the particular stresses engendered by special treatment environments.

* From Katon and Kleinman 1981: 261.

Focusing on illness problems makes care more patient-centered. It sanctions clinically applied anthropological assessment of the social and cultural dimensions of sickness, just as it sanctions assessment of the psychological and psychiatric dimensions of sickness. This should become a major field for medical social science research, in which ways to categorize and recognize problems are investigated and treatment interventions and management strategies are examined. The physician himself may not be competent to manage the entire range of illness problems, but he should be trained to refer them to appropriate experts and agencies. In establishing illness problem lists and priorities for patients and their families, the clinically applied anthropologist possesses a practical means for consulting on patient care problems. But such a formulation also enables the clinically applied medical anthropologist to teach and conduct research on the interaction between macrosocial structural constraints and microclinical issues. That is to say, concrete illness problem lists can be used to critique the economic, political and social structural determinants and consequences of ill health and poor care in a way that clinical students and practitioners find compelling.

3. *Negotiation*

Recently my colleague Wayne Katon and I have presented a negotiation model of therapeutic relationships that can be taught to health care professionals by liaison personnel as a guide to clinical care. It can also be applied by psychiatric and anthropological consultants to resolve staff-patient conflicts (Katon and Kleinman 1980, 1981). This model builds on the work of Lazare and his collaborators (1978) at the Massachusetts General Hospital as well as the Kellian school of psychotherapy (Bannister and Fransella 1974). This approach to the practitioner-patient relationship establishes a framework of genuine negotiation among colleagues as the model for care. The patient (and family) is viewed as ultimately responsible for making final decisions about care. The practitioner is viewed as an expert tendering advice. Where a negotiation approach is unacceptable on cultural grounds, it does not make therapeutic sense to alter therapeutic relationships along this line. The clinician also needs to determine if the patient, family, or both are the appropriate party to negotiation. Ethnic stereotypes are often mischievous and frequently do not apply in individual instances. The clinician who is sensitive to ethnic beliefs and norms concerning doctor-patient relationships can employ the explanatory model approach to determine if negotiation is feasible or not. Our impression is that simply showing an interest in the patient's perspective of the expected and desired form of clinical interaction has positive therapeutic consequences. Like the ethnographer working in an alien culture, the clinician needs to show the patient he is aware that there are likely to be differences as well as similarities in their ways of construing social relationships and that he is interested in determining what these are in order to minimize misunderstanding and maximize productive collaboration.

The stages in the negotiation approach are:

(1) The physician elicits the patient's explanatory model and illness problems.

(2) The physician, based on his knowledge of the patient's illness problems, and his biomedical knowledge of the disease problems, then clearly and fully presents in layman's terms to the patient his explanatory model of the disorder including his treatment recommendations. (He also invites questions from the patient to which he responds with as complete an explanation as is possible.) This step may involve patient education in biomedical knowledge, but where technically and ethically feasible the physician should translate his ideas into the patient's conceptual system and work within the idiom (psychosomatic, somatizing, social, cosmological, etc.) the patient employs to articulate his illness problems and treatment goals.

(3) Often the patient will respond to the doctor's explanations by shifting his or her explanatory model of illness towards the physician's model, thus making a working alliance possible. The reverse is also true, that the physician armed with a greater understanding of the patient's explanatory model and illness problems

may change his recommendations shifting more toward the patient's expectations of treatment.

(4) At times, however, the discrepancies in the patient's or doctor's expectations of treatment will remain. Here the doctor should openly acknowledge and clarify the conflict between the two. He can provide references and data to argue on behalf of his perspective and the treatment interventions it entails. He should also provide the patient and family with ample opportunity to present their alternatives and assess their arguments in support of them.

(5) Perhaps as a result of understanding one another's conflicting explanations the doctor, the patient, or both will change their position so that a mutually desired treatment can be agreed upon. We feel that this is the end result in most cases.

(6) Where a conflict cannot be resolved through such an understanding, the physician should decide on an acceptable compromise of treatment based on his biomedical knowledge, knowledge of the patient's explanatory model and illness problems, and his own ethical standards. Here the physician can call upon input from the family, other agencies or health professionals (social workers, ethnic and pastoral counselors, psychiatrists) to help implement the compromise. Similarly, patients must have the right to involve members of their social network and key others familiar with their case in the negotiation process, if they believe this to be important.

(7) Throughout this process it is essential to recognize that the physician's role is to provide expert advice and rationale for treatment recommendations but the patient is the final arbiter of whatever choice is made. There is nothing wrong with the physician arguing strongly on behalf of a particular course of action, as long as he clarifies to the patient and family that the ultimate choice is theirs. As in any negotiation the patient may counter the physician's offer with a counter-proposal and the physician must again decide with respect to his technical knowledge and ethical standards whether he should accept this offer or make another of his own. If a stalemate is reached in negotiation and the patient's decision remains unacceptable on biomedical or ethical grounds, then the therapeutic contract and alliance is broken. At that point referral to another physician should be offered. At any time, based on his explanatory model and value system, the patient himself may decide to abrogate the therapeutic alliance and seek care elsewhere. Rather than see this option as noncompliance or "doctor shopping", the physician must recognize it as an absolutely legitimate option for the patient — one that he should make the patient aware of and facilitate if the patient so chooses.

(8) Each negotiation must involve ongoing monitoring of the agreement and of each party's participation. Not only should the physician see this as his role, but he should encourage the patient and family to monitor the ongoing status of the doctor-patient agreement as well. Such monitoring may necessitate renegotiation of the key clinical issues at a latter date (Katon and Kleinman 1981: 270–271).

Like the explanatory model framework, the negotiation process can be expanded or contracted as needed. The fact that the negotiation process may take considerable time, although often it does not, should not exonerate the physician from participating. But it surely is a reason for the clinically applied anthropologist to identify structural constraints (e.g., organization of time, financial remuneration, etc.) that interfere with negotiation and seek to change them. The medical anthropologist's clinical orientation does not infringe his responsibility to analyze (and where feasible alter) how macrosocial structures constrain microclinical praxis in ways that negatively affect care. Indeed, as Case 5 demonstrates, the framework of negotiation substantially strengthens the anthropologist's chances for linking social structure and culture to patient assessment and evaluation of the biases, deficiencies and limits of clinical intervention.

4. Other Clinically Applied Anthropological Strategies

Elsewhere my colleagues and I describe *clinical social science rounds* as a teaching device in the training of family medicine physicians that brings together anthropologists, psychiatrists, and family physicians in the assessment of patient care problems (Smilkstein et al. 1981). Once monthly we meet in the Family Medicine Center at the University of Washington for one and a half hours to discuss a patient whose illness or care presents a major psychosocial or cultural problem for clinical management. The format is for a family medicine resident to briefly present the biomedical perspective on the case as well as several core psychosocial or cultural problems to focus the clinical case discussion. Thereafter the patient is interviewed before the group of residents, students, and other Family Medical Center staff. Where relevant and feasible family members are also interviewed. Following the patient interview, medical anthropologists, psychiatrists and family physicians discuss the case from different perspectives: cultural beliefs and values, illness behavior, network support systems, family dynamics, psychopathology, and so forth. Each discussant reviews basic concepts, applies them to the case under discussion, and suggests appropriate treatment interventions. A clinically applied medical anthropologist fellow summarizes the analysis and recommendations, often drawing on the explanatory model, illness problems and negotiation frameworks. When feasible, follow-up is obtained to assess efficacy of the clinical social science recommendations. Typical clinical problems discussed in these rounds have included tacit value discrepancies between ethnic patients and their physicians, family dysfunction and marital discord complicating chronic illness, somatization, maladaptive coping with chronic illness, overutilization of the clinic, particular kinds of staff-patient conflicts, and other serious patient management problems, especially in the care of patients labeled as "difficult". We have found this forum to be a convincing demonstration of the relevance of social science to clinical work and therefore an effective clinical teaching device.

Additional strategies may be found in the literature. For example, Pfifferling (1981) outlines several medical anthropological strategies to teach medical students and residents to overcome the ethnocentrism and cultural limitations of biomedicine. These include the cultural status exam of the patient, self-assessment of the cultural premises of the physician's world and their negative effects on care, and use of a physician problem list to evaluate the role of the care system in creating stressful problems in the lives of health professionals. The Goods (1981) present a clinical hermeneutic approach for training physicians to systematically interpret the meaning context of their patients' problems and their own practice. Zola (1981) views the problem of compliance as a key focus for sensitizing physicians to the difficulties patients must undergo in the medicocentric world of bureaucratic health care. These and other strategies are all appropriate for use on a psychiatric consultation-liaison service (cf. Eisenberg and Kleinman 1981). They provide a *vademecum* of practical educational and consultation techniques for the neophyte medical anthropologist beginning work in a clinical setting.

RESPONSES

Our attempt to integrate anthropology with consultation-liaison psychiatry and apply it to clinical care has been well received by medical students and residents. Third-year medical students on their required psychiatric rotations spend one afternoon per week making clinical rounds with me. Each week of their six-week rotation they interview a patient on the medical or surgical floors for whom a psychiatric consultation has been requested. They also speak with relevant staff members about the reasons for the consultation request and, when feasible, interview the patient's family. Afterward they present the case to me, and include in their presentation assessment of disease and illness problems, patient and staff explanatory models, and a comprehensive interpretation of the reason for the consultation request and the nature of the consulation problem as they see it. Strategies for managing the problem are recommended. Thereafter I interview the patient with them. I interdigitate psychiatric evaluation with elicitation of relevant ethnographic information. My interview focuses on the patient's perspective and how it compares to that of the staff. Following the interview, we speak to family members and staff members who are available, and then we retire to a conference room or my office where we have an open-ended discussion for approximately one hour in which we alternate between the particular problem before us and the general issues it raises.

During this discussion, I present relevant concepts and findings from both psychiatry and anthropology. I refer students to the appropriate literature, much of which is immediately available on our service. Where feasible I analyze the case problem and make treatment recommendations in terms of the framework of explanatory models, illness problems and negotiation presented in the preceding section. I introduce and explain concepts like sick role, illness behavior, help seeking, labeling, somatization, primary and secondary gain, and culturally constituted illness beliefs and values. The fellows in our clinically applied anthropology training program, at least one of whom accompanies me on rounds, and I attempt to demonstrate for each case how patient and staff differentially socially construct illness, and how these constructions lead to tacit discrepancies and conflicts which exert practical effects on care. We spend considerable time teaching students to concretely analyze the clinical reality socially constructed and legitimated in hospital wards and clinics. Students are encouraged to offer their own views of how distinctive clinical realities might influence care, in the particular cases under study and generally. We specially emphasize the potentially negative effects of these treatment settings, discussing methods to systematically recognize and respond to them. My purpose is not to train medical students to become psychiatrists or social scientists, but to make them aware of relevant knowledge from both fields and provide them with a sense that they can and should draw on such knowledge in a clinically practical way in everyday medical practice.

Students frequently report that these rounds are more useful to them than the rest of the inpatient psychiatry rotation, much of which strikes them as overly specialized and not relevant to primary care, the field of medicine most will enter. They usually let me know that this experience is more meaningful to them than the lectures I gave them in their first year on medical anthropology. While I have not been able to determine whether these rounds exert any lasting impact on their clinical behavior, I do know that in six weeks the medical students read through and discuss key materials in medical anthropology and clinical social science, and actually see these being applied in patient care. Furthermore, many tell me that this expeience has deeply influenced how they think about and approach patients. As a result, I myself feel these teaching sessions are the most important teaching experiences in which I have engaged. The enthusiasm and appreciation of students along with the obvious value of our approach for patients and staff have prevented me from "burning out" over the years. Indeed I look forward to my weekly rounds with the medical students as the high point of my academic week. Not the least valuable aspect of this work is the opportunity it provides to help fellows, residents and anthropologists develop skills in teaching medical students.

Residents' responses are usually positive too, but they tend to vary more and to be more complex. Primary care residents, especially those in family medicine, respond very positively to our clinical teaching activities. Psychiatry residents who are themselves strongly interested in consultation-liaison or cross-cultural psychiatry, or have had backgrounds in primary care and/or social science, uniformly report that their clinical experience has been enriched by our approach. But some psychiatric residents who are narrowly oriented either to descriptive (or biological) psychiatry or psychoanalysis appear to be threatened, at least initially, by anthropological and other social science concepts. They even occasionally actively resist such teaching. While their numbers are small, it is important to recognize that there is a group of trainees who are hostile to anthropology, and remain so even after clinically applied anthropological teaching. Not suprisingly, residents in tertiary care internal medicine and surgery are also often negatively predisposed, but when they recognize the practical clinical benefits in particular situations, they become more open to this approach, and a few even go on to develop a strong interest in it.

The psychology interns who attend my teaching rounds vary greatly in their responses. Those wedded to a behaviorist model are skeptical. Those who are pluralistic seem to find our strategies clinical common sense. Social workers tend to find clinically applied anthropology quite congenial.

But the responses that have meant the most to me have been those of fellows, residents and students for whom clinically applied medical anthropology became a major interest. Some undergo a genuine "Ah, Ha!" experience, finding that anthropological knowledge along with writings on the social construction of reality offer new and powerful illumination on aspects of clinical work and medicine that they previously found poorly explained by conventional psychiatric, psychological and clinical approaches. For these few, anthropology has the same liberating effect it had for me when I first systematically studied it as a Johnny-come-lately clinician in graduate school. I have been fortunate to work with a group of such residents and fellows who have gone on to make their own contributions to the development of clinically applied medical anthropology in psychiatric and primary care settings (see, for example, Blumhagen 1980, in press; Boken et al. 1981; Demers et al. 1980; Katon and Kleinman 1980, 1981; Like and Ellison 1981; Lin et al. 1981, 1982; Rosen et al. 1982). I think every teacher in a relatively small and new discipline needs at least a few such marvelous students to revivify his own commitment.

Finally, I have from time to time had anthropologists attend my clinical rounds – some from my own university, some from other American universities, and a few from abroad. The consultation-liaison setting, which places them immediately in the midst of clinical work, serves well as an example of the opportunities and difficulties of working in clinical contexts. Clinical rounds on our service – whether with students or residents, or in the Family Medicine Center's clinical social science conference – act as an effective immersion for both clinical ethnographic and teaching interests. It is an expeditious way to show other anthropologists what we are doing, and how we go about doing it. Conversely, the presence of other social scientists is a useful way to avoid stagnation, elaborate a self-reflexive criticism of our own work, and learn about the practical applicability of alternative social science teaching and consulting techniques.

The main conclusion that we draw from these responses is that to the extent we are successful in applying anthropological and other social science concepts to actual cases so as to better understand them and contribute to the resolution of clinical problems, we are able to convince trainees of the significance of medical anthropology and make them receptive to anthropological concepts and methods. Where we fail to make such clinical linkages, or inadequately demonstrate that we have done so, we lose the interest of our trainees and colleagues. Clinicians, not too surprisingly, are interested in clinical applications. Clinically applied medical anthropology like consultation-liaison psychiatry interests them because it is clinically useful. Whether that utility is more for physicians or for patients and their families does not matter. The central thing is that medical anthropology clearly contributes to clinical work, that trainees quite quickly become aware of this, and for this reason they find it more compatible and relevant than those social (or biomedical) sciences that are divorced from clinical reality. The ethnographic experience of the anthropologist trains anthropologists how to enter and take part in the alien setting of the clinic, a skill whose lack contributes to other social scientists' problems in medicine. It also provides an experience in which interviewing patients and becoming immersed in their life worlds and interviewing informants and observing and participating in their cultures are mutually seen as essential common ground, regardless of other obvious differences. Hence our notion that clinicalizing the anthroplogist is the basis for anthropologizing the clinician. That in turn is the royal road for the meaningful introduction of anthropology into medicine.

Anthropology in Psychiatry: An Addendum

Traditionally, social anthropology's main tie in the medical school has been with departments of psychiatry. Anthropologists have been active researchers in ethnographic studies of inpatient psychiatry units, and have taught psychiatry residents about culture and personality and transcultural psychiatry. They have more recently participated in behavioral science instruction of medical students. But besides occasionally being hired as program planners, facilitators and evaluators in community mental health centers, especially when these have a substantial ethnic clientele, anthropologists have not contributed in a major way to clinical teaching in psychiatry (in outpatient or inpatient settings). The consultation and liaison psychiatry service I have described in this paper, with its substantial anthropological input, is distinctly unusual, though I believe it is a paradigm for the future integration of anthropology and psychiatry.

Indeed, for all the decades of interest of anthropologists in psychiatry and psychiatrists in anthropology, anthropology has not had a major impact on psychiatric categories, which remain largely ethnocentric, medicocentric and insensitive to cultural differences. Yet psychiatry in the past has been more open to anthropology than any other medical school discipline save perhaps for departments of social, preventive and community medicine. But at the present time, psychiatry is undergoing a major reorientation with strong emphasis on its medical roots and the biomedical model. It is high irony, especially for a consultation-liaison psychiatrist, that biologically oriented psychiatrists are advocating a medical model which has been found overly narrow by primary care internal medicine and family medicine, where an integrated biopsychosocial model has attracted great interest, and which supports an approach to chronic mental illness that is less psychosocially sensitive than that advocated for chronic medical disorders. This reorientation has made some psychiatry departments less accessible to social science interests. As a result, today family medicine strikes me as more open to anthropologists and an anthropological approach than psychiatry, though there is still a strong interest in anthropology among social and cultural psychiatrists, psychoanalysts, and psychoanalytically oriented psychotherapists, who are rapidly becoming, however, a minority in academic psychiatry.

The picture presented in this paper should indicate to readers why primary care is a most suitable setting for clinically applied medical anthropology, whether or not that occurs in concert with consultation-liaison psychiatry. Within departments of psychiatry, I believe anthropologists can be especially effective in the type of clinical teaching sketched in this paper. But it will take perseverence and acceptance by supportive psychiatric colleagues to develop this in a major clinical teaching and research venue. No one should underestimate the difficulties for creating programs similar to the one I have described in more traditional psychiatric settings. Nonetheless I believe this is an extremely important direction for anthropological input into psychiatry aided by psychiatrists who either are themselves anthropologists or are substantially interested in the clinical application of medical anthropology.

There are, of course, other key involvements for anthropologists who work in psychiatry. Limitation on space prevents me from detailing all of these, but a few should be noted. Anthropologists can effectively instruct psychiatry residents in several didactic subjects: psychological anthropology, medical anthropology, and transcultural and international psychiatry. These subjects are best taught with a clinical orientation; for example, as lectures or seminars on cultural influences on schizophrenia, depression, or psychiatric nosology generally, or on ethnic influences on psychiatric illness behavior, labeling, help seeking, and therapeutic interactions among major American ethnic groups, or on anthropological assessment of transcultural psychiatric and psychiatric epidemiology studies concerning culture-bound disorders, non-Western cultures, folk healing, family and childhood disorders, and the like. Cultural sensitivity groups can be set up in programs with substantial numbers of ethnic patients or with residents from ethnic minorities and foreign countries. Special clinical case conferences and rounds can be developed either on an ad hoc or regular basis to cover cultural influences on psychopathology, doctor-patient relationships, and psychiatric practice that are organized around practical clinical problems. Several departments of psychiatry have established traditions for such rounds and conferences.

Anthropologists can effectively participate in community and social psychiatry training programs. Here they may occupy a very major role in organizing and implementing training, including teaching the social science foundations of community psychiatry, establishing curricula on the mental health needs and psychiatric care delivery issues for minority groups, the inner city and rural poor, the elderly, the mentally retarded, and the physically disabled. Not the least of this job is to act as translators of relevant concepts and findings from the social sciences for community psychiatry.

Surely there are other useful roles in psychiatry that anthropologists can and do play, such as program assessment. But one final area looms particularly large. A large number of American psychiatrists are centrally interested in psychotherapy. Because of this interest many find anthropological studies of healing of some importance. This is likely to be an abiding bridge between the two disciplines, one where anthropological writings and instruction will play a continuingly important part.

A final point is the relationship of anthropologists to cultural psychiatry and minority psychiatrists. Cultural (or transcultural or cross-cultural) psychiatry is conceptually weak, though its clinical and epidemiological methods are improving. It must strike many anthropologists as poorly founded in anthropology and social science theory and findings. It is the duty of those who teach or do research in psychiatric settings to improve this situation. But heretofore the principal change has gone the other way, with psychiatric anthropologists acquiring facility in psychiatric categories and methods to a much more sophisticated degree than psychiatrists master and use anthropological knowledge. Yet the fact that psychiatry is inseparable from meaning and social relations suggests that anthropology could contribute significantly to core clinical concerns of psychiatrists. Since in the short-run it does not appear that psychiatry – in a period of retrenchment, re-orientation, and financial scarcity – will open its doors to many anthropologists, it may well be that over the next few years anthropology will exert a greater influence via incorporation of the idea of culture into the mainstream of psychiatric theory. In that the Diagnostic and Statistical Manual No. III (DSM–III) of the American Psychiatric Association is virtually acultural, anthropologists and psychiatrists with anthropological training have their work cut out to offer a fundamental critique of psychiatric theory that can create a more anthropologically informed DSM–IV.

CONCLUSION

Impediments to the clinical application of anthropology arise from both sides of the border: medicine and anthropology (cf. Kleinman 1980: 375–388). As a late comer to the clinical domain, the anthropologist is viewed with some concern and suspicion by his clinical colleagues, who, in a era of scarcity, are protective of turf, time, positions, and general support funds. In some ways, his most natural allies (psychiatrists, psychologists, social workers) may feel most threatened, view-ing their world in the limited good mode that George Foster associates with peasant societies. Medical sociologists also may be threatened because they were often on the scene first and yet, because they lack or are uncomfortable with an ethno-graphic bridge to the clinic, have had to work harder to establish clinical contacts and credence. Negotiating the politics of medical schools and hospitals is a subject unto itself, but it is not made easier by those anthropologists who view anthropology as a *clinical practice*. This is most definitely not the way I view anthropology. There is a world of difference for anthropologists to be teachers and consultants, and for them to deliver care. Since there is nothing in anthropology *per se* that qualifies anthropologists as therapists, one would suppose that an anthropologist clinician would have to have additional training (e.g., medicine, nursing, social work, lay psy-chotherapy, etc.) to claim a primary care clinical competence. Yet if so, then surely it is this other discipline not anthropology which is the basis for his therapeutic involvement, and hence it is a mystification, and a mischievous one, for such a person to advertise himself as a *clinical* (in the sense of therapeutic) *anthropologist*. The movement to make anthropology a therapeutic discipline is, to my mind, wrong-headed; it will almost certainly provoke substantial resistance from clinicians, who see yet another field in competition with them for limited and shrinking re-sources, and therefore will make the teaching and consulting of *clinicially applied medical anthropologists* more difficult.

As we have seen, a large part of the anthropologist's dilemma in the clinical context is to take up a stance that is intrinsically divided: collegial, concerned with the practical resolution of clinical problems; and yet at the same time, autonomous, concerned with clarifying an independent anthropological theory of illness and healing that can stand on its own. Constantly shifting between patient and physician perspectives, the clinically applied anthropologist working in consultation-liaison psychiatry is an advocate for both. This inherent tension I take to be the source of medical anthropology's major contribution to clinical work. It offers a framework for interpretation that is broad enough to encompass all the major participants, and thereby is a more adequate guide to therapeutic choice. Indeed it is this inherently ethnographic ability to describe and compare distinctive cultural constructions of clincial reality that to my mind is the core contribution of anthropology to clinical consultation, teaching and research.

Nonetheless, it is also this divided stance that is the source of the clinically applied anthropologist's personal discomfort and professional unease. The clinician wonders, "Whose interest does this professional stranger support?" The patient and family look upon him with equal uncertainty. Each time he intervenes in the making of clinical decisions, the anthropologist feels the tug of divided loyalties. Not licensed to carry the therapeutic mandate, he is ambivalently situated between disinterested observation and committed participation. A practical philosopher in a land of atheoretical empiricists and the bearers of conventional commonsense, he is provoked to raise fundamental questions that challenge the taken-for-granted bases of everyday therapeutic action. If this shared symbolic structure of belief and behavior is crucial to placebo response and perhaps healing generally, as well it might be, can agnostic cultural analysis create untoward side effects, be iatrogenic? Caught up in the pull and push between macrosocial determinants and microclinical consequences, does the anthropologist's teaching about the form, not the substance, of social structure carry the possibility of paralyzing the clinician's judgment, alienating patients from sources of help now viewed as sources of oppression? How does one teach clinical students how to be more effective healers and at the same time challenge the ethnocentrism of their paradigm of care? Does cultural relativism, evolutionism, or universalism offer the most useful framework for working with patients and healers? In the hectic exigency surrounding sick people seeking help, does the anthropologist regard his contribution as marginal or central? Offended by the sometimes systematic inhumanity of biomedical training what does he say to colleagues, students, other anthropologists? The one member of his tribe in the midst of skeptical members of a tribe with a different world view, how does he learn to best make his points, remain silent when his words would be seen as useless, threatening or obstructive, and control his own emotional response to being disvalued and ignored? When he writes, who is his audience? The divisions go on and on. I have no answer to this dilemma. But I have found in my own experience that self-critical reflection on this divided stance can be the beginning of an authentic way of teaching and doing anthropology in the clinical world that has the potential to be immensely rewarding even if exhausting and lonely.

For if medicine is to be related to meaning in the actual practice of care it will take professional strangers like the anthropologist and the psychiatrist to be mediators. The mediating world of consultation-liaison psychiatry is a most appropriate place to systematically explore these possibilities and limitations of the clinical application of anthropology.

REFERENCES

Bannister, D. and F. Fransella
  1974 Inquiring Man: The Theory of Personal Constructs. Baltimore: Penguin.
Blumhagen, D.
  1980 Hyper-Tension: A Folk Illness With a Medical Name. Culture, Medicine, and Psychiatry 4: 197–228.
Bokan, J. et al.
  in press Tertiary Gain and Chronic Pain. Pain.
Demers, R. et al.
  1980 An Exploration of the Depth and Dimensions of Illness Behavior. Journal of Family Practice 11: 1085–1092.
Eisenberg, L. and A. Kleinman
  1981 Clinical Social Science. In L. Eisenberg and A. Kleinman (ed.), The Relevance of Social Science for Medicine, Dordrecht, Holland: D. Reidel Publ. Co. pp. 1–26.
Engel, G.
  1977 The Need for a New Medical Model: A Challenge for Biomedicine. Science 196: 129–136.
Good, B. and M. J. Good
  1981 The Meanings of Symptoms. In L. Eisenberg and A. Kleinman (eds.), The Relevance of Social Science for Medicine, Dordrecht, Holland: D. Reidel Public Co., pp. 165–196.
Hackett, T. and N. Cassem (eds.)
  1978 Massachusetts General Hospital Handbook of General Hospital Psychiatry, St. Louis: C. V. Mosby.
Harwood, A. (ed.)
  1981a Ethnicity and Medical Care. Cambridge, Mass.: Harvard University Press.
Harwood, A.
  1981b Mainland Puerto Ricans. In A. Harwood (ed.), Ethnicity and Medical Care, Cambridge, Mass.: Harvard University Press. pp. 397–481.
  (no date) Communicating About Disease: Clinical Implications of Divergent Concepts Among Patients and Physicians.
Holzner, B. and J. Marx
  1978 Knowledge Application: the Knowledge System in Society. Boston: Allyn & Bacon.
Inui, T. et al.
  1976 Improved Outcomes in Hypertension after Physician Tutorials. Annals of Internal Medicine 84: 646–651.
Katon, W. and A. Kleinman
  1980 A Biopsychosocial Approach to Surgical Evaluation and Outcome. Western Journal of Medicine 133: 9–14.
  1981 Doctor-Patient Negotiation and Other Social Science Strategies in Patient Care. In L. Eisenberg and A. Kleinman (eds.), The Relevance of Social Science for Medicine, Dordrecht, Holland: D. Reidel Publ. Co., pp. 253–282.
Katon, W. A. Kleinman, and G. Rosen
  1982 Depression and Somatization. American Journal of Medicine 72(1): 127–135 and 72(2): 241–247.

Kleinman, A.
1975 Explanatory Models in Health Care Relationships. *In* National Council for International Health: Health of the Family, Washington, D. C.: National Council for International Health, pp. 159–172.
1977 Lessons from a Clinical Approach to Medical Anthropology. Medical Anthropology Newsletter 8: 4: 11–15.
1980 Patients and Healers in the Context of Culture: An Exploration of the Borderland Between Anthropology, Medicine, and Psychiatry. Berkeley: University of California Press.
Kleinman, A., L. Eisenberg, and B. Good
1978 Culture, Illness and Care. Annals of Internal Medicine 88: 251–258.
Kleinman, A. and G. Smilkstein
1980 Psychosocial Issues in Assessment in Primary Care. *In* G. Rosen, et al (eds.), Behavioral Science in Family Practice, New York: Appleton-Century-Crofts, pp. 95–108.
Lazare, A.
1973 Hidden Conceptual Models in Clinical Psychiatry. New England Journal Of Medicine 288: 345–350.
Lazare, A. et al.
1978 Studies on a Negotiated Approach to Patienthood. *In* E. Gallagher (ed.), The Doctor-Patient Relationship in the Changing Health Scene, Washington, D. C.: USGPO, DHEW Publication No. (NIH 78–183), pp. 119–139.
Like, R. and L. Ellison
1981 Sleeping Blood, Tremor and Paralysis. Culture, Medicine, and Psychiatry 5: 49–64.
Lin, K. M. et al.
1981 Psychiatric Epidemiology in Chinese Cultures. *In* A. Kleinman and T. Y. Lin (eds.). Normal and Abnormal Behavior in Chinese Culture, Dordrecht, Holland: D. Reidel Publ. Co., pp. 331–355.
1982 Sociocultural Determinants of the Help-Seeking Behavior of Patients with Mental Illness. Journal of Nervous and Mental Disease 170(2): 78–85.
Lipowski, Z. J.
1974 Consultation-Liaison Psychiatry: An Overview. American Journal of Psychiatry 131: 623–630.
Manschreck, T. and A. Kleinman
1977 Introduction: A Critical Rational Perspective on Psychiatry. *In* T. Manschreck and A. Kleinman (eds.), Renewal in Psychiatry, Washington, D. C.: Hemisphere, pp. 1–41.
Manschreck, T. and A. Kleinman
1979 Psychiatry's Identity Crisis: A Critical Rational Remedy. General Hospital Psychiatry 2: 166–173.
Pfifferling, J. H.
1981 A Cultural Prescription for Medicocentrism. *In* L. Eisenberg and A. Kleinman (eds.), The Relevance of Social Science for Medicine, Dordrecht, Holland: D. Reidel Publ. Co., pp. 197–222.
Ries, R. et al.
1981 Psychiatric Consultation-Liaison Service: Patients, Requests, Functions. General Hospital Psychiatry 3: 204–212.
Rosen, G. et al.
1982 Somatization in Family Practice: A Biopsychosocial Approach. Journal of Family Practice 14(3): 493–502.
Smilkstein, G. et al.
1981 Clinical Social Science Conference. Journal of Family Practice 12: 2: 347–353.

Starfield, B. et al.
  1980 The Influence of Patient-Practitioner Agreement on Outcome of Care. American Journal of Public Health 71: 2: 127–131.
Zola, I.
  1981 Structural Constraints in the Doctor-Patient Relationship: The Case of Non-Compliance. *In* L. Eisenberg and A. Kleinman (eds.), The Relevance of Social Science for Medicine. Dordrecht, Holland: D. Reidel Publ. Co., pp. 241–252.

NOEL J. CHRISMAN

ANTHROPOLOGY IN NURSING: AN EXPLORATION OF
ADAPTATION

In 1970, Leininger argued that anthropology and nursing were "two worlds to
blend". Publications since that time have, in various ways, made the same kind of
point (Brink 1976; Bauwens 1978; Moore et al. 1980). One conceptual basis for
that argument is that the two areas are concerned with people from both scientific
and humanistic perspectives. Although this is a sound foundation on which to
structure the introduction of anthropology to nurses and nursing, a major difference
between the two poses all-too-real difficulties and challenges to the anthropologist
working in a school of nursing. The difference lies in this: anthropology is solely an
academic discipline — a structured approach to the search for knowledge; nursing,
however, is both a discipline and a human services profession. As a discipline, the
latter's objective is to build a science of nursing — a systematic and rigorous structure of enquiry regarding the health related aspects of human interaction with the
environment. But as a profession, nursing is a highly practical and well defined
service role for delivering care to patients (Donaldson and Crowley 1978). Anthropology, even in its applied form, does not have a socially sanctioned (and therefore
morally experienced) clinical, or service, mandate. Thus, because most teaching in a
school of nursing is to clinicians, anthropological understandings must be "translated" by the anthropologist so they are relevant to patient care. The challenge in
this translation process lies not only in discovering how to make concrete, practical
suggestions out of abstract concepts, but also how to introduce anthropology as a
scientific discourse within which such concepts form part of a system of ideas,
methods, data, and rather unique ways at looking at the world so that practicing
nurses can routinely use anthropological understandings in a disciplined rigorous
way as they engage in their professional duties.

The basic principle I use to accomplish this translation task in my teaching in
a school of nursing is to expand on the existing strengths of nursing as a discipline
and a profession. This makes explicit the value of what is being done already and
makes clear my readiness to aid nurses and nursing students in doing better what
they already do. To accomplish this, I need to identify central themes in nursing
thought and practice so that anthropological contributions to these domains of
knowledge can be clearly and effectively explicated as central to the interests of
nurses. The principal anthropological addition is a cultural perspective; one that
is relativistic and describes the lifeways of subcultures in the U.S. and abroad.

Identifying themes is no simple task when a national context is taken into
account. Many nursing schools build their curricula around the central perspectives
of one or another influential writer in nursing. For example, Sr. Calista Roy (1976)
proposed that the concept of adaptation is central in understanding client behavior
and designing nursing actions. Martha Rogers (1979) focused on the individual as

117

N. J. Chrisman and T. W. Maretzki (eds.), Clinically Applied Anthropology, 117–140.
Copyright © 1982 by D. Reidel Publishing Company.

a unified whole. Dorothea Orem (1980) has expounded on the concept of self care. And Leininger (1980a) supports a transcultural view of caring.

A key concept that I use is that of *care* or caring. Interestingly enough, the concept has not received a great deal of research and conceptual attention in the literature; though this is being remedied to some extent through the stimulus of annual conferences on "caring" organized by Madeleine Leininger (1980b). In nursing practice, care or caring seem to symbolize a quality of personal relationships that is infused with the work nurses do to aid patients to cope with health related aspects of everyday life – in the home, community, or hospital. The notion of caring carries with it a sense of personal concern for the client and has been differentiated into a number of caring constructs such as comfort, support, nurturance, and the like (Leininger 1978, 1980a). This personal concern is consistent with the anthropological tradition of identifying with informants and relating to them on a personal level.

As developed by Gaut (1979), the concept of care requires that the care-giver focus upon the nature of the subject of care, the patient. That is, for caring to occur, the interests of the patient must be served rather than those of the care-giver, no matter how altruistic the provider believes herself to be. Thus, the client's life style and health status must be understood relativistically from the client's point of view.

Initially, I chose to focus on care as a linking concept between anthropology and nursing on ethnographic grounds. That is, I noted that the term occurred frequently in conversations among nursing instructors when they talked about nursing practice or the behaviors of their students. I remember being struck by the similarity in both the amorphousness and centrality of the concepts of *care* and *culture* in nursing and anthropology respectively. I reasoned that, like culture, the unstructured but significant concept of care was probably learned by frequent exposure to role models – for nursing students, these models are their instructors and the clinical paradigms of good nursing they teach; for anthropology students, the models are the ethnographers and ethnological approaches in the paradigmatic books and articles we read.

Tied to the idea of care in the conversations of some instructors was the notion that care is facilitated when the nurse has a holistic perspective of the patient. One instructor who taught students in the hospital complained that her students were much too concerned about only assessing the pathophysiological qualities of patients and neglected an integrated and humanistic understanding of their patients. "How will they ever learn how to care for their patients when they don't understand them as people?"

Caring for and understanding the patient holistically underpin a particular conceptualization of the practice of nursing. In this perspective, nurses view their activities as aiding patients to cope with or adapt to their current life situation and health status. The nurse attempts to aid the individual to mobilize existing resources of daily living – including aspects of life style, community agencies, or hospital personnel – so that the demands of daily living can be met (Carnevali and

Patrick 1979). Holistic understanding is thus essential if demands and resources are to be accurately identified. In addition, since the concept of care, as I teach it, includes a relativistic understanding of the person from that person's point of view, the demands and resources must be those perceived by the patient.

Given the overwhelming importance of a biologically based, biomedical approach among health professionals, teaching the importance of the client's perspective is probably the most critical (and distinctive) contribution to be made by the anthropologist. The combined concepts of care, holistic understanding, and aiding the patient to cope with the current life situation provide a rationale *from within nursing* to introduce anthropological data and theoretical perspectives. Ethnography *is* a description of everyday life from a people's point of view. Anthropological concepts provide ways of categorizing these everyday life data so that cross-cultural comparisons and generalizations can be made. Moreover, anthropology's relativism can act as a counterbalance to the biological ethnocentrism of the health professions.

Anthropology's relativistic stance also causes a problem for clinical nurses. In order to evaluate and refine nursing interventions, the common, or universal, elements of nursing care situations must be identified (Peplau 1969). One of the purposes of nursing education is to introduce students to as many of those universals as possible. Yet anthropologists tend to shy away from making universal pronouncements, knowing how many factors provide variation. It creates a great deal of frustration when the anthropologist's answer to a general patient care question is "it all depends". The way I squelch my own impulse to use this phrase is to identify the major sociocultural concepts related to the type of case in question and to stress the need to adequately assess the individual patient in terms of these concepts.

Anthropology's strengths in a school of nursing include its scientific and humanistic approach to humanity, its repertoire of concepts to aid in analyzing patients' demands and resources in daily life, its wealth of ethnographic data that promotes greater understanding of people's ways of life, its liberating emphasis on self-reflexive assessments of personal and group bias and openness to alternative, non-orthodox viewpoints, and its focus on relating macro-social structural constraints with micro-social interpersonal situations. The primary weakness is that anthropology is not a clinical discipline and thus appears to be irrelevant in actual practice. The challenge facing an anthropologist in this educational setting is to provide clinical relevance without reducing the science of anthropology to a cookbook of sociocultural recommendations that yields thin stereotypes in place of thick interpretations. My own approach to this is crystallized in a proverb I tell my students:

Give a man a fish and he eats for a day. Teach a man to fish and he eats every day.

Teaching nursing students a set of conceptual perspectives that enables them to discover their patients' social and cultural backgrounds and to relate these to specific clinical problems provides a means for continually providing and monitoring culturally sensitive patient care that integrates other nursing knowledge.

THE NURSING AUDIENCE

Nurses' receptivity to an anthropological approach to patient care is most strongly influenced by the nature of their conceptual framework for engaging in nursing care and their past and current experience in nursing. The most influential conceptual framework in nursing is still the reductionist, pathophysiological biomedical perspective shared with physicians. This seemingly comprehensive and unified theoretical approach is learned early in the educational process and is consistently reinforced in patient care because medical outcomes are the most visible result of nursing care. Peplau points out that of the dual purpose of nursing, "first and foremost, the nurse favors the survival of the organism" (Peplau 1969: 346). Nursing students and practicing nurses tend to use this largely tacit framework to assimilate most nursing knowledge. It underlies their understanding of anatomical and physiological variation as well as variation in growth and development patterns and psychosocial qualities.

This same framework seems to be used to acquire sociocultural knowledge. Notions such as family, role relationships, and sickness are treated as *things*, amenable to single definitions and related to other things much in the fashion of the relation between kidneys and fluid and electrolyte balance. Students thus believe it is appropriate to learn concrete units of knowledge about American ethnic groups such as specific lists of food preferences among Hispanics, family characteristics among Blacks, or the pre- and post-natal practices of Asians. This trait list approach to cultural knowledge not only obscures the existence and importance of a behavioral science conceptual framework, it also promotes stereotyping and reifies esoteric cultural patterns as definitive aspects of ethnic group behavior. A second consequence of the tacit use of the biomedical framework is that sociocultural information is learned in terms of its relationship to the presence or absence of pathophysiology rather than to patterns of everyday life. Thus students frequently have difficulty learning the logic of folk illness systems because they make no sense in terms of Western biology. The strength of a Western biological perspective occasionally surfaces overtly in class with a question: "Your discussion of *susto* is interesting, but what is it *really*?"

In order to teach an anthropological approach to clinical care and not just a series of esoteric facts, it is essential to introduce it as part of a behavioral science conceptual framework. This can be accomplished efficiently by using statements from the nursing literature as a vehicle. For example, I have quoted Hildegard Peplau who noted that "when the life of the patient is assured, a second purpose guides the nursing practice. The nurse aids the patient to grasp the meaning of his health problem and to learn from his current experience with it" (Peplau 1969: 346). The focus of the quote is on the *patient's* meaning and experience, which can be contrasted with biomedical meanings through ethnographic examples, such as the meaning of "bug" for the man who refused to learn wound care because he could see none of the bugs that the student said would cause infection later. Or questions such as the one about *susto* above can be used to remind students of the illness-disease distinction and its centrality to the process of negotiating patient and professional meanings of sickness. Providing a rationale *from within nursing* that justifies an anthropological approach aids in heightening nurses' sensitivity to and interest in the meaning centered approach of anthropology that offers a systematic basis for conceptualizing patient experiences. The point needs to be made that just as biomedicine is much more rigorous than common sense knowledge of the biological basis of disease, anthropology is more rigorous, organized, and useful than the common sense most clinicians rely on for understanding the sociocultural context of illness experiences.

A second characteristic of the nursing audience that influences receptivity to an anthropological approach is the type of practice in which the nurse engages. Included in the nature of practice are (a) the range of settings for health care delivery and (b) the clinical specialty of the nurse. Settings range from highly structured instituions such as hospitals and nursing homes to less structured contexts such as hospital outpatient clinics, schools, and industry. A significant feature of setting for nursing practice is the locus of power or control in the nurse-patient dyad. In hospitals, nurses, like physicians, have a great deal of control over patient behavior. The highly structured environment forces patients into stereotyped molds. In contrast, when patients are on their own turf — in the community — they can avoid the control of the nurse more easily and their highly variable life styles become more salient for their health care. Thus, community based nurses tend to be much more attentive to how people live their lives since nursing care plans — including biomedical aspects — must be made with these lives in mind.

Experience in community settings underlies a much more positive view of an anthropological conceptual framework because the nurse has had to contend frequently with highly variable life styles. In addition, many of these nurses have constructed their own ideas of family variability, ethnic health beliefs, or social class variations and the ways these life style variables influence compliance and use of folk healers or folk medicines. It is a relatively simple step to replace or augment the experiential concepts with anthropological concepts that are more strongly grounded in the literature.

In contrast, nurses who practice in hospital settings experience patients and patient care differently. A much narrower range of patient behavior is evident and, except for flagrant examples of ethnic or other influences on patient behavior, there is less likelihood that the cultural qualities of patients have posed frequent problems. Exigencies of the situation such as very sick patients, a highly technological environment, and the primacy of the biomedical physician-oriented subculture decrease nurses' attention to patients' community life styles and their relevance to nursing care. Thus, anthropological knowledge and concepts about everyday life *seem* less important because the nurse is primarily concerned with daily life behavior in the hospital. As a result, nurses tend to want to know only about seemingly extreme responses to hospitalization such as depression, family visitors, sullenness, or ritual behavior, wondering whether these are "normal" for that subculture. However, hospital nurses respond favorably to anthropological analyses of role relationships such as the hierarchical structure of nurse-physician interactions, or of the "rituals" of patient care in the coronary unit or the operating room.

A second aspect of experience (or anticipated experience, in the case of undergraduates) that affects how nurses respond to an anthropological approach is the type of clinical specialty. To simplify the increasing complexity of nursing practice, I will focus on the major clinical areas of medical-surgical nursing, patient-child nursing, psychiatric nursing, and community health (or public health) nursing. Although this category is conceptually independent of setting, in actuality medical-surgical nurses are highly likely to be found in hospital settings, while community health nurses are not. The other two fall in between. Like settings, types of nursing specialties tend to imply a constellation of interests related to anthropological information. Medical-surgical nurses are likely to be the most focused upon medical chracteristics of their patients and usually consider sociocultural factors only insofar as they directly influence adaptation to hospital life. However, two sets of activities that are commonly part of this practice promote the nurse's need for knowledge of family and community life: patient education, usually preparatory to discharge, and rehabilitation. In each case, it is helpful (but frequently not fully recognized) to know the details of a person's life outside the hosptial.

The other three clinical specialties — parent-child nursing, psychiatric (or psychosocial) nursing, and community health nursing — are all strongly oriented toward the behavioral sciences. Although parent-child and psychiatric nurses are found in hospitals as well as community settings, the nature of their practices requires that they be able to take account of daily life factors in their assessments of clients' health statuses. As would be expected, parent-child nurses desire information on cultural variability in such areas as growth and development, pre- and post-partum practices, women's health, parenting, and birthing. With these clinical interests, nurses with a specialty in parent-child nursing tend to view anthropological data and insight in a positive fashion. In contrast, psychosocial nurses are most strongly influenced by psychology and sociology and anthropological contributions tend to be underrepresented. This is particularly interesting given the traditional link between anthropology and the medical specialty of psychiatry. I think that part of the reason for this discrepency lies in the nearly complete absence of anthropological analysis of mental hospitals, the historical clinical base for psychiatric nurses. The relatively recent shift toward community mental health centers has not altered the situation, though the work of Estroff (in this volume) for example, may promote change.

Of the nursing specialties, community health nursing tends to be the most positively oriented towards anthropology. This is partially due to the nature of the setting for practice, but the clinical activities of community health nurses are also strongly influential. Nurses with this specialty have primary responsibilities in the areas of disease prevention, such as administering immunizations; health maintenance, following discharged hospital patients, for example: and health promotion, which involves teaching individuals and families about nutrition, family planning, and the like. The continuing focus on the family also implies interests shared with parent-child nurses. These, and other activities, are closely tied to and frequently strongly constrained by people's life styles. Thus, community health nurses look to anthropology and the other behavioral sciences for help in unraveling the many frustrations of working with people in their own settings.

My growing understanding of conceptual relationships of anthropology and nursing, the nature of nursing audiences, and the importance of introducing an anthropological conceptual framework to supplement the biomedical framework has been useful in teaching nurses at various educational levels and in a number of situations. The remainder of the paper, however, will be concerned with only two particular examples: my experience teaching an undergraduate anthropology and nursing course and running a graduate program in cross-cultural nursing.

CROSS-CULTURAL NURSING AT THE UNIVERSITY OF WASHINGTON

Since 1976, all undergraduate nursing students have been required to take *Cultural Variation and Nursing Practice*, a course in which anthropology and nursing are integrated. The students are in the second quarter of their junior year. They have had one year of basic liberal arts courses, and increasing numbers have had much more than that. They have completed the first year of professional education which includes a basic nursing course with an introduction to nursing care in in-patient settings, two growth and development courses, and basic courses in psychosocial nursing, In the first junior year quarter, they complete half of the course in medical-surgical nursing. These students take the second quarter of medical-surgical nursing concurrently with the Cultural Variation course.

The qualities of these students as audience place rather stringent requirements on how the course can be taught. According to Olesen and Whittaker (1968), nursing students at the undergraduate level are strongly focused on the hospital as the setting for nursing care and believe, with justification, that the *real* focus of their education is on learning the knowledge and techniques of bedside care. Moreover, the implicit biomedical conceptual framework is strongly evident. Its value as a structure for assimilating knowledge in other courses reinforces students' already high level of interest in anatomy and physiology. Some students regularly point out that the cultural dimension is irrelevant; the students are accustomed to a course in which highly relevant "nursing" information is presented.

Responding to these, and other, audience characteristics, the course begins with an attempt to establish the logic of and need for an anthropological approach within nursing. First, I discuss the notion of care and caring, pointing out that in order to fully care for the client, the nurse should know the person's goals in the context of his or her life style so that those goals — not just those of the nurse — can be facilitated. Recently, I have added a brief review of human evolutionary history in order to suggest the importance of care within the family unit as an adaptive feature in human survival. Secondly, I discuss the potential dangers of taking only a biomedical approach to patients in hospital situations. One of the cases used for illustration was originally recounted in class by a student working in a hospital in which the current group of students will take a clinical practicum. Briefly, the case involves a Vietnamese baby brought to the hospital by her baby sitter with a severe cold and welts on her back. I point out that through ignorance of the Asian practice of scraping the illness out with a penny — producing the welts — the hospital staff began the process of removing the child from the custody of her "abusing" mother.

The third element in this introductory portion involves a discussion of an epidemiological perspective. Using the model of interdependent host-agent-environment interactions, I show how social and cultural features of daily life can contribute to host susceptibility and risk in the environment. The most complete example provided is one that some students will see in their later careers: infant diarrhea in a farmworker baby. This analysis focuses on the ineffectiveness of either primary care or hospital care for a baby who will return to the same poorly plumbed farm camp and experience a high risk of reinfection. The basic point is that narrow biological interventions are likely to have a low success rate when the sociocultural context is not given attention.

Most content in the course is an elaboration of the hidden sociocultural factors influencing nurse-patient interactions and the process of nursing care. To aid in understanding nursing, the subculture of nursing (Leininger 1970) in the U.S. and abroad is discussed. Many nursing behaviors are viewed in the context of major American value complexes such as efficiency, equality of treatment, man's technological control of nature, and the importance of work rather than play (Arensberg and Niehoff 1964). Behavior conforming to these values is shown, through example, to be sensitive or insensitive depending upon the similarity of values of nurse and client. For example, a highly technological approach is likely to be congruent with the values of middle class whites, but insulting or distant behavior in the eyes of Native Americans. In international settings, value differences emerge even more clearly and are shown to be related to culture shock.

Sociocultural factors influencing client perspectives are explored in great detail, emphasizing variability within and across American ethnic groups. Variability is seen to be related to sociodemographic concepts such as race/ethnicity, rural/urban residence, socioeconomic class, and the like. In this portion of the course I explicitly argue against what I perceive to be a widespread and dangerous set of beliefs in both nursing and medicine: i.e., that providing culturally sensitive care merely involves attending to a person's race — or, in current nursing terminology, "ethnic people of color" (Branch and Paxton 1976). These ideas are useful in sensitizing health practitioners to the fact that minority groups have special problems in the health care system. However, frequently the key factor examined is skin color; e.g., how to assess cyanosis among dark skinned people and that blacks live in extended families. In my view, this approach (a) obscures the very different meanings of race (a biological concept) and ethnicity (a cultural concept) and (b) inappropriately reinforces a biological, and potentially stereotypic, view of minority groups in American society.

Linking sociodemographic factors as sources of variability with cross-cultural patterns of health beliefs and practices provides a model of both similarities and differences in health related behaviors across populations (see Harwood 1981). For example, humoral pathology (Logan 1977) is presented as a major type of illness belief system with related health and illness practices. Cultural diversity wihin the type is related to the cultural contexts in which the system occurs: Chinese medicine, Hispanic medical beliefs, American folk medical beliefs, and the like. Students are thus exposed to world wide variability in a single type of system, allowing conceptualization of medical beliefs in their cultural contexts. In addition, similarities of belief cross-culturally are reinforced. Other belief complexes such as those related to magic, witchcraft, and sorcery, the germ theory, and spirit caused illness are also considered in a cross-cultural perspective.

Sociodemographic factors are discussed as they cross-cut health belief systems. For example, students learn that although Chinese medical beliefs are maintained among American Chinese, the degree of their importance to individuals and families is strongly influenced by occupation, education, and income (socioeconomic class), migration recency, residence, and social network, for example. I also teach the need to discover for particular individuals and groups which of the complex of Chinese beliefs have been maintained or rejected. The concept of *dual use* (Press 1969) is well demonstrated with ethnographic examples from Chinese-American populations (e.g., Gaw 1975). Emphasizing intra-group variability as well as inter-group variability and linking both to sociodemographic factors allows students to recognize the importance and interactions of both cultural and social variables in relation to health beliefs and practices. Among lower class and/or minority groups, maintenance of non-orthodox beliefs can be seen to be related to sociocultural features such as discrimination, variations in world view, and insular social networks rather than to the more simplistic basis of skin color.

Thus, the approach is grounded in theories of culture and society and not the reductionistic notion of color. Cultural and social factors are learned as they apply to all people's behavior and not just those of ethnic minority groups. In addition, attention is given to variation in health-related behaviors attributable to the contrast between "behavioral" and "ideological" ethnicity (Harwood 1981: 4).

This cross-cultural theoretical perspective provides the underpinnings of a culturally sensitive approach to nursing care. Patients' health beliefs and practices and their positions in society are discussed as the "sociocultural baggage" influencing their participation in nurse-client encounters. The translation of anthropological theory into clinical practice is keyed to the nursing process: assessment, plan, implementation, and evaluation. Through examples presented in lectures and a brief interviewing assignment, the students gain a rudimentary knowledge of how to ask questions that will elicit relevant socio-cultural data.

The anthropological conceptual framework is presented as the "cross-cultural nursing approach" and linked to the goal of being culturally sensitive in patient care. Students are taught that the traditional nursing approach tends to obscure culturally relevant facts and that an accurate assessment must include patient meanings and social characteristics. Students are encouraged to include cultural data in their plans for nursing care. For example, one student included a note in the chart on her Filipino patient's worry that the blood received in a transfusion would modify her personality or health. (She did not chart the woman's witchcraft belief concerning the etiology of her renal failure.) An extremely valuable teaching strategy has been the practice of using a cross-cultural graduate student as a teaching assistant. The T.A. spends time with students in their hospital based medical-surgical nursing course. In this way, we attempt to promote the idea that a culturally sensitive approach is necessary for all patients, not just those who are ethnic minorities.

During the final three or four weeks of the quarter, when students have become more comfortable with the many concepts they have been exposed to and with their practice skills in the hospital, they frequently share examples of folk health beliefs possessed by their patients and stories of culturally insensitive care they have observed. The folk belief examples are exciting for they demonstrate to the class that all that has gone before is not idle esoterica; people really do suffer because of God's will (Snow 1974); hot-cold imbalances really are included in people's explanatory models (Clark 1970). The insensitive care examples are disturbing because they expose the students' lack of power to do much about the cultural injustices of hospital care — though we always discuss ways of negotiating with other staff — and because students begin to see the enormity of the changes that will be necessary to promote culturally sensitive nursing care.

On these occasions, I discuss one of the "success" stories that are (or should be) included in the repertoires of all clinically applied anthropologists. One Sunday, a student called from the intensive care unit of the most conservative hospital in town. An extremely sick Gypsy woman was in the ICU totally disrupting their afternoon: she cursed; refused bath, medications, and intravenous fluids; she threw her infected sputum at any and all who entered the room; and all clinical indicators were at dangerously low levels. In addition, the doors were locked on the unit; there were two security guards in the hall; and the whole clan of Gypsies was camping downstairs in the waiting room. Not suprisingly, she asked if I had any suggestions. I asked what the patient was upset about. She said that the Gypsy woman was upset that hospital rules forbad her family being with her. (Hospital personnel believe, because of the storehouse of gypsy stories, that Gypsies congregate in the room in large numbers, disturb other patients, and steal equipment.) I suggested that the student attempt to negotiate with other staff so that two family members at a time be allowed to visit. Further, I explained that family ties are strong and sacred for Gypsies and this woman was at supernatural risk in her isolation. The next week in class, the student reported that the plan had worked, that the woman was getting better, and that the family was comfortable with the arrangement. Recently, I heard from a nurse at the hospital that a similar plan was instituted with repeated success.

Undergraduate student response to this class is mixed; although a majority enjoy it simply as a break from their primary commitment in medical-surgical nursing. Those students who are older, who have had more life experiences, or who were health practitioners prior to returning to college seem to perceive value in the ideas presented. They recognize the utility of being able to conceptualize patients' needs in the patients' own terms. Nurses returning for B.S. degrees, who work concurrently with the class, tell me that they use the approach in patient care and find it productive. However, a majority of the basic undergraduate students remain unconvinced of the usefulness of a cross-cultural approach. For them it appears peripheral to their real concerns. Later in their program of study, in the clinically oriented psychosocial nursing and community health nursing courses, the analytic concepts and the approach begin to take on more meaning. In part, this is due to growth in student abilities to understand and use abstract concepts; in part, it is due to greater relevance of a cross-cultural approach in the out-patient and community settings in which they work in these courses.

Even though the conflict in conceptual approaches makes it difficult to teach an anthropological perspective, it is worth the effort. By graduation, most students have begun the process of expanding their abilities to conceptualize human behavior and to integrate this knowledge into their own styles of nursing practice. Each quarter, a few seniors tell me that they have used the concepts in patient care and believe they are better prepared to provide more humanistic and culturally sensitive care. The personnel officer in one hospital told me that graduates of this program frequently mention the importance of culture-sensitive care in employment interviews and refer to the cultural variations course as influential in their philosophy.

GRADUATE STUDIES

The Graduate Program in Cross-Cultural Nursing at the University of Washington School of Nursing accepted its first graduate students in September, 1974. The program was built on almost a decade of preparatory work, beginning with a program that included the presence of an anthropologist as professor for, and consultant to nurses who were working for doctoral degrees in the Department of Anthropology. In 1969, Madeleine Leininger, a nurse-anthropologist, became Dean. Between 1969 and 1973, other anthropologists were hired and the ground work for a graduate program was put in place. In 1973, when I arrived, there were three anthropology and nursing courses: a seminar for the nurses working on anthropology doctorates (also taken by other graduate students), Leininger's specialty course on Transcultural Nursing, and an undergraduate child rearing course.

Final planning of, and later teaching in, the program was done by Elizabeth Byerly and me, in conjunction with the other anthropologists. We conceived of an overall plan containing three components: (1) a sequence of three seminars in which aspects of the anthropology of health as related to nursing would be taught, leading to a field experience in Summer Quarter. (2) A wide range of anthropology courses was recommended to provide breadth to student knowledge and to enable students to gain a sense of the major thrusts of anthropology as a discipline. (3) Students would be encouraged to do the research on which the Masters thesis is based on a sociocultural topic and among a population similar to the one served during the field experience.

The first program element — the seminars — was built on two existing seminars, the anthropology doctorate course and Transcultural Nursing, given in Fall and Winter. The other seminar, the field practicum, and a special topics course to be used as we needed it had to be written and shepherded through Departmental, School, and University curriculum committees. Engaging in this process introduced me to one of the stable features of curriculum development in nursing: course proposals must contain behavioral objectives, carefully written to reflect achievement of "graduate" levels of knowledge. (Howard Stein refers to this feature in medical education in his contribution to this volume.) Luckily we had a curriculum consultant available from whom we could learn by participant-observation.

Writing course descriptions (the only element of the process with which I was familiar from previous experience in an academic department), course outlines, and behavioral objectives was only the beginning of a long process of gaining approval for the courses and the program. Once the courses were written, I visited either department faculties (in Psychosocial Nursing and in Anthropology) or department heads (other nursing departments and Health Services in the School of Public Health) to obtain their suggestions for and concerns about the courses, and their agreement that the courses would not negatively impact their programs. Though tedious, this was a useful process because I learned about the interests of other programs in the University and they learned that I was willing to consult and was genuinely open to suggestions. The last step prior to approval by the University level curriculum board was a meeting with the School of Nursing curriculum committee. Experience gained in prior meetings was helpful in answering the questions posed in this body: e.g., why is anthropology important to nursing? What clinical experiences will students have and how do they relate to seminars? What is the knowledge to be examined and how does it contribute to better nursing care? I concluded that enthusiasm, confidence, and knowledge of what nursing educators considered important were as important as the substance of the courses. Like students, the professors needed to know that anthropology was not a threat to existing practice.

The basic structure of the program has remained largely unchanged during the eight years of its existence. The Transcultural Nursing seminar has been shelved temporarily to enable students to have an opportunity for more theory and practice in community health, the usual clinical specialty of cross-cultural graduate students. What has changed is my understanding of how the program works. Through working intensively with students, both the content of the classes and the ways material is presented have become more anthropology *in* nursing than anthropology *and* nursing. This change in content and presentation has been the result of an increase in my understanding of nursing, its theoretical bases and clinical practice. This ability to "talk the language" of the professionals being taught is critical.

Changes in how I teach the first seminar provide an example of this shift in thought. The first year, I taught introductory anthropological concepts using ethnographic data from around the world and some information about American ethnic groups. As frequently as I could (which was not often), I would suggest ways of applying this information, drawing mostly on my background in Public Health. In addition, many class discussions of application failed since none of us could stretch our minds enough to accomplish the task. Although student evaluations indicated that they enjoyed the class and liked anthropology, they were unanimous in saying that the class was irrelevant to nursing. (I might add that undergraduates reacted the same way the previous year when I taught an elective for them.) Slowly, through carefully listening to colleagues and students, I learned to understand what problems nurses face and were interested in solving. Through analyzing how nurses understood these problems in health care and by picking out their blind spots related to a lack of sociocultural knowledge, I began to teach how to fill in the blind spots. Thus, anthropology *in* nursing: the different viewpoint of anthropology fills in the blind spots.

For example, nurses and other health practitioners believe that patients should react "rationally" — where rationality consists of conforming to the practitioner's common sense reality. They also recognize that cultural factors can contribute to "irrational" behavior, but they do not have the conceptual tools to discover culture bound rationality — their own or their patients' — and thus become uncomfortable because of lack of knowledge. In one case discussed in class, a student said she was working with a "hysterical" woman about to give birth. The hysteria label derived from the woman's statement that a miracle had occurred through prayer — God told her that her birth canal had widened and a caesarean section would be unnecessary. The student already knew the importance of non-judgmental listening — taught with the concept of cultural relativism — but was seriously concerned that the woman was at risk for psychological (or spiritual) trauma when the expected vaginal birth did not occur. I suggested that the nurse request a new measurement, reasoning that even if it had not changed, the act would show the patient that her view was taken seriously. In this case, the woman was able to have a vaginal delivery.

In cases like this, the blind spot lies in the practitioner's certain knowledge that the biomedical construction of reality is the only possible one and that alternatives — no matter how non-judgmental the listener is — are not valid. On other occasions, patients' beliefs cannot be so easily correlated with biomedical reality and the nurse needs to know what to do then. The essence of what to do, as Katon and Kleinman (1981) point out, is to negotiate, accepting as many of the patient's beliefs as possible. Knowing that "irrational" beliefs can be understood on their own terms, that they are not all necessarily pathological, and that the nurse can work *within* the client's belief system rather than attacking it from the outside, reduces the discomfort health practitioners experience.

About five students are admitted to the program each year. They arrive with heterogeneous backgrounds, but share the innovative, and risky, interest in attempting to improve clinical practice and patient care through attention to people's cultural backgrounds. The number of years of nursing experience prior to entry has ranged from one to more than twenty. Two-thirds had had experience in intercultural settings, either within the U.S. or abroad. Most had worked in community health, but some had worked exclusively in hospitals.

In broad strokes, the core curriculum in the cross-cultural nursing program is organized around a sequence of objectives: (1) to be able to conceptualize social and cultural factors related to health concerns and how these factors influence health and illness behavior; (2) to conceptualize caring and nursing care cross-culturally using the literature in transcultural nursing; (3) to conceptualize the community as the context of people's health promoting, maintaining, and restoring activities, using ethnographic and theoretical literature on the community; (4) to use selected portions of this conceptual knowledge while practicing as a nurse in a community agency in order to begin the process of creating a clinical style based on a cross-cultural nursing approach.

The initial seminar, in which the first objective is addressed, is a critical socializing experience for the graduate students. The new conceptual framework is introduced both as an essential element in nursing practice and as a field of study with an intrinsic value. Students tend to be excited as they discover the literature that makes sense out of the previously inexplicable health practices such as talcum powder poultices for dehydration (fallen fontanelle) or magical object manipulations for infant viral infections. This excitement promotes the motivation necessary for the task of learning the numerous and complex models for understanding health related behaviors. Strong motivation is required not only because of the conceptual complexity, but also because previous learning was keyed to the use of one model rather than several. Once students begin to learn that conceptual approaches serve to facilitate their thinking in flexible, and culturally relativistic ways, the process becomes more enjoyable.

This course is organized to introduce anthropology as a field of study, then to examine the anthropology of health and illness in detail. The introductory portion shows the great variety of ways anthropologists attempt to understand social and cultural patterns. Using Beals, *Culture in Process* (1973) and the first half of Goodenough, *Cooperation in Change* (1963), we examine the nature of anthropological field work and the comparative method. Central concepts such as society, culture, value, belief, status and role, and the like are introduced, discussed, and related to nursing practice. The primary outcome of this part of the course should be two areas of student knowledge: the importance of cultural relativism in anthropology, and familiarity with the terminology and conceptual underpinnings that anthropologists use to understand cultural variation in common patterns of human behavior.

The second portion of the course is introduced with a discussion of the social science literature on health behavior, illness behavior, and sick role behavior (e.g., Becker 1974; Kasl and Cobb 1966; Mechanic 1978). This provides students with sociological and social psychological approaches to the study of sickness. This comparison of analytic concepts provides background against which students may evaluate anthropology's similarities and differences in approach with other behavioral sciences. The most significant concept in this literature for the students is the Health Belief Model (Becker 1974). Because the model is concerned with both illness and health, the nurses' traditional interest in and experience with health is reinforced and their perspectives expanded.

The remainder of the course is organized around the central conceptual elements of the health seeking process: symptom definition, role shift, lay consultation and referral, treatment action, and adherence (Chrisman 1977). Using this construct that was designed to facilitate a comparative view of illness episodes cross-culturally, the students have an overall scheme to aid in organizing the anthropological data and theory made available in the seminar. Weekly seminar meetings are devoted to each element in turn with three principal considerations to be discussed: (1) what is the breadth of the literature; what are the strengths and weaknesses; (2) what is the content discussed and how is this related to understanding illness episodes as they occur in a sociocultural context; and (3) how does this knowledge aid in better patient care. The symptom definition element, for example, provides the occasion on which folk and popular culture beliefs are examined and related to the sickness experiences of various ethnic groups. Network analysis and the mobilization of family and friends for support during illness are discussed during the seminar on lay consultation and referral.

One of the most important learning experiences in the course is the requirement that interviews be conducted and the data analyzed using concepts from the course. Interviews are assigned at three points through the quarter so the students will be able to recognize (a) that their expertise in conducting interviews grows along with their depth of theoretical knowledge and (b) that their conceptual understanding of what a person reports about being sick expands significantly. A core element in the two later interviews is the concept of explanatory model elaborated by Kleinman (1980) and his colleagues (Kleinman, Eisenberg, and Good 1978). This notion is related to the broader concept of clinical reality and the authors provide a list of questions that can be used by clinicians to elicit cultural understandings of illness from patients. Cross-cultural nursing graduate students have enthusiastically adopted the explanatory model approach in large measure because it systematizes and provides a theoretical rationale for what they had learned to do by experience. The interview assignments with analysis based on comparative anthropological concepts act to further combine experience with theory.

By the end of this course, the cross-cultural students have begun to perceive the value of anthropological concepts for nursing practice and to synthesize anthropology and nursing to achieve their goals in research and clinical practice. It is the foundation for their later educational experiences. On the other hand, graduate students from other nursing interest areas seem to achieve these beginnings to a lesser degree. This may be due to the fact that the course is an elective for them and not seen as central to their future careers. Concepts such as explanatory model and theoretical approaches such as the Health Belief Model are remembered and might be partially integrated with later thesis research. But the logic of integrating anthropology with nursing is usually not fully recognized. The conceptual framework for future advanced practice is, quite reasonably, expected to derive from core courses in their own interest areas. What this suggests is that regardless of the format used to introduce anthropological concepts, learner motivations are likely to be paramount.

In the second quarter of the cross-cultural nursing program, the basic under-standings generated earlier are reinforced, both in theory and in practice, and expanded with new content. Reinforcement in clinical practice occurs as the students carry small caseloads in community health agencies. This a time to test whether the theoretical perspectives aid in understanding their clients' goals more fully. Those working with members of ethnic minorities are able to observe some of the culture-specific patterns they had read about.

Reinforcement and expansion in the theoretical area occurs through considera-tion of the literature in transcultural nursing, primarily the work of Madeleine Leininger and other nurse-anthropologists. This literature varies the focus of cross-cultural health and illness behaviors toward the concept of caring as developed in nursing science. In this endeavor, the students examine the variation in the ways caring is carried out in a number of settings around the world. In addition, they are introduced to Leininger's theoretical perspective which differentiates nursing care into its components such as nurturance and succorance (Leininger 1978). These concepts are related to each other and to health care systems in an attempt to provide a better understanding of how nursing functions vary cross-culturally. Finally, using the experience of seminar participants and guest speakers, the students consider the roles of Western nurses who work in international settings.

The final theory seminar in the sequence is devoted in large measure to the concept of community and to strategies of instituting change in community settings. Again, the focus is upon multiple theoretical perspectives as they illuminate the many facets of community life. Much of the content is based in applied anthro-pology (Goodenough 1963). Various approaches to planned change in health and illness practices are considered and strategies discussed. The seminar concludes with speakers from community clinics in Seattle. The focus of these sessions is on the economics and politics of sustaining the community clinics so that students will have a knowledge base in health delivery that goes beyond the rather idealistic perspectives of traditional anthropology.

The culminating experience in the formal educational sequence (exclusvie of independent research) is a field practicum in Summer Quarter. Students are required to negotiate their own field placements, in part as an exercise in presenting themselves in their new roles as cross-cultural nurses. Field placements tend to be in the inner city clinics of Seattle including the Seattle Indian Clinic, the International District Community Health Center (Asian), Sea-Mar Clinic (Chicano), The Pike Market Clinic (downtown elderly), Pioneer Square Health Station (skid road), and a number of clinics serving low income, and largely Black, populations. In addition, students have chosen clinics on Indian Reservations and those serving rural migrant farm workers. One group worked in Monterray, Mexico in a small hospital serving the children of a squatter settlement.

The field experience is an opportunity to test the application of theoretical perspectives derived from nursing and anthropology in demanding but relevant practice settings. For example, three students have worked in the International District Community Health Center in Seattle's Chinatown. One of the tasks for all three (during different summers) was to help the clinic nursing staff and language translators prepare educational pamphlets for their clientele in areas such as nutrition, child birth and child rearing, and high blood pressure. In addition, they have helped in outreach case identification programs, blood pressure screening, and in clinic nursing. One of the students who worked in the Seattle Indian Health Board Clinic collaborated with a staff nurse to institute a foot care clinic for the elders who participated in a breakfast program. Another worked with the woman's health care specialist on family planning counseling. In these and other similar cases, the cross-cultural graduate students attempted to sensitize staff to cultural needs of clients that had not been attended to previously, to plan programs with staff, and to help in delivering the care.

A weekly seminar is conducted so that students exchange accounts of their experiences in order to assess similarities and differences. At least half of these seminars are devoted to examining difficulties in establishing a personally satisfying role in the clinic. Community colleagues and supervisors tend to be skeptical of student claims about their newly developed skills, emphasizing instead their need for additional help in the clinic. In most cases, however, clinic co-workers begin to recognize the unique contribution of the cross-cultural students to the operation of the clinic. Frequently, new and much more client centered programs or approaches to patient care are developed by the students and welcomed by the staff. Recognition of student conceptual abilities and knowledge of the literature leads to requests for formal inservice education from the cross-cultural nurses.

One of the most important outcomes of the field practicum for the students is the emergence of a sense that they now approach care in a qualitatively different fashion. Problems in failed appointments or lack of compliance are approached using a socioculturally informed understanding of the clients. Students report that client behaviors that had baffled staff previously can be placed in the context of client life styles and then understood by the staff. Participation in the seminar and the required practice of taking anthropological field notes throughout the summer provide the mechanism whereby students are able to judge the changes in themselves resulting from insights based on new conceptualizations of nursing practice.

An important generalization that has emerged from these summer experiences is that the clinic nurses who share an ethnic identity with their clients frequently do not differ significantly from their non-minority colleagues in the provision of culturally sensitive nursing care. In part, this is a consequence of the strongly biomedical orientation of the clinics that results from having physicians or health administrators in leadership positions and from the nature of funding; i.e., much of the support for these clinics derives from federal or state programs that are disease-specific. Another, and equally important, reason for the practice similarities of minority and non-minority nurses is the strength of the biomedical conceptual framework in nursing schools. My first introduction to this phenomenon occurred in 1975 when I gave a guest lecture on poverty, culture, and patient care to a seminar in parent-child nursing. Although I was using Chicano examples that day, showing the importance of attending to folk beliefs and the lack of monetary resources, the ideas were well received by a Native American nurse. She thanked me for reminding her of the importance of native health practices for her people, saying that she had not integrated these into her nursing practice at all. She had learned to know that what was "true" about health and sickness was the knowledge accumulated in scientific nursing and medicine.

Interestingly, students who have completed the program to this point are still not fully convinced that their new skills will be accepted in the job market. In part, this is due to the subtlety of their approach. In comparison to graduate students who will be cardiac or cancer specialists, the cross-cultural student cannot point to radically new technical skills; only to radically new ways of thought – still not fully accepted in the world of nursing. Moreover, few explicit career opportunities – such as an advertisement for a cross-cultural nurse – appear on bulletin boards in the school. On the other hand, when they have taken a regular nursing position, they find that their insight into client lifestyles is valued highly by their colleagues. An experience – not shared by all – that significantly aids in the process of accepting the identity of cross-cultural nurse is attendance at the annual Transcultural Nursing Conferences. At these gatherings, the students discover that others throughout the country actually do share their interests and excitement about providing culturally sensitive nursing care and conducting research on the social and cultural factors that influence health related behaviors.

Graduates of the Masters program in cross-cultural nursing are enthusiastic about their new approach to patient care and new understanding of nursing. In contrast with the undergraduates, the graduate students enter the program with a solid background in nursing. Moreover, they have frequently chosen the program because of frustrations experienced in taking care of patients whose cultural backgrounds contrasted with their own. These experiential qualities lead them to desire a new approach and to more easily recognize its value. A second quality that they share is a personal, temporal, and financial investment in making the program work for them as contributing members of the profession of nursing. These two qualities of experience and investment are strong motivating forces that underlie adoption of an anthropological perspective within nursing. Moreover, this motivation and confidence in their conceptual and clinical abilities underlie the risk taking in clinical settings when the graduates actively promote the anthropological perspective as beneficial and necessary to patient care.

DOCTORAL STUDENTS

Flexibility in approach to meet the various needs of different types of students is central to making anthropology "work" in nursing. Doctoral students require a fundamentally different style than do the undergraduate and Masters level graduate students in nursing. At these latter educational levels, the key is "translation" of concepts and methodology to meet the needs of people whose careers will be primarily as clinicians — either in practice or as teachers. In contrast, with doctoral students it is important to maintain the disciplinary integrity of anthropology, so that variations in the logic of discourse across disciplines can be made salient.

I work with nurses who are predoctoral students in the Department of Anthropology and in the School of Nursing. My association with the anthropology graduate students (who include non-nurses as well) arises, in part, from the fact that the Anthropology Department at the University of Washington does not have a formal medical anthropology program (a source of constant debate, but a program seems to be developing). Thus, the other medical anthropologists in the University and I (none of whom has a primary appointment in anthropology) become significantly involved in the education of anthropologists. Interestingly, I advise and teach anthropology students differently than the way I work with the graduate students in nursing. With exception that I am willing to consider non-traditional topics of research (American samples, social and health issues, and the like) I prefer a strong traditional (e.g., kinship, politics, religion) orientation among anthropology graduate students. My belief is that regardless of the fact that these students are nurses and may well teach later in nursing schools, their preparation must be fully anthropological. Only with such preparation can they contribute *as anthropologists* to nursing education. Anything less serves neither discipline well.

This approach, replicated in every other anthropology department that I know of, produces a "reentry" problem for the nurse-anthropologist who returns to nursing to work. That is, they feel a sense of "distance" from nursing resulting from immersion in anthropology that is similar to what is felt by non-clinician anthropologists in health science schools. Although their reentry is facilitated by their earlier experiences in the subculture of nursing, my impression is that they maintain some degree of distance and thus continue to be capable of providing an alternative perspective for colleagues and students.

With predoctoral students in nursing, I explicitly take the position that anthropology is a discipline, separate from and related to nursing, that potentially can contribute much to their own development in nursing science. This position requires that the initial question or focus of seminar or personal discussion derive from issues within nursing as a discipline. For example, one core seminar considering the ways families interact in and with society and the health outcomes of these interactions invited me to review some of the behavioral science literature on health care system utilization as it is influenced by family and other sociocultural variables. I also advise students about profitable anthropology courses to take as part of curricular requirements for preparation in cognate fields. In such cases courses are chosen on the basis of the extent to which the content of courses augments knowledge, but not necessarily the conceptual framework, needed in nursing.

PROBLEMS

I have found that the most pervasive problem I face in the school of nursing is the discomfort of being an outsider *and* of running a "deviant" (I usually prefer to say "innovative") graduate program. This discomfort was strikingly called to my attention about twice a year when a colleague would wonder whether the rumor was true that the cross-cultural program had been cancelled! Happily that has not happened again for two or three years, but the underlying issue continues, particularly in these days of diminishing funding levels in higher education. One important attempt at reducing the vulnerability of the cross-cultural program has been to integrate it with other specialty areas in advanced community health nursing. This has been beneficial in that the program looks less deviant now and the students are receiving more extensive educational experiences in a traditional focus of nursing practice. There have also been costs: one seminar has been temporarily dropped, reducing the intensity of the curriculum as originally conceived; the students have a more complex set of course requirements than previously.

Personal feelings of being an outsider have now reduced to such an extent that I frequently must consciously remember that I am not a nurse. My involvement on the curriculum committees for both the undergraduate and Masters level programs increased my knowledge of how the educational process works in the school. In fact I have authored sections of reports and planning documents in these areas. I am also heavily involved in the continuing development of the doctoral program as my department's representative to the governing body.

I view these, and other, commitments as essential elements in the process of promoting an anthropological perspective: (1) I have been able to teach the faculty what I teach and to show them how it fits with other curricular elements in an integral fashion rather than deviant fashion. (I have also given workshops on content for faculty members to accomplish the same end.) (2) Through inclusion in this important communication network, I have learned about student interests and cocerns and have had the opportunity to discuss these in class. (3) I have been able to defend the undergraduate course and the Masters program when questions of their validity or importance arose.

The costs of consistent committee participation are extremely high because of the time commitment. Nursing schools seem to be overcommitteed anyway, and two other processes exacerbate the problem. One of these is the concern with explicating and writing the rationale – philosophy, mission, goals, objectives – for nearly every activity of the school. Once written, such documents must then be subjected to a long editing and approval procedure. In this lies the second problem: my colleagues seem to believe that nearly complete (preferably unanimous) consensus must exist around every decision. For example, a faculty decision that was passed by only 3 votes was not implemented until more of a consensus was reached.

Another problem relates to the prevalent themes in the "research culture" of the school. Most of the faculty have Ph.D. degrees in the behavioral sciences and thus the natural science bias found in schools of medicine is not as strong. However, there is the belief that research should be conducted in which there are large samples, quantifiable variables, and sophisticated statistical analyses. Although I have benefitted greatly from the intensive exposure to this type of perspective, I continue to be frustrated that there is so little commitment to understanding the value of descriptive, qualitative, ethnographic research. One colleague asked me to clarify the differences between anthropology and "scientific" research, with quantifiable elements. One consequence of these beliefs about research is a reluctance, sometimes antipathy, on the part of graduate students to believe that they could ever carry out a research project. The word "research" seems to carry with it the connotations of "difficult, if not impossible, to do" or "drudgery and certainly never fun". One of my thesis advisees expressed her amazement in the acknowledgement of her thesis that I had made research fun.

A final problem to mention concerns the nature and level of discourse, both in seminars and among colleagues. A self-critical and disciplined discussion of issues is common and expected in anthropology and other disciplines, but nearly foreign to the health science professions. For health professionals, "philosophical" discussions about the logic and assumptions embedded in thought are consistent with neither the action orientation that is so prevalent, nor the strong pressure to adhere closely to accepted standards of practice. Professional style and demeanor are simply different.

Scholarly debate, therefore, is not usually expected and frequently is seen as a personal threat. For example, I remember a meeting concerning a curricular issue in which a colleague (with doctoral preparation in sociology) and I engaged in a heated, and very enjoyable, debate over concepts. Some of the majority of clinically prepared faculty at the meeting spoke to me privately later to express their sympathy with me about the "ordeal" I had undergone. In order to partially counter the negative image of debate and to expose students to the existence of legitimate differences of opinion about research perspectives, one sociologist and I regularly argue the advantages and disadvantages of quantitative and qualitative research methods. Happily, the University of Washington School of Nursing, like the schools in other major universities, includes a large (and growing) proportion of faculty with Ph.D. Degrees – mostly in the behavioral sciences. As a consequence of this, the level of discourse has been rising over the years. Frustration continues, however, when conceptual issues are ignored in favor of personal anecdotes about nursing practice.

CONCLUSION

Anthropology does share a great deal with nursing – the practice and the discipline. In part, this is demonstrated by the presence of at least one anthropologist (and now six) in the school for nearly two decades. The health promoting and maintaining interests of nurses fit better with anthropology than the curative orientation of physicians. This should, and does, make life a little easier. Anthropology still seems deviant though: our research methodologies are "soft" and are a source of concern to the other social scientists on the staff. Recognition of the importance of cultural patterns – of both patients and nurses – has been slow to emerge, is unequally distributed across the country, and may only be focused on minority groups or skin color. A biomedical conceptual framework is prevalent and persuasive. Finally, I think anthropology makes life uncomfortable by challenging existing assumptions about practice; and because our approach is personal and holistic, like that of nursing, perhaps we sometimes hit close to home.

The foundation of my integration of anthropology with nursing is an analogue of participant-observation. I have participated fully in the life of the school, but frequently try to step back to comment as an outside observer. In curriculum development and teaching, I have tried to make anthropological perspectives, methods, and data be part of nursing — an elaboration, expansion, improvement of what is; but anthropological insight based on a strong scientific and humanistic tradition is also presented for self criticism and change.

The experience has been frustrating and challenging — and rewarding. From students and colleagues I have learned about nursing. In trying to meet their anthropological needs, I have also learned more about anthropology. The most excitement, however, has been generated at a more encompassing level: across the university in nursing, anthropology, public health, psychiatry, and family medicine; and in activities involving patient care, teaching and research. The excitement lies in synthesizing a clinically applied anthropology from such diversity.

ACKNOWLEDGEMENT

This is a substantially revised version of a paper given at the Sixth Annual Transcultural Nursing Conference, September, 1979. For their substantive and editoral comments, I would like to thank Madeleine Leininger, JoAnn Glittenberg, Arthur Kleinman, and Maxine Binn.

BIBLIOGRAPHY

Arensberg, Conrad and Arthur Niehoff
    1964 Introducing Social Change. Chicago: Aldine.
Bauwens, Eleanor E. (ed.)
    1978 The Anthropology of Health. St. Louis: C. V. Mosby Co.
Beals, Alan R.
    1973 Culture in Process, Second Edition. New York: Holt, Rinehart and Winston.
Becker, Marshall H. (ed.)
    1974 The Health Belief Model and Personal Health Behavior. Thorofore, New Jersey: Charles B. Slack, Inc.
Branch, Marie F. and Phyllis P. Paxton
    1976 Providing Safe Nursing Care for Ethnic People of Color. New York: Appleton-Century-Crofts.
Brink, Pamela J. (ed.)
    1976 Introduction. In Transcultural Nursing: A Book of Readings. Englewood Cliffs, New Jersey: Prentice Hall.
Carnevali, Doris and Maxine Patrick
    1979 Nursing Management for the Elderly. Philadelphia: J. B. Lippincott.

Chrisman, Noel J.
  1977 The Health Seeking Process: An Approach to the Natural History of Illness. Culture, Medicine, and Psychiatry 1: 4: 351–377.
Clark, Margaret
  1970 Health in the Mexican American Culture. Berkeley: University of California Press.
Donaldson, Sue K. and D. Crowley
  1978 The Discipline of Nursing. Nursing Outlook 26: 113.
Freidson, Eliot
  1970 Profession of Medicine. New York: Dodd, Mead.
Gaut, Dolores
  1979 An Application of the Kerr-Saltis Model to the Concept of Caring in Nursing Education. Unpublished Ph.D. dissertation, University of Washington.
Gaw, Albert C.
  1975 An Integrated Approach in the Delivery of Health Care to a Chinese Community in America: The Boston Experience. In A. Kleinman, et al. (eds.), Medicine in Chinese Cultures. Washington, D.C.: Fogarty International Center. DHEW (NIH) Publication #75–653.
Goodenough, Ward
  1963 Cooperation in Change. New York: Russell Sage Foundation.
Harwood, Alan
  1981 Introduction. In A. Harwood (ed.), Ethnicity and Medical Care. Cambridge: Harvard University Press.
Kasl, S. U. and S. Cobb
  1966 Health Behavior, Illness Behavior, and Sick Role Behavior. Archives of Environmental Health 12: 246–266.
Katon, Wayne and Arthur Kleinman
  1981 Doctor-Patient Negotiation and Other Social Science Strategies in Patient Care. In L. Eisenberg and A. Kleinman (eds.), The Relevance of Social Science for Medicine. Dordrecht, Holland: D. Reidel, pp. 253–282.
Kleinman, Arthur
  1980 Patients and Healers in the Context of Culture. Berkeley: University of California Press.
Kleinman, Arthur, Leon Eisenberg, Byron Good
  1978 Culture, Illness, and Care. Annals of Internal Medicine, 88: 251–258.
Leininger, Madeleine
  1970 Nursing and Anthropology: Two Worlds to Blend. New York: John Wiley and Sons, Inc. Chapter 5.
  1978 Transcultural Nursing: Concepts, Theories, and Practices. New York: John Wiley and Sons, Inc. Chapter 3.
  1980a Caring: A Central Focus of Nursing and Health Care Services. The Ohio State University Distinguished Professorship Lecture.
Leininger, Madeleine (ed.)
  1980b Caring: A Human Helping Process. Proceedings of the Three National Caring Conferences.
Logan, Michael H.
  1977 Anthropological Research on the Hot-Cold Theory of Disease: Some Methodological Suggestions. Medical Anthropology, 1:4.
Mechanic, David
  1978 Medical Sociology, Second Edition. New York: Free Press.
Moore, Lorna G., et al.
  1980 The Biocultural Basis of Health. St. Louis: C. V. Mosby Co.
Olesen, Virginia and Elvi Whittaker
  1968 The Silent Dialogue. San Francisco: Jossey-Bass.
Orem, Dorothea
  1980 Nursing: Concepts of Practice (Second Edition). New York: McGraw Hill.

Peplau, Hildegard
    1969 Professional Closeness. Nursing Forum 8: 4: 342–360.
Press, Irwin
    1969 Urban Illness: Physicians, Curers, and Dual Use in Bogota. Journal of Health and
          Social Behavior 10: 209–218.
Rogers, Martha
    1979 Theoretical Basis for Nursing. Philadelphia: F. Davis.
Roy, Sr. Calista
    1976 Introduction to Nursing: An Adaptation Model. New Jersey: Prentice Hall.
Snow, Loudell
    1974 Folk Medical Beliefs and Their Implications for Care of Patients. Annals of Internal
          Medicine 81: 82–96.

CHERYL RITENBAUGH

NEW APPROACHES TO OLD PROBLEMS: INTERACTIONS OF CULTURE AND NUTRITION

INTRODUCTION

Teaching anthropology outside the confines of anthropology departments presents a challenge in translation. The perspectives of anthropology must be couched in terms relevant to the new audience. Fortunately, the relevance of anthropology to the understanding of human diets and eating behavior is not difficult to illustrate. Eating is a perfect example of the biocultural interface: culture conditions the range of choices, but there is biological feedback regarding the long-term suitability of any particular set of choices. For the individual, suitability is measured in terms of adequate growth, health, and reproductive competence; for the population, the measures are demographic stability and persistence through time.

The following pages describe a course developed originally at Michigan State University within the departments of Anthropology and Nutrition and Food Science. The first section of the chapter defines the audience for the course, and the course goals. It covers the basic instructional model, and a discussion of the theoretical aspects of anthropology found to be relevant to the audience. The second section of the chapter provides an in depth illustration of the anthropological approach to a nutrition problem developed in much the same way as for the class. It deals with the problem of obesity, provides source material on the topic, and demonstrates how the anthropological approach differs from those approaches routinely used by health care professionals.

I. THE COURSE

The course resulted from the combination of a "Food and Culture" class from a nutrition department and a "Nutritional Anthropology" class from an anthropology department into a jointly-taught "Interaction of Culture and Nutrition".[1] Both courses had been designed for seniors and beginning graduate students, and this educational level was maintained. It has been jointly listed and truly team-taught, with the physical anthropologist and community nutritionist sharing most lectures. In spite of this structure, the course has remained primarily one of translating and applying anthropological principles and analyses to food-related problems.

Students came from two quite distinct scientific subcultures: nutrition, one of the natural sciences, focusing heavily on molecular and cellular interactions; and anthropology, one of the social sciences, concerned with human and societal interactions. These contrasting backgrounds presented a series of challenges in teaching. First, the students had contrasting biases, growing out of the method

N. J. Chrisman and T. W. Maretzki (eds.), Clinically Applied Anthropology, 141–178.

and theory of each discipline, and out of the natures of the applied components. Second, the students often lacked basic data in the other field, presenting problems in designing a course which would truly be an integration. The following paragraphs will describe the students in more detail and present our solutions to this basic problem in course design.

Nutrition Students

The course was one of two options to fill a requirement in the dietetics program; thus the bulk of our students always came from nutrition. The background of a senior or beginning graduate student in nutrition generally focuses heavily on the natural sciences. It is likely to include, for example, math, physics, inorganic and organic chemistry, biochemistry, anatomy, and physiology. (Often, majors are required to take one or two classes in the social sciences, but these are usually the most basic freshman level courses and are taken in the junior or senior year, crammed in between the more "important" science courses.) Some students also take food courses, which focus on the chemical reactions involved in preparation, preservation, and so forth. Texture and color of food are understood in terms of chemical structure. Reference is made to what sensory attributes are most appealing, but such data are presented in a very limited context. The methods and theory of the nutrition learned by these students are thus overwhelmingly rooted in the deductive portion of the experimental method, providing (and selecting for) a rationalistic approach. Students tend to carry this approach with them into issues of human behavior.

Many nutrition students at the time the class began tended to view behaviors only in the context of their biological effects. Thus eating became, in this view, a way of maintaining adequate nutriture. Interestingly, most of these students admitted that their own eating patterns were not based on scientific principles; however, they thought that they probably should be. An extension of this ratio-nalist "culture of science" view of eating behavior assumes that any problems associated with eating "improperly" can be remedied through education: if people know what is the healthy behavior, they will follow it.

There is one other bias shared by students trained in nutrition programs in the United States. That is a tendency to have considerable knowledge of the nutrient composition of diets based on major American farm products (predominantly of western European derivation), but to have little idea of whether or how diets composed of very different foods can meet basic physiological requirements. We found, for example, that many of the students have learned about the Basic Four Food Groups so many times in their schooling that the students imagine the Basic Four to have been "engraved in stone". It did not occur to them that fully adequate diets can exist which do not follow this pattern very closely. In fact, they usually did not understand that the "Basic Four" used to be the "Basic Seven" (Ahlstrom and Rasanen 1973), and is only a nutrition education tool to help Americans choose a reasonable diet from the most abundant American foods. Other countries have devised other schemes to deal with local food issues.

The applied component of nutrition — dietetics — focuses predominantly on pathologies either caused by dietary imbalances or treated through dietary change. Because of this focus on the associations of diet and health, nutrition scientists and nutritionists are often somewhat cautious about general nutrition intervention. One common concern voiced is that the recommendations for change will be followed to an extreme by some individuals. Potentially deleterious, unforeseen consequences are also feared in the realm of individual physiologic idiosyncracy: recommendations correctly followed may for some individuals prove to be harmful. The focus is entirely on the individual and on biological issues.

Anthropology Students

Anthropology students entered the class with a very different set of assumptions and concerns. The subject matter of their education has been cultural systems, with an emphasis on variety and complexity. They have learned enormous amounts of detail regarding the rituals, beliefs, behaviors, and rules of cultures, and often come to see human behavior as hopelessly complex, and possibly beyond the power of any single individual to alter. They were less attuned to common biological needs of humans and more sensitive to the variety of alternative practices. Probably because of the self-selection that takes place both in studying social sciences and in choosing this course, our social science students often entered the class convinced that American diets are terrible, and that diets virtually anywhere else are more healthful ("natural and/or pure"). They were often quite unaware of the depth of knowledge in modern nutritional science.

By their last year in college, anthropology students have generally acquired another bias growing out of the nature of the discipline. Anthropology is, for the most part, a research field, with only a relatively small applied component. This emphasis on research encourages students to question and analyze, but to be reluctant to make recommendations (decisions) with "inadequate" information. And of course, in their opinion, the information available is always inadequate. The applied component of anthropology with which they are most familiar is that which evaluates why programs have failed. Such applied analyses (post-mortems) often emphasize the complexity of and interaction of cultural systems by showing the causal links between an intervention and apparently unrelated (and certainly unforeseen) negative consequence. Thus anthropology students are cautious about recommending intervention because they are certain that unforeseen (apparently unrelated) and deleterious consequences will follow at the cultural or societal level; other changes will occur in response to the recommended one which will be more problematic than the original situation. The assumption underlying most interventions is that the change agent is more knowledgeable than the local personnel; anthropologists tend to question this assumption, instead seeing the change agents and recipients as possessing different kinds of information. This leads anthropology students to perceive the desirability of establishing partnerships rather than super-ordinate-subordinate relationships.

The Problem of Prerequisites

Thus the entering students had quite different assumptions, and had fairly minimal or non-existent backgrounds in the other discipline. Since we did not want to require that all students complete introductory classes in both fields prior to taking the class, we designed a pair of prerequisite tests covering what we considered to be basic information in the two fields, approximately equivalent to what one might be expected to learn in an introductory class. (See Appendix.) Our philosophy regarding these tests is that we wanted all the students to have this basic information; we did not want their class grade affected by how quickly or slowly they learned it and we did not want to waste class time on remedial material. The following arrangements were accepted by the university curriculum committee. First, all students had to pass both tests at 70% to pass the course. We operationalized this to mean that students had to pass the tests before the final drop date (about three weeks into term) or drop the class. Second, the students could take the exams any number of times in order to pass and exams were only graded pass/fail. We provided handouts which, in conjunction with a nutrition text and an anthropology book, provided all the answers. Once students knew what sort of knowledge we considered prerequisite for the course, passing the pretests was not difficult.

Construction of the nutrition pretest was relatively straightforward. It involved reviewing the material to be discussed for the term, identifying the basic nutrition information required, and consulting the introductory course to determine what level of knowledge was expectable. A key was then constructed for the test providing page numbers where the information could be found in each of several texts. Most nutrition students passed it on the first attempt, or the second after some minimal review. The anthropology students had more difficulty, but none considered it unfair.

Construction of the anthropology pretest was more problematic. Introductory anthropology courses vary enormously and could not be readily used as models. We finally decided to develop a list of terms and concepts to which we would refer throughout the course, and to provide this list with definitions as a handout. The test involved definitions and examples. A scoring method was devised so that memorizing definitions without adequate understanding — as illustrated by examples — did not result in a passing grade. Anthropology students generally passed on the first attempt. Nutrition students found it easy after doing the reading and studying the terms. They found the reading interesting and the test fair.

In addition to student response to the individual tests, there was a more general response that should be mentioned. Virtually all the students were, in the end, pleased that this pretest system allowed the course to be given at the appropriate level of sophistication. Many had been disappointed previously in taking "advanced" courses in which some students were inadequately prepared and the whole course slowed down to accommodate them. They appreciated being given a mechanism (and being required) to overcome their own background weaknesses.

Course Goals

Our course goals were developed based on two sets of evaluations: (1) our evaluations of the biases the students brought with them to class, as discussed above; and (2) our evaluation of the probable career directions of the students. Based on our own teaching experiences it appeared to us that many of the nutrition students would find jobs as nutrition counselors, dieticians, or nutrition educators, trying to translate their knowledge of biochemical nutrition into behavioral recommendations that might be helpful to real people. In contrast, it seemed likely that most anthropology students would end up doing something other than full-time anthropology, and thus would need to learn how to apply anthropological information or approaches in non-academic settings where anthropology concepts and jargon are not understood.

The nutrition students, who constituted the bulk of each class, began the term with some strongly held opinions about correct behavior and solutions to dietary problems. Our goal for them was to widen their assessment of the components of problems to include the behavioral and socio-cultural factors. Practically, this meant their learning how to use consultants and their working toward more creative and broadly-based solutions. It is interesting to note that while nutrition education specialists often see their task as convincing their clients of the association between proper diet and health, our task in this class has been to convince our students (future nutrition educators) of the interrelatedness between diet and issues other than health, including many aspects of culture and population biology.

The social science students generally entered the class appearing hostile towards any interventions (for the reasons mentioned above) and appearing unwilling (or afraid) to assume responsibility for assessment and recommendations. Our goal for them was to develop their skills as consultants, encouraging them to assess the behavioral and socio-cultural components of the problem, and to generate a range of alternative interventions with the possible drawbacks of each indicated.

THEORETICAL ASPECTS OF ANTHROPOLOGY UNFAMILIAR TO NUTRITIONISTS

Anthropologists operate under a number of premises, at different levels of abstraction, that affect their approach to issues of diet and nutrition. In teaching anthropology to students of nutrition, it was necessary to make the relevant premises quite explicit at the beginning of the class. Interestingly, the anthropology students found this review equally helpful.

One of the most basic components of anthropological thinking is the evolutionary perspective. I have discussed the evolutionary development of human dietary patterns in detail elsewhere (Ritenbaugh 1978a, b; Ritenbaugh 1981) and will only briefly review it here.

Anthropologists tend to think in terms of the time depth of the human species or of particular cultures. The study of the last two million years of human evolution is increasingly becoming the study of human behaviors and biocultural interactions rather than of biology alone. For humans more than other species, the behavioral content of the process of adaptation is of primary importance. Most of the terms which identify stages in human evolution refer to patterns of food procurement and consumption. The earliest hominids, the Australopithecines, were probably the first primates to systematically collect meat, although whether or not they actually hunted remains an open question. The appearance of the upright posture charac-teristic of hominids was probably somehow related to this dietary change. Early hominid social organization, consisting of family groups in base camps, was prob-ably a development contemporaneous with increased meat consumption. Killed animals provided a concentrated nutrient source most efficiently consumed by groups (Lovejoy 1981). Thus from human beginnings, diet, biology, and social organization were intimately linked, and food served both physiological and social functions.

Hominids spent the longest period as hunter-gatherers, followed by a consider-able time as big-game hunters. The next stage was a short one of intensive localized hunting and collecting, and was followed by the agricultural revolution. At each of these stages, the food base changed (initially toward increasing meat consumption, but after the big-game hunting period fairly consistently toward decreasing annual meat consumption) along with changes in settlement patterns (first the seasonal coming together of larger and larger groups, and then increasing sedentization) and the accompanying necessary changes in social organization and religious beliefs. The sense of great time depth and continual change exemplified here is central to the anthropological perspective.

If we examine a variety of "traditional" diets today, there is considerable evidence that adjustments in food choice and technology over time have resulted in dietary improvement. For example, many traditional staple food combinations provide complementary amino acid patterns. Maize processing techniques, which involve soaking the dried kernels in an alkali solution, improve the amino acid pattern and niacin availability of the consumed product in addition to improving the ease of grinding (Katz 1974). Some foodstuffs widely consumed today (manioc) or previously (acorns) require considerable processing to be edible, and appropriate technologies have been developed to cope with them. These dietary behaviors can be considered evidence of behavioral adaptations (see also Haas and Harrison 1978). While all behaviors that appear to have great time depth are not necessarily adaptive, the ramifications of long-term behaviors need to be examined in some detail before such behaviors are dismissed as foolish, harmful, or old-fashioned, as well as too readily accepted as adaptive. Recent changes in other facets of culture, environ-ment, or diet may serve to render some formerly adaptive behaviors harmful; understanding the former advantage (if any) and the current situation requires careful analysis.

A basic concept of anthropology that must be explained to nutrition or other non-anthropology students is that of "culture". One definition which is often understandable to students unfamiliar with the concept is that culture is the body of shared and learned assumptions, beliefs, symbols, and ways of behaving which characterize a human society (Harrison and Ritenbaugh 1981). Culture is what enables us to make sense of our surroundings and the behavior of people around us and to behave in ways which make sense to them. It provides the individual with a set of rules for behaving and interpreting the behavior of others. In the words of Goodenough (1963: 250–259), "Culture consists of standards for deciding what is, what can be, how one feels about it, what to do about it, and how to go about doing it." The knowledge that one acquires as a member of a culture can be likened to a cultural grammar, or set of rules, for the interpretation of behavior. In fact, many linguistic anthropologists have pointed out the parallel relations of culture to behavior and language to speech. There are four consequences of this concept which are important in food-related issues.

First, it is clear that like the rules of language (grammar), the rules of culture cannot always be recognized or verbalized by the bearer. However, whenever someone breaks a cultural rule, even if we are not entirely conscious of it, we feel uncomfortable because we cannot interpret his/her behavior. For example, it is well-known that the appropriate distance between people in social situations varies cross-culturally. Two people, whose unconscious assumptions about appropriate interpersonal distance differ, may find themselves vaguely uncomfortable together as one moves closer and the other retreats. Neither may be aware of the source of the discomfort, although each may feel the other to be either pushy or "unfriendly". Similarly, table manners vary tremendously between cultures, so that what is considered appropriate to one group is seen as a sign of vulgarity or crudeness to another.

A second consequence of the existence of cultural maps, or rules for behaving and interpreting behavior, is that, despite the culture bearer's lack of conscious awareness of all the rules, they can be made explicit, studied, and learned. Thus cross-cultural communication is possible. A third consequence of this notion of culture is that individuality in behavior, perception, and feelings is taken into account. It is not necessary for everyone in a given society to share exactly the same cognitive map, only that everyone shares enough component parts to make behavior mutually intelligible.

Finally, like a linguistic grammar, culture is generative. Given a set of linguistic rules, we can produce sentences that have never been produced before and expect them to make sense to the listener. Given a set of cultural assumptions and rules, we can produce specific behaviors that do not repeat earlier acts and expect them to be interpreted correctly. New cultural elements can be introduced or invented (often as variations on, or combinations of, existing elements), tried out, and accepted or discarded or modified. For example, there has recently been a proliferation of types of food available at "fast food" establishments. A number of these are completely new foods (e.g., fried chicken patty on hamburger bun) that can best be understood as extensions of the "hamburger" class of food in terms of shape, condiment, and consumption patterns.

How can these implications of a definition of culture be related to issues of food consumption and U.S. culture? Food related behaviors (choice of foods, preparation style [recipes], meal composition, feasts) are not public behaviors requiring the same level of uniformity across the country and between individuals as are, for example, language, interpersonal distance, or table manners. Food is usually prepared and consumed within the household or among friends or close acquaintances. In contrast, when food is consumed in large groups or with total strangers (e.g., army, college), little individual choice is possible and complaints are widespread.

Because food related behaviors are relatively private and family-centered, ethnic patterns of eating can be maintained, sometimes several generations removed from the geographic source. Such ethnic patterns may be interpreted by those following them today as "the way our family does it" or "the way my mother cooks" with no awareness of the source of the behavior except as individual idiosyncracy. For example, it was only when I visited England as an adult that I became aware of the overwhelmingly English pattern of my family's (and my own) food consumption. Although I knew of our English ancestry (and in fact visited relatives there), and I knew that my grandmother occasionally cooked classic English dishes such as steak and kidney pie, I did not recognize that virtually my entire meal pattern — what I considered appropriate foods for breakfast, lunch, dinner, for combating colds and flu — was of English derivation. Only then did I begin to understand, for example, my vague sense of unease when a dinner did not end with something sweet.

Developing students' awareness of their own cultural values, whether they were derived from foreign heritage or associated with mainstream America or their contemporaries today, is an important step in developing their ability to deal with clients who differ from them. Clearly once the cultural content of their own behaviors becomes apparent, they are in a better position to begin to learn about those that differ. Students should also understand that there is considerable individual variability possible within any cultural system. It is primarily within the realm of individual variability (that is, *within* each culture) that psychology, sociology, and perhaps education carve out their own areas of interest.

The final implication of the definition of culture — its generative potential — is very important for nutrition students who are, of course, the diet counselors and nutrition educators of the future. With some creativity and an understanding of their own and their clients' cognitive maps, new food-related behaviors can presumably be suggested to clients that meet the professional goal of improving health while being acceptable within their clients' conceptual and behavioral framework. Clearly, behavioral change occurs all the time. The role of culture in shaping food-related behaviors can be mistakenly construed as implying that change is impossible. In contrast, we hoped students would see that some understanding of the role of culture can facilitate working toward behavioral change.

Two general perspectives of anthropology become apparent when one begins to discuss definitions of culture and to use the evolutionary perspective. The first is the concept of holism. Anthropologists see human functioning within a complex system (see Figure 1) that includes all of the basic biological parameters, as modified by stage of life and environmental factors. It includes the environmental

AN ECOLOGICAL MODEL
FOR NUTRITIONAL ANTHROPOLOGY

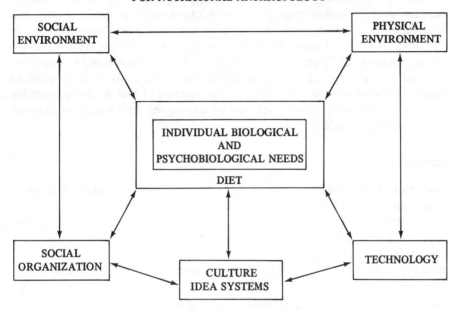

Fig. 1. From 'An Ecological Approach to Nutritional Anthropology', N. W. Jerome, G. H. Pelto, R. F. Kandel. In *Nutritional Anthropology*, N. W. Jerome, R. F. Kandel, G. H. Pelto (eds.), Redgrave Publishing Co., Pleasantville, N.Y., 1980. p. 14.

parameters that affect what is available for humans to interact with, and the technology that shapes the interaction. It includes the social factors, the belief systems, and continuous interaction throughout the system. While as anthropologists we clearly do not command detailed knowledge of all aspects of human functioning, the ideal of holism tends to guide analytic attempts. Anthropologists recognize that an item as central to human biological functioning as food has also been central to social functioning since the Australopithecines.

The second general perspective is that of cultural relativism. Anthropology as a discipline views all cultures as equally "good", although different. While individual anthropologists maintain their own idiosyncracies, this overall tone remains. Anthropology is interested in functional integration, in understanding what role a behavior plays (even a behavior such as cannibalism) in the maintenance of a cultural system. Because we view culturally patterned behaviors from a vantage point of integration, we minimize judgment and maintain a posture of cultural relativism.

A consequence of this viewpoint is that behaviors of individuals which might be initially construed as aggressive or unfriendly (as with interpersonal distance differences), for example, can be recast in a neutral context. We can intellectualize, as it were, and shift out of a negative emotional response to one of "understanding" or "learning". This ability to shift can be an extremely important one for individuals working in health care settings. Some health care workers do this intuitively, and they are probably among those more satisfied with their jobs. Others can learn. In the realm of nutrition, students can begin to learn that different eating behaviors are not "wrong" or "dumb" or "disgusting", but just different, and perhaps even interesting. This shifts the professional-client relationship a little from the standard superordinate-subordinate relationship in the direction of that of partners working toward change. Finding a dietary solution for a particular client becomes a challenge akin to solving a puzzle.

Instructional Mode

With these basic anthropological concepts in mind, then, the course became an opportunity to teach students how to operationalize the notion "Interaction of Culture and Nutrition". The course focused not on cultural particulars — which many students expected to be required to memorize, and in fact would have preferred — and not on nutritional data, but on biocultural interactions. The goal of the class was for students to learn how to ask appropriate questions of a given situation so that they might identify the interactions, and in so doing, have confidence in developing appropriate interventions or recommendations.

When the course was originally designed, there were not many useful books available in nutritional anthropology. That situation is rapidly changing. There is now a general work by Farb and Armelagos (1980) which is a popular view of the interactions between humans and their food (Ritenbaugh 1980b). A collection entitled *Nutritional Anthropology* (Kandel, Jerome, and Pelto) provides a good theoretical chapter and some useful case studies (Ritenbaugh 1980a). Greene and Johnston (1980) have compiled an excellent set of more biologically-oriented papers on the general topic. Other useful works are those by Fitzgerald (1976), Margen and Ogar (1978) and Jerome (1981).

As organized, the course was designed less to teach anthropology than to teach students how to approach problems as anthropologists might. To accomplish this, our course design was based upon detailed examination of problem areas encountered in nutrition. Each involved conflicts between "pure" biochemical nutrition on the one hand and socio-cultural issues on the other. Our team-teaching strategy has been to use the nutritionist and anthropologist instructors to model for the students how these complex problems might be approached in a holistic way. Whenever possible we have attempted to take into account both the evolutionary and historic backgrounds and provide adequate analyses of the biological (nutrition and population), social, and cultural components.

Five problem areas were chosen: obesity, lactose intolerance, pica, infant feeding, and changing the dietary behavior of groups. Each of the analyses took 3–6 hours of class time and involved such general questions as: What range of factors might be interacting? What beliefs/behaviors/biological parameters are involved? Are unusual behaviors harmful, neutral, or advantageous? How unusual are these behaviors on a world-wide basis? Should they be changed? Table I provides a brief resume of some of the relevant questions for each of the five topic areas, and a limited set of readings. More detailed outlines for two of the others (pica and

TABLE I

Problem	Evolutionary and historical factors	Nutritional issues	Cultural issues	References
Obesity	Body shape, environmental factors, and adaptation/ Changing definitions	Negative health correlates (but correlation ≠ causation)/ Difficulty of altering body composition	Stigma and power of body size and composition/ Cultural definitions of beauty, health/ Women's roles	See text
Infant feeding	History of infant feeding here and abroad/Breast milk composition and evolution/ Birth control	Infants should receive optimal nutrition — what is it?	Urbanization and employment of women? Insufficient milk syndrome/Breasts and sex	See outline, also: Edson (1979), Jelliffe and Jelliffe (1975), Raphael (1980).
Dietary change: Planned and unplanned	History of human diets/Dietary change and acculturation, technology, economics	What foods are "good", "bad"? For whom? In what quantities? Why?	Relation of eating patterns to economy, beliefs/ Politics of dietary recommendations	Ahlstrom and Rasanen (1973), Food and Nut'n. Jerome (1980), Kolasa (1978), Olson (1980), Passmore et al. (1980), Harper (1980), USDA (1980).
Lactose intolerance	Genetics of adult lactase sufficiency/ Herding and natural selection	Lactase deficiency vs lactose intoler- rance: biologic variation and diet	Orientation of federal programs, dairy industry to universal milk consumption/ Dietary ethnocentrism?	Almy (1975), Barr (1979), Harrison (1975), McCracken (1971), Lebenthal (1979), Mitchell (1977), Paige (1977), Rorick (1979), Simoons (1978), Johnson (1981)
Pica	Definitions/ Distribution/ Cultural adaptation?	Does it interfere with nutrient intake, absorption? Is it a sign of pathology?	Cultural differences between providers and clients/ Biomedicine vs folk medicine.	See outline

infant feeding) are provided in the appendix. These outlines are not exhaustive, but rather are designed to provide a guide to the broad range of issues which can be explored under these topics. The issue of obesity is more fully developed in the second section of this chapter. It is clear that this approach is not associated with a syllabus which contains much nutritional anthropology *per se*. On the contrary each problem becomes a study in nutritional anthropology, and thus the course involves doing rather than reading nutritional anthropology.

To complement the instructional model being used in the didactic portion of the course, the students were assigned a teamwork problem instead of the usual term paper as the major written assignment. Teams each composed of three or four students were assigned to solve the problems presented in an illustrative paper case (see Appendix). These cases were composed by the teaching staff (faculty and graduate assistants) based on our own experiences or experiences related to us. They did not come out of any particular references, so there was no way for students to find already completed analyses. The students presented their solutions as team papers. To assign students to teams, we used information on students' background and experience which they provided to us on cards filled out during the first class meeting. We attempted to balance teams, with all students of about equal competence so that no one student would be the obvious leader. Further, we attempted to include on each team of three at least one student who had substantial social science background. Each team, then, usually represented as diverse interests as possible.

Students were encouraged to create their own detail for each case where it was lacking — these fictional details then determined how they approached and ultimately solved the cases. Because of the latitude available in each case, no two papers have ever been the same. We have produced enough different cases (12 now) so that in none of our classes have more than two teams undertaken the same case.

In approaching each case, students are referred back to a diagram such as Figure 1. They are encouraged to consider all of the peripheral components indicated in the figure (e.g. social environment, physical environment) as well as the central ones. For each case, the student team must identify and clearly define the nutritional and sociocultural components of the problem. Although many of the cases are couched in terms of a particular individual or family, students are encouraged to think more generally about the categories of people affected, and about structural (policy) solutions as well as individually-tailored ones.

Many of the resulting papers have been highly creative and have shown considerable insight developed by the students as they have learned about the variety of details potentially related to their cases. The papers have also frequently been quite long; we have found over the years that while length is no guarantee of quality, very short papers almost always reflect inadequate reading, thinking, and discussing. Graduate students have done better on cases not directly in their own areas of expertise. Apparently they find it easier to think creatively in new rather than in already familiar territory.

The variety of approaches possible can be illustrated by the range of papers we have received in response to the case of Mrs. Homer, Example Case A. In different years, she has been a Pima (because they have the highest prevalence of diabetes), a Navajo (because one of the team members had worked there), and Chippewa from northern Michigan (because one of the team members was interested in native wild plants of the region). The papers differ vastly as students tap their own most readily available sources for information.

Student response to the team paper assignment must be described longitudinally. In spite of our warnings to the contrary, most students initially expect a team paper to be easier than a single-authored paper because there are more people to share the work. With the due date approaching, however, complaints begin to surface about team members who are not doing their share or meeting team deadlines. We often hear the comment, "It would be easier to do the whole thing myself!" In spite of this, there are few serious breakdowns in team functioning (about one per term), and these are readily handled on an individual basis. After completion of the term, many of the same students who have complained return to tell us that they greatly valued the experience. In retrospect, they find that they have learned a great deal about themselves, about working with others to complete a task, and about solving problems.

CONCLUSIONS

In attempting to teach anthropology in a clinically applied setting, we used a problem-solving approach structured in an anthropologically holistic framework, and containing a strong dose of cultural relativism. In this class, the emphasis has not been on ethnographic detail but on how to use an anthropological viewpoint to improve data collection and analysis of nutrition problems. For the anthropologists who find themselves in such a class, it provides an opportunity to learn what skills and approaches they have which might be useful outside of anthropology *per se*, and how they might need to translate their own ideas in order to communicate. For faculty, it has been an exciting opportunity to watch students mature as they tackle problems more similar to those they will encounter beyond the university.

II. OBESITY IN AMERICA: ANTHROPOLOGICAL ANALYSIS OF A NUTRITIONAL PROBLEM

Obesity, one of the five major topic areas of the course, provides a particularly apt illustration of how problems were approached in the course. There is good information available to support both nutritional and anthropological analyses. But more importantly, the topic is culturally charged: there is a general concern in the contemporary U.S. about corpulence and all health professionals will be affected in some way. It is an important social issue with a long history and has obvious biological components. Moreover, it is a topic on which virtually every American is an expert, whether by virtue of professional training, personal experience, or extensive reading (ranging from *Readers Digest* through self-help advertisements to professional journals). The following pages provide an analysis of this issue in the framework that would be used in the course just described. That course was taught jointly by a community nutritionist and a physical anthropologist; the material presented here illustrates how the issues might be approached by an anthropologist in early 1981 based on the available literature.

Evolutionary and Historical Information

Humans have come in a wide range of body shapes throughout their history. Among the earliest pictorial evidence of corpulence is found in the Venus of Willendorf and other clay figurines ("fertility goddesses") dating to about 20,000 years ago in northern Europe (Beller 1977). The well-known Venus figurine, although not having facial detail, is highly accurate in its portrayal of a corpulent female figure, probably pregnant. In fact, the figurine shows evidence that its living model had knee damage from excessive weight-bearing – the knees are caved inward as from massive obesity today. Most archeologists interpret the figurines as evidence of a high value placed on that body shape during a hunting-gathering period in a cold climate.

Physical anthropologists in this century (Roberts 1953; Newman 1975; Steegman 1975; Dugdale and Payne 1977) have explored in some detail the possible adaptive advantages of various body shapes under particular environmental circumstances. Fat serves two separate functions: first, it provides insulation and serves to conserve heat; second it represents storage of food energy. These two functions do not always relate neatly to each other. For instance, energy storage may be needed in hot climates where extra insulation could be dangerous. The converse is that stored energy may need to be utilized in cold climates where depletion of insulation could lead to dangerous heat loss. In these two types of circumstances, apparently, other aspects of body shape have been under selective pressure to partially offset the problems. In hot climates, for example, some populations have developed very localized fat storage depots (particularly in the buttocks) which do not increase overall body insulation. In cold climates, there seems to be a greater preponderance of stocky bodies which, by shape, improve heat retention capabilities; of course, adult body shape is not under complete genetic control, but rather is the outcome of the complex interaction of genes and environment throughout development. This is obvious in light of some of the major changes in body shape that have accompanied acculturation to Western diet and lifestyles (these will be discussed below). One other, perhaps more directly genetic, aspect of body shape that may be important in temperature regulation is the shape of the body of the arm and leg muscles. Populations of northern (cold climate) ancestry are more likely to have the body of the muscles extend over the length of the limb, providing insulation (and resulting in the configuration known as "thick ankles"). Populations with long histories in hot climates have the body of the muscle located very close to the trunk on each limb, with tendons extending to the joint. This shape maximizes the heat radiation capacities of the limb, as well as facilitating rapid movements such as sprinting or jumping.

Human populations also differ greatly from one another in their recent (last 10,000 years) history of exposure to regular periodic food shortage. Many anthropologists today might hypothesize that there are likely to be differences in efficiency of energy storage related to that history (Dugdale and Payne 1977). At this time the understanding of physiological differences between individuals and between populations in this regard is in its infancy; in the future this seems likely to become much clearer (DeLuise et al. 1980; Bondy 1980).

Another aspect of body fat that has been the center of debate in the past decade is its relationship to female fertility. It has been observed under a number of conditions that the rapid onset of extreme leanness in females (through anorexia nervosa, marathon training, ballet practice) is associated with the cessation of menstruation. Frisch (1974, 1978) has suggested that a critical amount of body fat — about that necessary to sustain a pregnancy — is required for females to begin to menstruate and to maintain menstrual cycling. This has been expanded into an explanation of lactation amenorrhea and population fertility control. Others (Chowdhury et al. 1977 and 1978; Ellison 1981; Nimrod and Ryan 1975; Quandt in press) have countered that the association is a statistical one, and that fatness is not the causal variable at the physiological level. At this writing, Frisch's position seems the most tenuous. What is clear, however, is that female fatness and fertility have probably been linked cultural symbols since the first "Venus" figurines.

Biocultural Interactions

Prior to this century, some degree of fatness seems to have been valued world-wide. There are several biological reasons why fatness would have been advantageous. The most obvious advantage it provided the individual was some protection against periods of food scarcity, which might occur on yearly (seasonal shortages) or multi-year (e.g., crop failure) basis. Additionally, some extra storage of energy is probably important in the successful recovery from illnesses which include extended periods of fever and anorexia, especially in the absence of antibiotics. Certainly extra fat stores were usually an indication that nutritional status was adequate to maintain immunological competence. One of the most feared diseases — tuberculosis — has a pattern of expression apparently linked to undernutrition. The most common cycle of tuberculosis is to have it transmitted from an older individual with active disease to a child, who is immunologically competent and successfully walls off the infection within his or her body (but does not eliminate it). At some later time, when the body's immune system is less competent, the disease becomes active, and transmission to another non-immune person occurs. The reasons for the reactivation of the disease may include undernutrition, along with other kinds of stress. Certainly individuals with the active disease generally were thin, thus leading to a perceived association of protection from tuberculosis with adequate fat stores. Prior to this century, children contracted a wide range of standard "childhood diseases", each with a high caloric cost due to fever and anorexia. Children of marginal nutritional status even today do not survive those illnesses, although increasing numbers of children never contract them due to the widespread use of immunizations.

Thus it is clear why, prior to very recent times, fatness in varying degrees was a sign of wealth, of status, and of health. Only in this century, the exact date varying with local conditions, has the symbol inverted, with wealth now associated with thinness ("You can't be too thin or too rich"). Several developments make such an inversion possible. This century has been characterized by unbelievable improvements in sanitation (clean water supplies, waste disposal, etc.), the stability of the food supply (transportation, agricultural technology, etc.), and in the last 40 years, medical care (especially antibiotics and immunizations). Tuberculosis has also declined tremendously, especially in the middle and upper classes, and is readily treatable today when it appears. As a result, to be rich means to have the luxury of being thin. It signifies that one need not worry about periodic food shortages, exposure to debilitating transmissable diseases, or lack of good medical care. Even infants and children can "afford" to be slim.

These changes in attitude have been taking place throughout the world, but the rate of change varies with geographic area and social class. One of the factors that has apparently played a role in the world-wide spread of the value of thinness, particularly among women, has been the spread of Western clothing and values among the upper classes. Body shapes that were fully acceptable in the loose traditional garments are less so in form-revealing Western styles. In spite of this, there is still considerable variation in attitudes toward body shape; and within countries which have a thin-conscious upper class, there are segments of the population that do not share this ideal. For example, in rural Yucatan today, a woman who would be considered "obese" by United States standards is termed "substantial", a word conveying the same information about body shape but with a positive connotation (Jordan, personal communication). In urban Colombia, among the middle and upper classes, the slim body is valued among young women, but beyond age thirty-five, everyone expects that body weight will increase with age. In fact, individuals beyond that age who are counting calories or in other ways attempting to maintain the youthful look are considered somewhat vain and certainly to be wasting their time. A person worrying about eating too much might be told: "With all the things there are to worry about, why fuss about gaining a few pounds? At your age (anything beyond 35), it's just normal." Further evidence of the basic lack of concern is the almost complete absence of bathroom scales. Although people who can eat what they want and remain thin are considered lucky, virtually the only individuals concerned with dieting are those who have recently been to the U.S. or who have relatives there (M. Sandefur, personal communication; see also Baylor 1972).

Nutrition Issues

The topic of obesity has been discussed here thus far without clear definition in order to convey the notion that definitions of what is fat, much less what is "too fat", occur on a continuum, with values varying among different populations.

Similarly, the means and distributions of actual body shape vary. Thus any criterion or set of criteria to define obesity must be arbitrary and specific to the culture that constructs the definition.

A person becomes increasingly fat as he or she stores excess energy for later use; thus obesity is due to repeated consumption of more energy than is used. In this country, the emphasis until recently has been on the intake side of the equation with much information being published on how to eat less and lose weight. Changes in the American diet over the last few decades have probably played some role in promoting a perpetual, if low-level, excess of intake over expenditure. For example, since a pound of body fat consists of about 3,500 kilocalories of energy, a daily intake of only 20 kilocalories in excess of expenditures over a year would result in a gain of about two pounds; one teaspoon of sugar contains almost 20 kilocalories. Although this analysis is in all likelihood too simplistic since scientists are only beginning to understand regulation of intake and efficiency of storage, it does illustrate how minor changes in diet might lead to slow accumulations of body fat.

The two changes in the U.S. diet of potential importance are (1) the reduction in dietary fiber, and (2) the increase in protein consumption (Donald et al. 1981). First, the reduction in dietary fiber means the reduction in the volume of food that can be consumed for the same number of calories. To the degree that satiation is associated with volume consumed, reduction in bulk is likely to lead to increased consumption of calories. The second change may be significant in light of a recent study of the effect of differences in diet on the body composition of adult rats. Two groups of adult rats ate diets of exactly the same caloric level, but one rat group consumed the normal protein levels, and one consumed twice the normal levels. The group on the high protein diet became substantially fatter and heavier than the normal group during the course of the experiment in spite of the similarities in energy intake (Donald et al. 1981). The exact applicability of this study to humans is not clear, but it is suggestive and indicates important directions for future study.

In spite of the concern with consumption of excess calories, recent analysis of the 1977 United States Department of Agriculture Nationwide Food Consumption Survey indicates that adult women are, on the average, eating only about 1,600 kilocalories per day. Based on the U.S. food supply and the usual intake patterns, it is probably not possible for an individual to be well-nourished on this intake without supplements. Thus it seems likely that interest is currently focused on the wrong side of the energy equation. Rather than reducing intake, attention should be on increasing the level of energy expenditure in the population.

Throughout human evolution, people have had to use their upper bodies for strenuous work, and their lower bodies to do considerable walking. Today in the U.S., the use of cars for transportation as well as the use of "energy-saving" devices (they save human energy but use electricity) in the home and the workplace have greatly reduced the amount of energy expended in a day, in most cases without decreasing to the same degree the amount of time required to complete the tasks.

Thus people are using fewer calories, but often are not saving enough time to permit other activities, perhaps recreational, which would provide the same degree of exercise. The recent increase in interest in exercise (jogging, tennis, health clubs, spas) indicates the growing awareness of the need for increased energy output.

Considerable controversy and confusion surround attempts to specify criteria for deciding whether or not someone is obese. The standard definition has been one based on weight, and the result is more appropriately termed "overweight". This classifies as obese anyone who is 120% or more of ideal or desirable weight for height. Several problems arise with this definition. The first is the issue of weight standards. This issue will be dealt with in more detail below, but the standards most widely used are those derived from the Metropolitan Life Insurance "blood pressure and body build study" in 1958. A second problem with any weight criterion is that one who is "overweight" may not necessarily have excessive fat. Muscle weighs more than fat for an equal unit of volume — athletes, particularly male athletes, tend to be heavy but with relatively little body fat. They can more readily be in excess of 120% of ideal weight without being fat.

The best method we have of measuring body fat is densitometry or underwater weighing. The principle behind this is that most of the lean body mass weighs approximately the same as water per unit volume, while fat is lighter. Thus, after corrections are made for residual lung volume, intestinal gas, and skeletal mass, comparing dry and underwater weights permits an estimate of percent body fat. However, densitometry is time-consuming and requires a large tank. It is neither portable nor convenient.

The alternative noninvasive measure of body fat is the measurement of fatfold thickness using special calipers. While the equipment is portable and the measurement relatively quick, there are problems with measurement error. Additionally, as we all know, the distribution of fat differs from one individual to another. Thus measuring fatfolds at only one site means that the likelihood for over- or underestimation of total body fat is increased. The analytical problems involved in measurement at multiple sites are currently being addressed by physical anthropologists and exercise physiologists, but their solutions are beyond the scope of the non-professional concerned with his or her body fatness. Recent television ads for a supposedly dietetic breakfast cereal challenged people to see if they could "pinch an inch" at their waistlines. (Answers in the affirmative were supposed to indicate that they were too fat, and needed to diet, starting with buying the cereal. This probably included 75% or more of the adult population!) While the aforementioned indicates a move in the direction of focusing concern on fat rather than weight *per se*, which is probably a useful shift, a problem exists in using fatfold measurements beyond those mentioned above. The problem is "how much is too much?" Little of the current longitudinal prospective research on overall or cardiovascular morbidity or mortality has included such measures. Until such data are available, most researchers are using the 85th percentile of the nationwide HANES (Health and Nutrition Examination Survey) as a study criterion. The usefulness of this in individual decision-making for clinical treatment is not known.

This distinction between body weight and body fat is an extremely significant one in terms of dieting. In terms of body fat stores, that is, in terms of energy balance, a person can probably only lose a pound of body fat by burning on the average of 3,500 more calories than are taken in. If, every day for a week, someone eats 1,000 calories less than are used (and remember that the average woman of stable weight only consumes 1,600 per day), he or she will only lose two pounds of body fat per week. Then, what occurs when diets promising losses of "7 pounds in 7 days" are followed? The additional *weight* loss is through dehydration; it represents a loss of "water weight" rather than body fat.

This loss of water occurs through three mechanisms. First, as caloric consumption does not keep pace with energy output, glycogen stores are depleted. The average person can, under special circumstances ("carbohydrate loading"), store up to 2,500 grams of glycogen; a more normal range is probably 1,000 to 1,500 grams. For every gram of glucose stored as glycogen, 3 grams of water are also retained. Thus, for example, as 1,000 grams of glycogen are used, 3,000 grams (6.6 lbs.) of water are excreted. The second mechanism is that of ketosis-induced dehydration. When the body no longer has glycogen stores to draw upon, and the diet does not provide adequate carbohydrate for energy, fat begins to be used as an energy source. The body cannot be completely efficient in fat utilization with limited carbohydrates, and the result is increased levels of ketones — the breakdown products of fats — circulating in the blood. The excess is excreted in the urine by the kidneys, and take with it extra water. A third, perhaps more speculative, mechanism is that while on a weight-reduction diet, sodium (salt) intake often declines. In part the amount of water retained is a function of the total body sodium; thus as total body sodium declines, some additional water is lost. The large contribution of water loss to the total weight lost on short term diets is one of the main reasons why weight is often quickly regained after the end of the diet. The popular confusion of excess weight with excess fat perpetuates the problem.

Health Issues

Health care professionals would not be so involved with issues of obesity if they did not consider there to be legitimate health concerns involved. With specific conditions, there is a direct relationship between weight and disease severity (Larsson et al. 1981). For example, among patients with adult-onset diabetes who are obese, reduction to "normal weight" will often result in normal or near-normal glucose tolerance. Similarly, hypertensive patients are often obese, and weight reduction among such patients will often result in the lowering of blood pressure. Some hyperlipidemias are improved in obese patients following weight loss. In addition to these chronic conditions, obese patients have increased risks from surgery in three areas. First, fat has a poor blood supply; thus wound healing is delayed or may not occur at all, and wound infection is more likely in these patients. Second, obese individuals are at a higher risk from the anesthetic since many anesthetics are fat soluble, and this absorption of the drug into the fat makes blood levels of the anesthetic more difficult to regulate. Third, obese surgical patients are more prone to thromboembolic and pulmonary complications.

The previous paragraph discussed problems which exist and can be directly assessed among individuals who are already obese. But these are, for the most part, not the main reasons given for considering obesity to be a major health problem today. The reasons most frequently cited for the health concerns about obesity are: (1) it decreases life expectancy, and (2) it is an important cardiovascular disease risk factor. These two assertations need special examination.

The belief that overweight leads to earlier death has been considered a fact for most of this century. To understand the source of this belief and the problems inherent in it, one should know its history and how it has been operationalized. This has been summarized by Ancel Keys, a noted nutrition scientist, famous for his work on obesity and starvation. The following is abstracted from his presentation as the prestigious Atwater Memorial Lecturer at the Western Hemisphere Nutrition Congress in Los Angeles, August 11, 1980 (Keys 1980a).

In the early 1900s the actuaries began to find that their death claims were indicating excess mortality among their heaviest policy holders. In 1912 the Association of Life Insurance Medical Directors and the Actuarial Society of America published their *Medico-Actuarial Investigation*, the analysis of death claims which showed that the men in the top of the distribution of weight for given height and age had an excessive death rate. So, life insurance companies began to charge extra premiums for gross "overweight"; the extra charge commonly being applied to men who were 25 to 30% above the average weight of American men of their age and height who had applied for life insurance.

As the years passed, the death claim experience justified the extra premiums demanded by the actuaries; persons who paid extra premiums because of overweight proved to have unduly high death rates. But, as has been pointed out repeatedly, the life insurance data are seriously flawed. In general, only 2 or 3% of life insurance applicants have been required to pay extra premiums because of overweight; but all independent surveys show that the actual frequency of the corresponding degree of overweight in the population is around 6 or 7%. Obviously the overweight persons who apply for life insurance are a self-selected sample. Among persons so overweight as to be subject to extra premiums on that account only, a minor percentage apply for insurance. Why? It is well known in the insurance industry that the insured tend to "select against the insurer". Commonly, the insurance applicant does not disclose extra risks he may know or suspect. It is highly probable then, that many persons "rated" because of overweight are bad risks in other respects unknown to the insurance company.

Another major objection about the data of the life insurance companies is the fact that many of the heights and weights recorded on the applications do not represent measurements. When the Society of Actuaries reexamined their data in 1959 they were pleased to conclude that as many as 80% of the weights recorded were actual measurements – with the applicants "as customarily dressed", including shoes. Further, there is no information about the frequency of cases in which weights or states of health were falsified. Economic persuasion being what it is, falsification does occur. The difference between an ordinary life insurance premium and the one rated because of overweight or indication of disease is substantial. The insurance agent is paid according to his success in selling policies that are accepted by the underwriter. The examining physicians whose reports may result in policies declined by the company or the applicants are shunned by the agent.

The Metropolitan Life Insurance Company, with the leadership of its chief actuary, the late Louis Dublin, has been a major source of propaganda about the evils of overweight. That was the source of the tables of so-called "ideal weight", later less presumptiously called "desirable weight", based on the notion that after growth in height and ossification is completed in the early twenties, there is no physiological reason for further increase in body weight. But the fact is that in all but a few primitive peoples the average body weight continues to increase into middle age so the great majority of people aged 40 would be labelled grossly overweight by that standard.

Dublin considered that the "ideal" weight should be the average weight for given height and sex of applicants in their mid-twenties for insurance policies issues. But when he examined the data on the weights of his policyholders in their mid-twenties he found a great range for persons of the same sex and height. He thought in part at least, that wide distribution reflected differences in body shape or "frame", as he called it. There are no data on body shape or frame type – and this lack continues today – but Dublin created three frame "types" very simply. At given height he divided the distribution of body weights into thirds and labelled these "small", "medium", and "large", frame, alternatively called light, medium, and heavy frame. The average weights of those thirds of the distribution were then termed "ideal" weights for those frame types.

The fact is that the tables of "ideal" or "desirable" weight are arm-chair concoctions starting with questionable assumptions and ending with three sets of standards for "frame" types never measured or even defined. Unfortunately, those tables have been reprinted by the thousands and are widely accepted as gospel.

Average weights of men, aged 40–55, applying for insurance today are on the average 12% above the published "desirable" weights. Other studies indicate that in the U.S., average men in middle age are 12–17% above the "desirable" weight. It is this statistic that has led to statements about the epidemic of obesity in the U.S. and has been cited as the cause for the "coronary epidemic" (Keys 1980a; Lasagna 1980).

In contrast to the poor quality of research involved in the Metropolitan study, there have been a number of carefully designed retrospective and prospective longitudinal studies designed to determine what risk factors are associated with premature death or coronary artery disease among adult men. The results of the studies are surprising in light of popular notions about body weight.

In a longitudinal prospective study of coronary heart disease among middle-aged males in 15 populations in 7 countries, Keys (1980b) found no overall correlation between average body mass index or average fatness and coronary heart disease incidence or mortality. Within populations the simple relationships of body mass and fatness to overall mortality or mortality from coronary heart disease were highly variable; in only one country (Italy) were heavier and fatter men at higher risk. In more sophisticated analyses of total mortality with blood pressure statistically held constant, curvilinear relationships were found in most cases: the leanest and heaviest were at higher risk than those individuals in the middle. The average weight male did not experience excess mortality from overweight (average was generally more than 10% above "ideal" weight by the usual analysis); in fact, the lowest mortality was at a weight above the average. It might be countered that each of these samples was biased because men already ill might appear lighter. However, each sample population was chosen to only include healthy men, and bias does not seem a likely explanation for these consistent results.

In the same type of analysis done for mortality from cardiovascular disease, the results are similar (Keys 1980b). In addition, other studies have shown that of patients admitted to the hospital with acute myocardial infarction, those who are slightly fatter than average do better. In a prospective study by Keys of 286 healthy men begun in Minneapolis in 1949, to date 143 have died, 62 of cardivascular disease. Controlling for height, those who have died from all causes weighed 2.6 pounds more than the survivors. And those who died from heart disease weighed 5 pounds more than the survivors. The results are in the direction expected by the "obesity is bad" model, but are non-significant statistically and without clinical meaning (Keys 1980a, b; see also Andres 1980). As Larsson et al. (1981) summarize findings from 43 studies: "the impression sometimes given that obesity constitutes the predominant and most important single health problem in industrialized societies can hardly be considered correct".

It would appear from these studies that: (1) within a broad range of weight for height (± at least one standard deviation from the U.S. population mean, or for 70–80% of the population) there is essentially no association between weight and coronary heart disease mortality or total mortality; and (2) the ideal weight for height of the 1958 Metropolitan standards are associated with *higher* mortalities than are somewhat greater weights (12–20% heavier). We lack studies on the role of weight or fatness on morbidity and mortality among women and among younger men. We have learned, however, that being able to run a marathon does not indicate immunity from early death, and training for and running a marathon does not reverse coronary heart disease. Given the data presented above, it is not so surprising that the extremely lean marathon runners are not as well protected as previously thought.

In sum, from a medical/nutritional point of view, it appears that for each individual there may be a wide range in weight which is consistent with health. The upper limits may be defined by the appearance of abnormal glucose tolerance, hypertension, bone and joint problems. (With regard to hypertension and diabetes, we are not yet certain that excess body weight causes them.) The lower limit may be definable by a number of criteria of undernutrition. The point is that these limits may differ greatly from one person to another, and within one person at different ages. Evidence of reaching the limits at either end is prima facie evidence that diet and exercise and thus body weight manipulation is in order. This, then, is the group who presumably should form the dieting cohort.

Cultural Issues of Obesity: United States

Obesity in the U.S. today carries considerable stigma. Since body fat is accumulated under conditions in which energy consumption exceeds energy output, the particular cause of individual obesity is generally attributed in a judgmental way to overeating (gluttony) or underexercising (laziness), or both. Thus in this country, body shape is seen as an indication of personality and character attributes as well as physiological balance. The stigma is manifest in many ways, including decreased employment opportunities, promotions, admissions to graduate and professional schools (particularly health and nutrition-related), and alteration of interpersonal relationships. Allon (1975) provides an excellent overview of the cultural associations of obesity. He shows how obesity is variously characterized today as sin through indulgence (see above), crime (overconsumption of food, medical care, space), disease, and ugliness (not conforming to the thin norm). Groups such as Fat Power (Louderback 1970), and magazines such as Big Beautiful Woman (BBW) are attempting to alter this stigmatization, and in this way they confirm its existence.

One of the consequences of obesity is, for many, the requirement of perpetually trying to reduce. In spite of the apparent tremendous interest in diets, exercises, behavior modifications, and other regimes, the five-year "success" rate of any weight reduction intervention is around 5%. This suggests three possibilities, not mutually exclusive: (1) the underlying physiological drive toward maintenance of a particular body weight is tremendous (Mahan 1981); (2) people are (virtually) incapable of permanently changing obesity-promoting lifestyles; and (3) people who diet do not find that their new body shape provides what was promised. For example, many women who undergo gastrointestinal surgery to limit their food consumption (gastric stapling) or absorption (ileo-jejuneal bypass) find that they experience extreme disruption in their personal lives, with many divorces following such procedures (see Kleinman in this volume). It has been conjectured that this is good, that these marriages must not have been very strong in the first place. Whatever the case, though, this phenomenon suggests that many aspects of life are balanced around body shape. It is possible that these formerly obese people will find their new lives to be all that they had hoped; it is more likely that they will not. In spite of the apparent stigma of obesity, a number of eminent women have sensed a reduction in their impact and personal power as their weights decreased; they have for this reason consciously chosen to return to their larger proportions. Similarly, one male lawyer found that his success with juries diminished as he reduced his body size. When he realized that his smaller size was not as forceful, he chose to regain the lost weight (Cassidy, personal communication). These cases (each of individuals of high achievement) would probably be classified in diet programs as diet "failures"; in fact, they indicate that large body size may, even in the U.S., have important positive attributes that are being overlooked in the emphasis on slimness. Apparent diet failures may need to be analyzed from a new perspective.

What are the cultural forces that help to promote the extreme value placed on thinness in our society? Several are probably operating simultaneously. The first has been, of course, the overall emphasis on youth, which became very significant in the early 1960s as the post-war baby boom generation began to be a force in the market place. The emphasis on youth continued throughout the 1960s and early 1970s ("You can't trust anyone over 30") and brought with it a desire to continue to appear young, and therefore slim. One can only await with interest the aging of the baby boom cohort, and perhaps the diminution of this emphasis on youth. (A review of commercials for jeans suggests that the emphasis on youth may have nearly bottomed out.)

A social change coinciding with the youth culture has been the change in women's roles: the simultaneous entry of women into the workplace and the drop in the birth rate. The expected increasing plumpness of women as they grow older has been associated with the motherly look, and in fact for many women increasing body fat is associated with each subsequent pregnancy. As the birthrate has dropped, motherhood has been devalued, so that appearing "motherly" has become more of an insult than a compliment. With women only experiencing one or two pregnancies, this component of increased storage of body fat is minimized. Working women are also more in the public sphere, where in many cases there are social advantages in not appearing maternal. Available clothing emphasizes body shape; thus the requirement of an "acceptable" body shape throughout adulthood for women has developed.

The cultural norms, values, and attitudes discussed above do not occur independent of the economic structure, particularly in the United States. Two major industries heavily influence American attitudes toward body shape and obesity: the advertising industry and the diet industry. The two are not independent, but for the purposes of discussion, I will attempt to separate them, dealing with advertisements first. In the U.S., ads are our major source of cultural symbols. The visual media — television, magazines, newspapers, billboards — bombard us daily with images of the ideal body type. We generally are not aware that these images are not just pictures of real people, but rather manipulated photographs and artists' renderings. For example, photographs are regularly airbrushed to remove unwanted excess body size and make the person portrayed appear slimmer. A perhaps apocryphal but illustrative story was circulated that photographs of the U.S. Women's Swim Team which were printed in a national magazine had been retouched because the females portrayed appeared to have too much muscle to suit editors. Similarly, a close examination of apparent photographs of women in cigarette advertisements indicates that the pictures are in fact composites of a number of shots taken from different angles; the result is a female body which is extremely slim and is in a position that the intact human body cannot attain.

When one examines the types of female figures used in advertisements, it becomes clear that specific body types are used to sell specific products. Cigarette ads directed at women often include extremely thin models, apparently subliminally reinforcing the use of cigarettes to alter metabolism. Cars, liquor, and perfume generally include somewhat more fleshy models who could be considered "sexy". Carbonated beverages, whether low-calorie or not, are only advertised by the slimmest, most active-looking models. In the case of the low-calorie version, the viewer rarely asks why a person of that build would need a no-calorie beverage (besides water). The high-calorie drink is similarly consumed by a thin person, thus absolving the beverage from any role in the gradual increase in body fat over time. "Motherly" figures are only associated with household products (especially oven cleaners) or baked goods (which cause dirty ovens). It appears that even a normal (average) amount of body fat is only acceptable if it is associated with the preparation of high-calorie food for others, and in these situations, such foods are generally equated with love.

Men fare somewhat better in visual advertising. Since athletes (and former athletes) come in a variety of body builds, there is a much wider range of role models for men than women (see for example the men's underwear ads, featuring Pete Rose). This discrepancy in the range of acceptable builds between men and women can also be seen in the wide range of builds among actors who have leading roles, in contrast to the range among actresses.

The other important aspect of advertising is that it is designed to entice people to consume particular foods. How advertising works is succinctly summarized by Henry (1965), but in the context of obesity it is useful to note that foods receiving the greatest advertising push are generally those with the highest profit margins. They tend to be highly processed foods of the snack variety, adding many calories to an average diet but often few nutrients. In fact since they add to a meal pattern, often not substituting for any usual food, they generally represent a net addition to intake. One of the most successful behavioral changes brought about by advertising has been in the response to thirst: today when someone is thirsty, they tend to think of opening a refrigerator and a can or bottle rather than opening the tap. The net infusion of calories into Americans by the substitution of sweetened beverages for water is astounding (net per capita annual consumption in the U.S. is now 600 cans/year! [Calloway 1981]). The other aspect of food merchandising of increasing importance is the promotion of fast food chains. While the food provided in these establishments is certainly not harmful *per se*, the limited choice often makes it difficult or impossible to choose a moderate calorie, low fat, moderate bulk meal, which is still a possibility in most regular restaurants. Furthermore, published information on the number of hamburgers, etc., sold suggests that such food has become a staple rather than a "treat" for a large number of Americans.

An extremely important component of our understanding of U.S. attitudes toward obesity is the diet industry. This industry, which includes publishing (books, magazines), foods, drugs, salons and fat farms, and a variety of other gimmicks, has been described as being one of the biggest industries in the U.S., worth over $10 billion in 1973 (Allon 1975). One need only look at the amount of advertising space devoted to solutions to obesity to realize what an enormous impact this industry has on our awareness of the problem. For example, in some months virtually every issue of womens' magazines available in grocery stores has a new diet or exercise regimen that promises to eliminate many pounds per week or unsightly bulges (see Table II). It is difficult not to continually appraise one's need for such advice with constant exposure to the magazines. Even people not purchasing such magazines are still confronted by the headlines and the message that obesity is an issue of overwhelming importance. In this situation, we see a positive feedback loop in operation. Having helped to create a market, the magazines must continue to complete with each other in that market. And since diets by and large do not work as well as suggested (and the readers blame themselves or the particular diet but do not question the importance of the issue) the market is perpetual. Diet plans become expendable commodities rather than permanent purchases, and thus the market does not become saturated.

TABLE II
Headlines on Magazine Covers: March, 1981*

Journal	Headline
Woman's Day	"Eating to Live Longer"
Cosmopolitan	"Wasting Away: Why You Can Be Too Thin" (followed by "Instant Pasta Magic")
Family Circle	"Exclusive Diet and Exercise Plan from Weight Watchers' New Spa"
Ladies Home Journal	"New! 2-Week Diet from Weight Watchers"
Good Housekeeping	"How I Lost 125 lbs." (followed by "Special Treat Cookbook: Fancy but Easy Main Dishes and Desserts")
US	"Lose 30 lbs. on the New Swimsuit Diet"
Harper's Bazaar	"Dr. Linn's Shortcut Shape-up Diet: Lost 7 lbs. in 7 Days" (also: "Drink Wine and Live Longer – Special Health Report")
People	"The Diet Doc Killing"
Glamour	"The Diet/Binge Seesaw: How I Got Off"
Redbook	"Try Our New Money Diet" (an article about saving money)
New Woman	"An Amazingly Simple Way to Lose 10 lbs. Without Dieting"
Globe	"8-Meals-A-Day Diet: The Easy Way to Lose 12 lbs."
National Enquirer	(none, but there is usually a story about a dieting star)
Star	(none, but previous week covered Liz Taylor's most recent diet)

* This list includes every magazine that was available in the check-out aisle area of a major food chain supermarket, except for news magazines.

In the case of other kinds of products, autos for example, we understand quite clearly how advertisements and other aspects of media coverage create a demand which is then met by the producers. The same economic, symbolic, and cultural forces are at work in regards to body shape and weight reduction behavior. In this case, I suggest, the demand that has been created is for a body shape unattainable by most individuals given basic biological realities and the other aspects of American lifestyle that govern overall caloric intake and energy output.

Synthesis

What implications does this type of analysis have for health care providers? First, it suggests that clinical concerns are shaped not only by carefully collected bio-medical data but also by the cultural milieu. The Metropolitan standards have been accepted with fewer questions and countervailing data have been ignored more consistently than can be explained on purely scientific grounds. Health care providers are good members of their cultures, and respond to the same general societal forces as their clients. The same is also true of biomedical researchers, who structure their research according to assumptions and grant allocations, the politics of which accord with those of the granting bodies.

A number of incongruities should have raised our suspicions about the purely medical nature of the perceived problem of obesity. First, while the risks associated with obesity are usually discussed in relation to heart disease, this is primarily a health hazard for men, and most of the concern with dieting is among women. Second, the "problem" is a virtually intractable one, and the lack of success of most regimes tried might begin to suggest that the problem is as much in the definition of the problem as in the treatment. Third, concern with obesity is supported by enormous industries — both diet and advertising — which thrive on its continued existence. This thorough integration of the supposedly treatable problem into the economic structure makes it suspect. Fourth, obesity is imbued with considerable social meaning — the stigma of obesity, its reflection on personality, etc. Each of these four factors alone is associated with other conditions, but the combination suggests that this situation may be in a different realm, more of a cultural issue than a biomedical one.

One aspect of the emphasis on dieting which is interesting is its relationship to American ideals of equality and democracy. We have been faced in this country with adjusting to many kinds of plurality — racial, ethnic, religious, gender, age, even sexual preference — about which we want to avoid discrimination, because presumably the categories are immutable. A person "can't help" being black, or female, or gay. Body shape, however, would appear to be something which is infinitely modifiable, given the "right" combination of diet, exercise, reducing machines, and so forth. Thus, theoretically any person can choose how to look, can change at any time, and therefore it is fair to judge them based on their current condition. Perhaps this is the reason it is almost imperative for many women to be perpetually and publicly on a diet even though their body shape may remain stable for long periods. They are sending the message that their ideals conform, even if their bodies do not.

Dealing with obesity is a special problem for health professionals. First, health professionals have been well socialized into mainstream culture and their training has often included little or no attention to social and cultural factors. In many ways, they operate with the same biases as our entering nutrition students. Second, health professionals as a group may be more likely to be the type of people who have learned to deny themselves things — free time, vacations, sleep — because of the nature of the demands of the educational process they go through and of the job situations which they encounter. Thus they may lack patience with evidence of behavior that they consider indulgent, that is, with obesity. They may also be, by their training, more likely to believe what they read of the negative consequences of any particular behavior or body type and less likely to believe contradictory evidence. They are accustomed to thinking in terms of "disease," and in the recent past a number of former moral flaws (e.g., alcoholism, drug addiction) have become labelled as diseases (Engel 1977; Fabrega 1975). (Perhaps it is more relevant that some conditions formerly labelled "diseases" have moved into other categories through the conscious effort of the individuals "afflicted", for example, homosexuality and physical handicaps.) It is by an extension of the disease concept that editorials are written such as one in a recent issue of Medical Tribune entitled "Operation Obesity: A National Challenge" (Lasagna 1980) which calls for a "national commitment to correct a derangement, control of which has prophylactic and therapeutic import for millions of Americans" (see also Bray 1979). I would suggest that we need to look very carefully at social impact and economic issues before using the Metropolitan Life Insurance Weight for Height standards (which Lasagna uses as evidence of the epidemic) to define over a third of the adult U.S. population as "sick".

Summary of the Obesity Problem

Clearly, the preceding discussion has only begun to explore the myriad of relevant social and cultural issues surrounding body shape and dieting in this society. Those mentioned might be visualized schematically as in Figure 2, a modification and

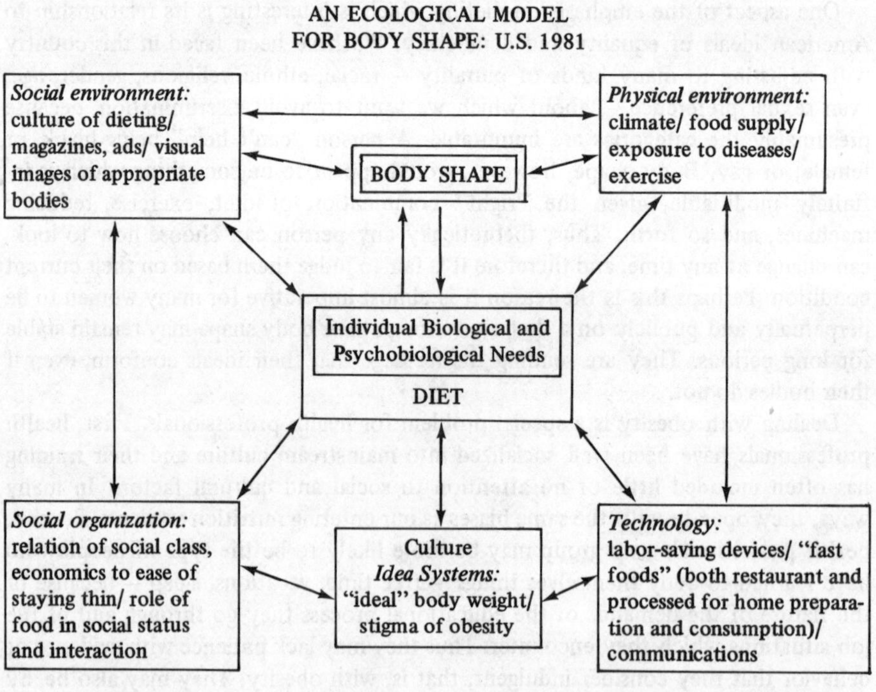

AN ECOLOGICAL MODEL
FOR BODY SHAPE: U.S. 1981

Fig. 2. A modification of Figure 1 to illustrate interactions of some of the components affecting body shape.

elaboration of Figure 1. Yet this paper has not addressed, for example, the great difference within the U.S. between ethnic groups in their beliefs and behaviors regarding obesity, nor the differing impacts of the visual representations of appropriate body shape on different age and sex groups. This whole topic has been little discussed in the literature, although there are a few excellent articles (Allon 1975; Tobias and Gordon 1980; Hirsch 1975; Dwyer and Mayer 1975).

APPENDIX

PREREQUISITE TEST: NUTRITION

1. Define "food fad".
2. Define Recommended Dietary Allowance (RDA). Include in the definition the segment of the population for whom the RDA is applicable.
3. What are the calories per gram of: (a) carbohydrate; (b) vitamin; (c) fat.
4. Name the fat soluble vitamins.
5. Name two macrominerals.
6. How is weight loss achieved? For a dieter, what is the recommended weight loss (in pounds) per week?
7. Define "lactose intolerance".
8. Nutrients are classified in six groups. Name the groups and each group's general function.
9. In general, nutrients function in the body: as a source of to promote and in of body processes.
10. Name the Basic 4 food groups. Give the recommended number of servings per day for each group.
11. What are the differences, generally, between protein from plant and from animal sources?
12. The following is a list of deficiency diseases. Describe the symptoms of the disease and name the nutrient in short supply. (1) xerophthalmia; (2) rickets; (3) scurvy; (4) goiter; (5) kwashiorkor.
13. Is cholesterol a fat: yes or no?
14. Define "calorie".
15. What percent overweight is considered "obese"?
16. Name three high carbohydrate foods and three carbohydrate-free foods.
17. Name at least one factor to be considered when determining if a child should be breast- or bottle-fed.

PREREQUISITE TEST: ANTHROPOLOGY

1. Define the term "culture" as used by anthropologists.
2. For the following terms, provide the definition as used in anthropology, and two examples. One example should apply to this country, and one should be from the reading when appropriate.

(a) cultural relativism; (b) ethnocentrism; (c) enculturation; (d) endogamy; (e) genotype

3. For each of the following social categories, give an example which demonstrates its effect on food choice. Explain each example.

4. Define the term "taboo". Name two common American food taboos (these items should be considered appropriate food elsewhere). Name two religious food taboos and the associated religions.

5. Define the term "adaptation" as used in anthropology. Give an example of a biological adaptation and an example of a cultural adaptation.

Case A

At the Indian Health Service Clinic, a physician has just examined Mrs. Homer, who complained that she "just wasn't feeling well". Mrs. Homer is a 35-year old full-blooded American Indian. Clinic records show that she is 158 cm. tall; today she weighed 73 kg.

She has 5 children and has become diabetic during each pregnancy. Her glucose tolerance returned to normal after the birth of each previous child, but it has not done so since the birth of her youngest, who is now 8 months old. The physician believes that Mrs. Homer's glucose tolerance is now "borderline".

Mrs. Homer lives in a small 2-room house on the reservation with her husband, her children, and her aunt. Their house has no indoor plumbing and is considered "sub-standard". Federal funding which was supposed to help the reservation build new housng has never come through.

Neither Mr. nor Mrs. Homer is employed, so there is little money coming into the household. Most of the Homer family's food is purchased at the reservation store. Mrs. Homer dislikes buying food there but their only income is in the form of goods the trader at the store gives in exchange for craft items they make. They also receive surplus commodity foods. Neither Mrs. Homer nor her husband knows much about any wild plants available that they might eat to supplement their diets, though an anthropologist visiting the reservation recently did ask them about wild foods.

Mrs. Homer is frightened about being a diabetic, since her mother died from complications of diabetes several years ago.

1. What is the distribution of adult-onset diabetes among American Indians?

2. What is the distribution of obesity among American Indians?

3. Describe the living conditions on her Indian reservation, including physical environment, employment, education. Describe the economic situation and programs of the tribe.

4. What is Mrs. Homer's diet likely to be? What has her diet history been? What are the social, cultural, and economic factors affecting her diet?

5. How would you counsel her to change her diet? Why? Be sure to take into account:

    (a) Availability of foods.
    (b) Preferences.
    (c) Motivation.

6. Discuss her prognosis without dietary modification.
7. What organizational or policy changes could help avert or ease similar problems for others?

Case B

The outreach worker at a congregate meal site (Nutrition Program for the Elderly) in a small rural town is responsible for seeing that the program attracts those people who need it the most. She has found several older people who are reluctant to participate although she is sure their cupboards are nearly bare. The following case is an example:

Mrs. Wilson is 75 years old and lives in a small rented house on the edge of town. She finished the 8th grade and has been a housewife all her life. Her husband was a janitor at the local grade school, but he died several years ago leaving her to live on a small savings account and her monthly social security check. She does not have a car because she doesn't drive, so getting to the store is a problem. A friend takes her along shopping once a month and she can walk to a nearby small grocery store where the food is expensive. She used to have a small garden, but she doesn't have enough energy now to keep it up. She rarely sees her old friends, many of whom are now gone or confined to their homes. Her appetite is not very good and she has lost interest in food preparation with only one person to cook for. Consequently, she uses what little money she has to buy things that are easy to eat and require little preparation.

Mrs. Wilson's record shows that she is underweight and that she is mildly bothered by diverticulosis for which the doctor suggested she eat a bland diet when she last saw him six years ago. She hasn't been to the doctor since because she doesn't like to go to the doctor and hasn't been really sick. She has a vague feeling that she is not up to par and would see the doctor if she didn't have to watch her money so carefully.

The outreach worker has tried to get Mrs. Wilson to come to the Senior Citizen Center for the meals and activities, but she has refused in spite of urging, saying she doesn't need the meal.

As the nutritionist for the county Nutrition Program for the Elderly, you are responsible for seeking a solution to this problem.

1. Describe the food behavior patterns that are typical of an older person like Mrs. Wilson.
2. Discuss the ways in which her eating habits might be related to diverticulosis. Discuss the therapeutic diet the physician prescribed. What would he advise today? How might she respond?
3. Discuss the possible reasons for Mrs. Wilson's reluctance to participate in the program.

4. How has the Nutrition Program for the Elderly affected the lives and health of American citizens since 1974?
5. What are your suggestions for solving the problem? How would you make them work?
6. What policy or organizational changes would you recommend?

PICA

(1) *Definition*: the regular consumption of non-food items, or of foods in an abnormal way; the most common forms are clay-eating (geophagia) and starch-eating.

(2) *Distribution*: Geophagia is practiced all over the world, often as a nutritional supplement or medicament (e.g., Maalox, Kaopectate are marketed U.S. examples). Starch-eating is predominantly a U.S. phenomenon. Many other unusual substances are consumed today in the U.S.; the best examples published involved pregnant women (See Snow and Johnson 1978; Lackey 1978).

(3) *Cultural history*: (See Hunter 1973). There is a widespread trade network in sub-Saharan Africa to manufacture, distribute, and market uniformly and distinctively shaped geophagical clays. These are mined from the sub-soil zone, where the minerals leached from the thin tropical soils above have been concentrated. Analyzed clays have shown no evidence of toxic minerals; they have high concentrations of required minerals. Apparently slaves transported to the U.S. continued this practice with the available local clays that looked or tasted similar to preferred African ones. Urban migrant Blacks within the U.S. South continued to receive gifts of clay sent from home; migration to the North led to the replacement of clay-eating by starch-eating. Argo Laundry Starch is particularly valued for its crunchy/slippy taste, and the sweet taste that remains in the mouth after eating it. It's eaten to relieve general stress, and particularly during pregnancy. Clay eating is also common among Mexican-Americans who may eat "beneficial little jars" of unfired clay; in Mexico, the clay is often taken from the churchyard (often an ancient burial ground) and is therefore high in calcium.

(4) *Nutrition problem*: Clay and starch eating are associated with iron-deficiency anemia, but it is not known which is the cause, which is consequence, or if the association is coincidental. Some clays do bind iron, especially if eaten at the same time as iron-rich foods. Starch has many calories, but no other nutrients, thus it may replace iron-rich foods in the diet (Ansell and Wheby 1972).

(5) *The Conflict: What should the health care provider do*?: Geophagia and starch-eating and other forms of pica are usually considered normal by informants themselves, but they recognize that these practices are frowned upon by the health professionals, who in fact consider them bizarre and in need of correction. Thus the information about consumption is often not sought, and is certainly not volunteered. When is consumption of these non-food items a problem? A benefit? Neutral? And what is the appropriate role for the health provider?

INFANT FEEDING: ISSUES IN THE UNITED STATES

(1) *Background information*: Human milk is a species-specific product, apparently adapted to the needs of the growing human infant. It provides nutrition, anti-infective properties, and direct drug action. The composition, in comparison with that of other mammals, suggests that it is for an infant who nurses very frequently and who has relatively slow body growth compared with brain growth. The milk is available in a positive-feedback loop, in which increased demand leads to increased supply. The composition changes during a feed (higher fat content at the end may be related to satiety), through the day, and as the infant matures. When everything works "properly", human milk alone should provide adequate food for the first 6–9 months of the infant's life. Milk available to the infant is mediated by two hormones released by the pituitary. Prolactin, which controls production, is affected by number of feeds and strength of infant's suckling. Oxytocin, which stimulates the milk ejection reflex, is strongly affected by central nervous system factors, and its release can be inhibited by stress and anxiety. (Jelliffe and Jelliffe 1978a and b).

(2) *History of infant feeding*: The traditional pattern was true demand feeding, with the infant carried by the mother, and the breast continuously available day and night. Nursing continued for two to three years or until the next pregnancy; solids were introduced gradually beginning in measurable quantities around six months. Records for the Middle East and Europe suggest that women have been trying to find alternatives since at least the Egyptian dynastic period, including use of special containers for artificial feeds and wet nurses for those who could afford them.

(3) *Nutrition issue: The infant should receive optimal nutrition.* When the mother can successfully breast-feed the infant for an extended period, this is the most desirable state. However, not all infants grow "adequately" on their mother's milk alone — are the standards wrong or is the milk "inadequate"? Infants are known to grow "well" on infant formula. But allergies and infections (especially diarrhea) are more common among formula-fed infants. Does breast-feeding improve mother-infant bonding? If so, how important is it? In spite of the pro-breast-feeding recommendations, what practices of the health profession hinder it — prenatally, in the hospital, postnatally (pediatrician)? What about breast milk contaminants? (Aykroyd 1977; Cunningham 1977; Jelliffe and Jelliffe 1978a and b; Mosher 1980; Sauls 1979).

(4) *Cultural issues*: How do the sexual symbolism of the breast and standards of public modesty affect women's decisions to breast-feed? Infants are unwelcome in many public settings in the adult-centered U.S. society. What role does employment play in making breast-feeding difficult, including lack of paid nursing leave, nursing breaks, or child care in the place of employment? How much does the infant lose through a mixed formula/breast strategy? How has the loss of female-transmitted

information on the common problems and solutions regarding breast-feeding affected success, including the "hostile mother-in-law" effect? How many women experience insufficient milk syndrome? What are its causes? What does the experience do to the mother in terms of guilt, disappointment? (Gussler and Briesemeister, 1980; Niehoff and Meister, 1972; Jelliffe and Jelliffe, 1978b).

(5) *The conflict*: What do you recommend to the future mother? How hard do you push toward breast-feeding? What factors do you include in your analysis? How much does feeding mode really matter? How can you best support her in her decision?

NOTES

1. This course was taught between 1976 and 1980 at Michigan State University, East Lansing, Michigan. A modified version of this course has also been presented by K. Kolasa, the nutrition co-professor, as an NSF Chatauqua-type short course entitled, "American Food and Nutrition Hassles."

REFERENCES

Ahlstrom, A. and L. Rasanen
  1973 Review of Food Grouping Systems in Nutrition Education. Journal of Nutrition Education 5: 1: 13.
Allon, N.
  1975 The Stigma of Overweight in Everyday Life. *In* George Bray (ed.), Obesity in Perspective, DHEW Publication # (NIH) 75–708, pp. 83–102.
Almy, T. P.
  1975 Evolution, Lactose Levels, and Global Hunger. New England Journal of Medicine 292: 1183–1184.
Andres, Reubin
  1980 Effect of Obesity on Total Mortality. Int. Journal of Obesity 4: 381–386.
Ansell, J. E. and M. S. Wheby
  1972 Pica – Its Relation to Iron Deficiency: A Review of the Recent Literature. Virginia Monthly 99: 951–954.
Aykroyd, W. R.
  1977 Is Breast-feeing Best for All Infants, Everywhere? Nutrition Today, Jan./Feb.: 15.
Barr, R. G. et al.
  1979 Recurrent Abdominal Pain in Childhood Due to Lactose Intolerance. New England Journal of Medicine 300: 26: 1449–1452.
Baylor, Byrd
  1972 Yes is Better Than No. New York: Charles Scribners and Sons. (Fictional account of an urban Papago woman in Tucson. Some preposterous events, but overall positive attitudes towards substantial body size are instructive.)
Beller, Anne Scott
  1977 Fat and Thin: A Natural History of Obesity. New York: McGraw Hill.
Bondy, Philip K.
  1980 Metabolic Obesity? New England Journal of Medicine 303: 18: 1057.
Bray, George A.
  1979 Obesity in America: An Overview of the Second Fogarty International Center Conference on Obesity. Int. Journal of Obesity 3: 363–375.

Calloway, Doris
    1981 Controversies about Nutrition. Paper presented at the Nutrition Update Conference, University of Arizona, Tucson, Arizona, 5 March, 1981.

Chowdhury, A. et al.
    1977 Malnutrition, Menarche and Marriage in Rural Bangladesh. Social Biology 24: 316–320.
    1978 Postpartum Amenorrhea: How is it Affected by Maternal Nutritional Status? Science 200: 1155–1157.

Cunningham, C.
    1977 Morbidity in Breast-fed and Artificially Fed Infants. Journal of Pediatrics 90: 726–729.

DeLuise, M., G. L. Blackburn, and J. S. Flier
    1980 Reduced Activity of the Red-cell Sodium-potassium Pump in Human Obesity. New England Journal of Medicine 303: 18: 1017–1022.

Donald, P., C. C. Pitts, and S. L. Pohl
    1981 Body Weight and Composition in Laboratory Rats: Effects of Diets with High or Low Protein Concentrations. Science 211: 185–186.

Dugdale, A. E. and P. R. Payne
    1977 Pattern of Lean and Fat Deposition in Adults. Nature 266: 349–351.

Dwyer, J. and J. Mayer
    1975 The Dismal Condition: Problems Faced by Obese Adolescent Girls in American Society. In G. Bray (ed.), Obesity in Perspective. DHEW Publication # (NIH) 75–708.

Edson, L.
    1979 Babies in Poverty – the Real Victims of the Breast/bottle controversy. The Lactation Review 4: 1: 21–38.

Ellison, Peter T.
    1981 Threshold Hypotheses, Developmental Age, and Menstrual Function. American Journal of Physical Anthropology 54: 337–340.

Engel, G. L.
    1977 The Need for a New Medical Model: A Challenge for Biomedicine. Science 196: 129–135.

Fabrega, Horacio
    1975 The Need for an Ethnomedical Science. Science 189: 969–975.

Farb, P. and G. Armelagos
    1980 Consuming Passions: The Anthropology of Eating. Boston: Houghton Mifflin Company.

Fitzgerald, T. K.
    1976 Nutrition and Anthropology in Action. Assen, Netherlands: Van Gorcum and Company.

Food and Nutrition Board, NRC, NAS
    1980a Staff Report: The New Recommended Dietary Allowances (RDAs). Reproduced In Nutrition Today, September/October, 1979.
    1980b Toward Healthful Diets. (Published as Pamphlet.) Reproduced In Nutrition Today, May/June: 7–11, 1980.

Frisch, R. E.
    1974 Menstrual Cycles: Fatness as a Determinant of Minimum Weight for Height Necessary for Their Maintenance and Onset. Science 185: 949–951.
    1978 Population, Food Intake and Fertility. Science 199: 22–30.

Goodenough, W. H.
    1963 Cooperation in Change. New York: Russell Sage Foundation.

Greene, L. and F. Johnston
    1980 Social and Biological Predictors of Nutritional Status, Growth, and Development. New York: Academic Press.

Gussler, J. D. and L. H. Briesemeister
  1980 The Insufficient Milk Syndrome: A Biocultural Explanation. Medical Anthropology
       4: 2: 140–164.
Haas, J. D. and G. G. Harrison
  1977 Nutritional Anthropology and Biological Adaptation. Annual Review of Anthro-
       pology 6: 69–101.
Harper, A.
  1980 Critique of the British Prescription. Nutrition Today, September/October: 28–29.
Harrison, G. G.
  1975 Primary Adult Lactose Deficiency: A Problem in Anthropological Genetics. American
       Anthropologist 77: 4: 812–835.
Harrison, G. G. and C. Ritenbaugh
  1981 Anthropology and Nutrition: A Perspective on Two Scientific Subcultures. Federa-
       tion Proceedings 40: 11: 2595–2600.
Henry, Jules
  1965 Culture Against Man. New York: Random House.
Hirsch, J.
  1975 The Psychological Consequences of Obesity. In G. Bray (ed.), Obesity in Perspective.
       DHEW Publication # (NIH) 75–708.
Hunter, J.
  1973 Geophagy in Africa and in the United States: A Culture-Nutrition hypothesis. Geog.
       Review 63: 170–195.
Jelliffe, D. B. and E. F. P. Jelliffe
  1975 Human Milk, Nutrition, and the World Resource Crisis. Science 188: 557–559.
  1978a The Volume and Composition of Human Milk in Poorly Nourished Communities: A
       Review. Americal Journal of Clinical Nutrition 31: 492–515.
  1978b Human Milk in the Modern World. New York: Oxford University Press.
Jerome, N. W.
  1980 Diet and Acculturation: The Case of Black American In-migrants. In N. Jerome,
       R. Kandel, and G. Pelto (eds.), Nutritional Anthropology. Pleasantville, New York:
       Redgrave.
  1981 U.S. Dietary Pattern from an Anthropological Perspective. Food Technology 35: 2:
       37–41. (This volume includes a symposium on related topics.)
Johnson, R. C., R. E. Cole, and F. M. Ahern
  1981 Genetic Interpretation of Racial/Ethnic Differences in Lactose Absorption and
       Tolerance: A Review. Human Biology 53: 1: 1–13.
Katz, S. H., M. L. Hediger, L. S. Vallery
  1974 The Anthropological and Nutritional Significance of Traditional Maize Processing
       Techniques in the New World. Science 184: 765–773.
Keys, Ancel B.
  1980a Overweight, Obesity, Coronary Heart Disease, and Mortality: The W. O. Atwater
       Memorial Lecture, Western Hemisphere Nutrition Congress VI in Los Angeles,
       August 11, 1980. Reprinted In Nutrition Today, July/August: 16–22, 1980.
  1980b Seven Countries: A Multivariate Analysis of Death and Coronary Heart Disease.
       Cambridge, Mass.: Hartford University Press.
Kolasa, K.
  1978 I Won't Cook Turnip Greens if You Won't Cook Kielbasa: Food Behavior of Polonia
       and Its Health Inplications. In E. Bauwens (ed.), The Anthropology of Health. St.
       Louis: Mosby.
Lackey, Carolyn J.
  1978 Pica – A Nutritional Anthropology Concern. E. Bauwens (ed.), In the Anthropology
       of Health. St. Louis: Mosby.

Larsson, B., P. Björntorp, and G. Tibblin
   1981 The Health Consequences of Moderate Obesity. International Journal of Obesity 5:
      97–116.
Lasagna, L.
   1980 Operation Obesity: A National Challenge. Medical Tribune, October 1. (This is an
      extreme example of the "obesity as illness" viewpoint. Other such examples are prob-
      ably readily available in current newspapers or magazines.)
Lebenthal, E.
   1979 Lactose Malabsorption and Milk Consumption in Infants and Children. American
      Journal Dis. Child. 133: 1: 21–30.
Louderback, L.
   1970 Fat Power: Whatever you Weigh is Right. New York: Hawthorne.
Lovejoy, Owen C.
   1981 The Origin of Man. Science 211: 341–350.
Mahan, L. K.
   1981 Obesity: New Knowledge and Current Treatments. In B. S. Worthington-Roberts
      (ed.), Contemporary Developments in Nutrition. St. Louis: Mosby.
Margen, S. and R. Ogar (eds.)
   1978 Progress in Human Nutrition, Volume 2. Westport, Connecticut: Avi Publishing
      Company.
McCracken, Robert
   1971 Lactose Deficiency: An Example of Dietary Evolution. Current Anthropology 12:
      479–517.
Mitchell, J. D., J. Brand, and T. Halbisch
   1977 Weight Gain Inhibition by Lactose in Australian Aboriginal Children. Lancet 1: 500–
      505.
Mosher, M. R. and G. Moyer
   1980 PCB's and Breast Milk. Nutrition Action, November: 10–13.
Newman, Russell W.
   1975 Human Adaptation to Heat. In A. Damon (ed.), Physiological Anthropology. New
      York: Oxford University Press.
Niehoff, A. and N. Meister
   1972 The Cultural Characteristics of Breast-feeding. Journal of Trop. Ped. and Environ.
      Child Health 18: 1: 16–20.
Nimrod, A. and K. J. Ryan
   1975 Aromatization of Androgens by Human Abdominal and Breast Fat Tissue. Journal
      of Clinical Endocrinology and Metabolism 40: 376–372.
Olson, Robert E.
   1980 Statement to the House Agriculture Committee on Domestic Marketing, Consumer
      Relations, and Nutrition. Reproduced In Nutrition Today, May/June: 12–19, 1980.
Paige, D. M., T. M. Bayless, and G. G. Graham
   1977 Milk Programs: Helpful or Harmful to Negro Children? American Journal of Public
      Health 62: 11: 1486.
Passmore, R., D. Hollingsworth, and J. Robertson
   1980 Prescription for a Better British Diet. Nutrition Today, September/October: 23–
      37.
Pelto, G. H., N. W. Jerome, and R. F. Kandel
   1980 Methodological Issues in Nutritional Anthropology. In N. Jerome, R. Kandel, and
      G. Pelto (eds.), Nutritional Anthropology. Pleasantville, New York: Redgrave.
Quandt, Sara
   in press Changes in Post-partum Adiposity and Infant Feeding Patterns. American Journal of
      Physical Anthropology.

Raphael, Dana
    1980 Give Us Feeding Choices: Third World Women. And Move to Legislate Breast-Feeding
         Soon. (Also other articles.) The Lactation Review 5: 1: 1–4.
Ritenbaugh, Cheryl
    1980a Human Foodways: A Window on Evolution. In E. Bauwens (ed.), The Anthropology
          of Health. St. Louis: Mosby.
    1978b Model Course IV: Nutritional Anthropology. Medical Anthropology Newsletter 9: 2:
          23–29. Reprinted in H. Todd and J. Ruffini (eds.), Teaching Medical Anthropology,
          Washington, D.C.: Society for Medical Anthropology, 1979, pp. 41–53.
    1980a Review of Nutritional Anthropology, N. W. Jerome, R. F. Kandel, and G. H. Pelto
          (eds.), Pleasantville, New York: Redgrave. Ecology of Food and Nutrition 10: 125–
          126.
    1980b Review of Consuming Passions, P. Farb and G. Armelagos, Boston: Houghton Mifflin.
          Journal of Nutrition Education 13: 1: 33–34.
    1981 An Anthropological Perspective on Nutrition. Journal of Nutrition Education 13: 1:
         suppl. 1: 12–15.
Roberts, Derek F.
    1953 Body Weight, Race, and Climate. American Journal of Physical Anthropology 11:
         533–558.
Rorick, M. H. et al.
    1979 Comparative Tolerance of Elderly from Differing Backgrounds to Lactose-containing
         and Lactose-free Dairy Drinks: A Double-blind Study. Journal of Gerontology 34: 2:
         191–196.
Sauls, H. S.
    1979 Potential Effect of Demographic and Other Variables in Studies Comparing Morbidity
         of Breast-fed and Bottle-fed Infants. Pediatrics 64: 4: 523–527.
Simoons, F.
    1978 The Geographic Hypothesis and Lactose Malabsorption. A Weighing of the Evidence.
         American Journal Digestive Dis. 23: 11: 963–980.
Snow, L. F. and S. M. Johnson
    1978 Folklore, Food, and Female Reproductive Cycle. Ecology of Food and Nutrition 7:
         41–49.
Steegman, A. T., Jr.
    1975 Human Adaptation to Cold. In A. Damon (ed.), Physiological Anthropology. New
         York: Oxford University Press.
Tobias, A. and J. Gordon
    1980 Social Consequences of Obesity. Journal of the American Dietetics Association 76:
         4: 338–342.
USDA, USDHEW
    1980 Nutrition and Your Health: Dietary Guidelines for Americans. (Available as pamphlet)
         Reproduced in Nutrition Today, March/April: 14–18, 1980.

WITCH DOCTOR'S LEGACY: SOME ANTHROPOLOGICAL IMPLICATIONS FOR THE PRACTICE OF CLINICAL MEDICINE

The purpose of this paper is not to descry the faults of modern medicine while holding up the "witch doctor" or folk curer as a proper example of healer. My purpose, rather, is to raise some of the problems faced by biomedical practitioners as they represent a medical system which may fill only part of the healing needs of its patients. Where there is a problem, the fault does not lie with the individual physician or nurse, but rather in the disjuncture between medical and social or cultural systems. However, in that control over healing and allocation of health resources lies squarely in the hands of the practitioner and his science, I am arguing that the opportunity and responsibility for ameliorating the problem can only lie in these hands, rather than the patient's. We must begin with sensitizing the biomedical practitioner to the cultural and social concomitants of disease, and to the ways in which other types of healers (representing other types of systems) cope with them.

INTRODUCTION

It is not my goal to offer specific techniques for anthropological sensitization of clinical practitioners. There are too many variables involved in the process of teaching and applying anthropology within clinical and medical school settings. My purpose is to offer a set of arguments and general principles which can be used in either classroom or clinical teaching to impress upon medical students and clinical physicians the utility of anthropological insight in enhancing therapeutic relationships and medical outcome. In that our expertise lies with the symbolic, rather than somatic elements of disease and healing, it would seem that one of our major tasks involves achieving legitimacy for such symbolic phenomena in the eyes of biomedical practitioners. The other task involves the manner in which we translate our expertise into clinically relevant suggestions and interventions. This expertise is largely built upon a foundation of cross-cultural data and comparative analyses. All too often it is quite exotic in nature, and too bound to specific sub-cultures for general clinical application (particularly with "non-ethnic" patients). Needed are guidelines and suggestions for translating the lessons of exotica into examples and techniques for general use by clinical medicine.

The following is divided into two parts. The first discusses arguments for symbolic healing and cultural sensitivity that may be useful in persuading beginning clinical physicians to be sensitive to cultural phenomena. The second part attempts to derive generally applicable lessons for clinical practice from folk healers' styles and techniques. Because anthropologists are engaged in so wide a variety of clinical teaching roles, this paper is written as though directed less to them than to the

N. J. Chrisman and T. W. Maretzki (eds.), Clinically Applied Anthropology, 179–198.

clinical physician or staff member relatively unfamiliar with anthropological principles and examples.

I

In recent years there has been growing concern with biomedical care, motives, and effectiveness. Critics such as Illich (1976); Szasz (1962), Knowles (1977), Freidson (1971), Dubos (1950) and others join in condemning biomedicine's impersonality, pecuniarity, unintelligibility, monopoly, and downright ineffectiveness in many instances. Much is said of biomedicine's abandonment of concern for the "whole person". Definitions of the "whole person" vary wildly (not just widely), and include an array of elements from the mundane to the astrological. By and large, they revolve around the behavioral and symbolic/psyschological concomitants of disease – which many social scientists refer to as "illness".

Physicians who recognize the disease/illness distinction nonetheless tend usually to interpret "illness" in strictly behavioral terms – perhaps of interest in the reduction of anxiety, but of little relevance to the curing of the disease itself. In truth, of course, attending to the "illness" does far more than ameliorate anxiety and "behavioral" symptoms produced by the "real" (somatic) disease. The sensation of symptoms, the severity of disease, the decisions to seek professional care, the presentation of symptoms to the health professional, and the actual physical healing process are heavily affected by symbolic elements. This is the case regardless of the patient's ethnic background or social class.

Every patient – whether ethnic migrant or upper class majority member – conceptualizes and expresses sickness (both behaviorally and symptomatically) in a symbolically laden manner. Furthermore, *every* named and known disease comes equipped with an image and reputation that affects the sufferer's response in some manner or other. Colds, flu, hernias, hemorrhoids, arthritis, and high blood pressure have clear reputations and implications for sufferers. Cancer and TB are examples of diseases whose rich literary careers have significantly affected the public's response to health seeking and treatment (Sontag 1978). This response includes outright alteration of symptoms as well as stereotyped treatments and prognoses by physicians. Fabrega suggests that "the *bulk* of medical complaints that physicians practicing in *industrialized* nations are called upon to treat" are "subject to considerable cultural masking or distortion" (Fabrega 1972: 189; emphasis mine).

Now, culture is not merely a significant element in the sensation, identification, expression, and interpretation of symptoms. What can cause and shape symptoms may also significantly influence their remission. There is no reason to doubt that symbolic phenomena may affect the brain's ability to stimulate production and dispersal of chemicals such as interferon or endorphins. Nor is there reason to doubt that pain abatement induced by placebo effect is due to the production of endorphins via symbolic triggers. There is increasing evidence that symbolic stimuli may trigger biochemical mechanisms capable of diminishing cancer. Patients trained in imaging techniques may experience diminution or stabilization of malignant growth. Using biofeedback techniques, researchers have demonstrated the body's ability to produce specified brain waves, lower blood pressure, and stabilize heart beat (cf. Blanchard and Young 1974; Kamiya 1976/77). All of these internal body changes are induced via conscious thought — that is, via symboling, which is a 100% cultural act.

Moerman has recently suggested that "The symbolic component of [medical] treatment is significant" (Moerman 1979: 60). Some studies, he argues, have demonstrated that a placebo is fully 30 to 60% as effective as an active medication (Moerman 1979: 62). Thus, he reasons, perhaps half the effectiveness of *any* medication may be due to what he calls "general medical treatment" — i.e., symbolic concomitants of the healing act. The remaining half is due to "specific medical treatment" by the active medication or manipulation (Moerman 1979: 63). His conclusion is that "the *form* of medical treatment can be effective medical treatment" (Moerman 1979: 62). Kleinman and Sung speak of the phenomenon of "cultural healing" which occurs automatically when any medical system gets to work by defining the disease, mobilizing defenses and administering treatment (1979). At the same time, of course, the patient must have some degree of receptivity to the symbolic elements of the system. Small wonder that many ethnics in U.S. cities still exhibit minimal or tentative commitment to biomedicine, and are thus less receptive to biomedical treatment (cf. Weidman 1978: 848ff; Schensul and Bymel 1975).

It cannot be reiterated enough that cultural healing and symbolic manifestation of disease are characteristic of *all* human episodes of sickness. Middle and upper class WASPS, Jews, or Catholics, no less than Cambodian, Chicano, or Haitian migrants, *always* clothe their diseases in symbolic dress, and are *always* susceptible to symbolic stimuli — both as cause and as aid to cure. Thus it is that the realm of medical anthropological insight embraces far more than the exotic or variant migrant and his odd health beliefs and behaviors.

How can the physician or other biomedical health practitioner be sensitized to the cultural/symbolic aspects of health and illness, modify customary techniques accordingly, and enhance both general and specific healing?

II

Some suggestions require the physician to become an ethnographer, highly knowledgeable about the health beliefs of various ethnic groups (Stein 1979). While there is nothing wrong with the basic idea of such sensitivity, in practice it is impossible to implement. The physician would need advanced training in anthropology, including the ultimate sensitizer of field work requiring intensive interaction with a culture distinct from his own. Furthermore, in an ethnically mixed patient constituency, the clinician would ideally need to be familiar with the health beliefs of a number of distinct groups. Clearly, this is too unrealistic an expectation.

General sensitization of physicians to cultural health differences is difficult for another reason. Aside from rather obvious phenomena such as ethnic heterogeneity, the biomedical paradigm simply does not have a ready place in it for cultural input to health and medical practice. Certainly, the concept of "bedside manner" and frequent references (in literature and teaching) to the "art" of medicine (i.e., the subjective, interpersonal aspects of physician-patient interaction) tell the clinician that behavioral elements are important to health delivery. But these are generally expressed in terms of paternalistic, "gentle insistence" on the physician's part when dealing with patients. This art or manner is something the doctor learns "on the job" that contributes to medical personality.

The confusion — and equation — of the traditional art of bedside manner in medicine with *cultural* sensitivity is common. When delivering a lecture to first-year medical students I was assured by them that they were perfectly capable of developing the required sensitivity to patients' cultural and symbolic needs. "A little practice" was all that is required. Good will, "compassion", and "understanding" could be developed by anyone, and a Ph.D. in Anthropology was certainly not necessary — nor special training of any length, for that matter. At another medical school, I was told by first-year students that medicine "naturally selects individuals who are more sensitive to interpersonal aspects of health." That this is reinforced by their subsequent training is indicated by the paucity of cultural-sensitizing courses (or even modules) in medical school curricula.

Physicians as a group tend to share common modes of logic, and sets of priorities distinct from those of their patients. By and large, physicians are recruited from a fairly homogeneous sociocultural pool. This is true in almost all nations. The middle to upper class majority (whether white, brahmin, latino, ruling tribe, etc.) provide the bulk of physicians. They bring to their calling a view of family life, of social behavior, of achievement, of conformity to majority standards, and of acceptance of the industrial world view that clearly colors their approach to medicine. Often, this means that physicians are as ignorant of the variants within their own culture as they are of significantly different cultural traditions.

Lorraine Zimmerman (personal communication), for example, reports that most of her medical students who specialize in family practice bring with them to medical school an idealistic view of the American family as a whole, warm, supportive unit whose atmosphere neatly augments the physician's ministrations and promotes a context of healing. When she attempts to inform them of the fact that a significant portion of adult Americans do *not* live in families (singles, divorcees), and that many families are not whole (due to abandonment, death, divorce, unmarried pregnancies, etc.), and that many "whole" families are anything but warm and supportive units — barely a fifth believe her. One can easily imagine the depth of the difficulty faced when these practitioners must deal with patients from significantly different cultural traditions.

After all that has been said, therefore, how can the physician amend the *form* of his practice of medicine so that cultural/symbolic elements of healing are enhanced? General principles are fine — such as the charge to "be sensitive to the cultures of your patients" — but how is this to be put into operation? There is, of course, a relatively large body of literature on the health beliefs and practices of a number of cultural and ethnic groups. Some good suggestions are available for treatment of Latino patients with strong hot-cold food beliefs. If, for example, your patient believes that diarrhea is a "cold" disease, and that penicillin is a "cold" — and therefore inappropriate — medicine, then by dissolving penicillin in a "hot" substance (such as orange juice or chocolate), the ostensible exacerbating effects of penicillin's "coldness" can be moderated (Logan 1973). But this is a highly specific phenomenon. It may be meaningless to many Latinos who were raised with different hot/cold beliefs, or none at all. And other ethnics may refuse penicillin for entirely different reasons. Similarly, it might be useful to know that lowerclass Colombians, who believe that Tuesdays and Fridays are especially propitious for healing acts, would likely experience enhanced peace of mind — and perhaps enhanced healing as well — if surgery were scheduled on these days. Some blacks believe that a menstruating woman may become ill if she is exposed to cold or gets wet. Snow suggests that hospitalized women with such beliefs will experience less anxiety if they are not required to bathe while menstruating (Snow 1974: 95). But again, unless the average U.S. physician deals regularly with Colombian, Mexican, or working class black patients, he has little need for such specific knowledge.

III

I believe that a useful guide to the enhancement of cultural healing lies in the role and general stylistic characteristics of the folk curer. I am not suggesting that curers themselves be utilized. This could (and indeed, has proved to be) practical where the patient constituency is largely mono-ethnic (Chicano, Puerto Rican, Navajo, etc.). However, in that all folk healers derive their paradigm and practice from specific cultural traditions, the use of such practitioners in culturally heterogeneous medical settings is inefficient. There is also the problem of recruitment. Most urban curers, for example, are not "formal" professionals, but rather neighborhood residents with part-time practice and limited clientele. The problem of locating and legitimizing curers for biomedical training or consultation becomes difficult.[1]

Unfortunately, wherever folk healers are employed within the biomedical framework, their skills and concepts are almost invariably limited to treatment of behavioral ("psychiatric") problems. Often, such "problems" represent simple noncompliance with the biomedical regimen. Ordinarily, folk curers are not allowed to treat *somatic* disorders, and it goes without saying that they are used almost exclusively for treatment of "ethnic" patients (an exception to the latter might be the utilization of faith healers and other non-ethnic curer types in a limited number of pain clinics). Where folk healers are employed by the biomedical establishment, it is usually in tribal reserve clinics or, less frequently, inner city mono-ethnic health centers. In such situations, *financial support* of curers is usually underwritten by grants or by the agency itself. Professional folk curers tend to charge for their services, and the costs can be high. Haitian *hungans* in Miami ask upwards of $50 for a consultation, and ritual paraphernalia (particularly in cases of suspected sorcery) may run into additional hundreds of dollars. Medical insurance will not recognize and reimburse expenses for most non-biomedical healers. Who, then, will underwrite the curer consult?

A more practical way of utilizing the folk curer's style is to derive certain general practical principles from this style, for use by biomedical personnel themselves in the clinical setting. Even where the stylistic or societal differences are too great to allow transfer or generalization, it can be argued that simple awareness of these differences can sensitize the biomedical practitioner to the critical limitations of our medical system and the roles that operate within it. Such sensitivity may help the practitioner mitigate some of the stresses built into the very soul of our health delivery paradigm and organization.

Anthropologists have long suggested or implied that appropriate sensitivity to symbolic/personal aspects of disease (i.e., the illness) is exhibited by folk curers. Much of the curer's pharmacopoeia and many physical techniques are not empirically effective in themselves. Thus, their utility is clearly enhanced when delivered in symbolic context. A number of curers have told me that at base, the efficacy of a treatment depends largely upon "whether the patient believes". Usually, the patient *does* believe, precisely because his medical system has evolved to maximize symbolic healing. All medical systems, furthermore, have developed etiological theories consonant with local world view, technological competencies, and social structure (cf. Press 1980). The healer — whether calling upon the help of the supernatural, performing a complex "sociopsy" designed to reveal the broken threads in the social fabric, gazing into a glass of water to endow it with his own grace, or reading the print-out of a blood-gas analysis — automatically reflects the cultural/symbolic functions of the medical system of which he is part.

Not all folk curers are highly personal in their approach to patients, or know the patient's own medical system well. Elsewhere, I have stressed that urban curers may be as impersonal as their biomedical counterparts (Press 1971). Furthermore — and this is a most significant point — the majority of *all* curers' patients (whether in tribal or urban settings) come with mundane somatic complaints (as opposed to supernatural or exotic "socio-ritual" problems): generalized chronic pains, arthritis, obesity, indigestion, fever, wounds, ulcers, sores, and whatnot. I am now convinced that the long personal interview by any curer in any setting is the exception, rather than rule, and that the folk curer's general efficacy lies in other, less exotic (though still symbolically significant) directions. Some of these directions may be consonant with the goals and capabilities of biomedical practitioners.

Though folk curers vary incredibly in etiological and technical approach, there are some stylistic elements which are fairly generalizable, and from which, coupled with our discussion thus far, we might derive insight to applications in biomedical practice.

(1) Folk curers share significant parts of their constituency's world view and health concepts. They share the patient's etiological beliefs, particularly insofar as these picture man and his health as bound to nature, community, cosmos, and other men.

Explanations of disease are meaningful to the patient at the patient's common level of understanding and experience. There are no sharp differences between patient and curer knowledge of, and labels for, parts of the body and categories of disease.

In peasant Mexico, for example, the division of diseases is typically broken down as follows:

(a) Natural diseases (arthritis; obseity; "liver"; "fallen fontanel"; get obstruction; "airs", etc.).

(b) Supernatural diseases (God's will; punishment of gods or God; Saint's will).

(c) Interpersonal diseases (sorcery; evil eye).

(d) Emotional diseases (susto; bilis. The former results from a fright or emotional shock; the latter from uncontrolled anger).

Though such clean categories are not overtly utilized by the peasants, the divisions are derivable from differential responses to their constituent ills. The point to be made here is that these categories reflect real-life concerns and experience. All have well-recognized causes and cures that most community members can name. Disease concepts and cures are developed from *within* the community, and *must* have meaning to the patient constituency in order to continue in the common repertoire of beliefs and practices. There are no other outside sources of knowledge or legitimacy for diagnoses and cures. Very frequently, curers take cues from the family about "desirable" diagnoses. Here they corroborate lay diagnosis, rather than produce unanticipated analyses of obvious or invisible symptoms. Fabrega (1971) finds little difference in healer and layman knowledge of disease categories, body parts, disease symptoms, and remedies. The difference, rather, lies in the curer's personal grace which (like the biomedical physician's state license to practice) legitimates his diagnoses and creates confidence in his ability to cure. He is thus the one to validate the family's suspicions of witchcraft or simple arthritis. Countermanding the family or patient's suspicions is ultimately self-defeating. Unlike the biomedical physician, folk curers have no external, independent mandate to practice. They are more susceptible to community opinion and must please their constituency. Their diagnoses and manner of cure must fit contemporary community morals and stresses. If working mothers and over-eager utilization of Anglo behaviors or contacts are frowned upon among Mexican American groups in Los Angeles or South Texas, then such phenomena can become causes of illness, and curers are quick to pick up cues from worried (threatened) parents and spouses (see Edgerton et al. 1970; Madsen 1964).

Implications for Biomedical Practitioners

It must be stressed again that lay people's ignorance of biomedical concepts does *not* mean lack of complex beliefs and patterned behaviors relating to disease and healing. Furthermore, the highly specialized training required of physicians precludes even the most educated or sophisticated of middle or upper class white "majority" patients from even approximating official biomedical knowledge. It can be argued that where patients can fit the disease and its explanation into their

personal world view, they will experience less anxiety and be more receptive to
treatment ("compliant"). Patients' explanatory models may be essential to their
general defense mechanisms. Thus, by reflecting acceptance (in part, whole, or in
principle) of the patient's explanatory model, and by recognizing the importance or
meaning of the illness to the patient and his family or community (as opposed to its
meaning for biomedicine) — the physician may be activating a powerful symbolic
tool for healing. Waitzkin (1979) provides a clinical example in which a patient
"believed that her chronic thrombophlebitis was caused by anesthesia that she had
undergone during a hysterectomy". The physician attempted to correct her by
insisting that it was more likely due to prolonged bed rest than to pentathol. Here,
the patient associates bed rest with healing and renewal, and would prefer not to
learn that it could be dangerous. Here, too, the physician assigns blame to the
patient (for being in bed, and perhaps not moving around enough). The patient
would obviously like the fault to lie elsewhere. To categorically deny the possible
effect of the anesthesia upon blood clotting is unnecessary, and possibly counter-
productive. While the physician is certainly under no obligation to agree with the
patient, it would seem that some satisfaction could be given by saying: "Well, it's
unlikely that the pentathol contributed to the phlebitis. It's more likely that in this
case the nurses were at fault for not getting you to move around and exercise more.
And if you don't like this anesthetic, maybe next time you're put under, we can use
a different kind". At Miami's Jackson Memorial Hospital, it is not uncommon to
find that a black diabetic has postponed biomedical treatment by self-treating his
"sweet blood" with oral doses of vinegar, lemon juice, or aloe (sour substances).
This belief and related practice is most logical (and deeply rooted) and must not be
ignored when attempting to explain insulin treatment and diet to the patient. Easy
as it is to deny the efficacy of lemon juice in reducing blood sugar, it is just as easy
to say that "it doesn't reduce the sweetness of the blood in a case like yours". An
unsweetened citrus beverage can even be written into the diet by the hospital dietician. Recall also Logan's previously-cited example of hot-cold beliefs and penicillin
use. *It must be stressed that the physician's job is not to defend or teach patients
the essentials of the biomedical paradigm.*

At the same time, physicians need not admit to the existence or efficacy of
sorcery, or God's will. Yet, where patients believe in these phenomena, it is not the
physician's job to deny them categorically. Distrust can result. There are two ways
of handling this problem. One is to take the supernatural or bizarre into account —
and then discount it. For example, a 16 year old Haitian boy was brought into
Miami/Jackson's emergency room with severe abdominal pain and blood in his
stools. It was soon determined that he had an ulcer. He, however, produced two
possible alternative explanations. His mother had diagnosed his problem as "fallen
sternum" and treated it with a poultice of orange leaves. He also entertained the
possibility that he was suffering from sorcery worked by a woman for whom he had
baby sat. He leaned toward the sternum explanation, yet worried about the sorcery.
He was successfully relieved of this worry by being assured that his problem "was
definitely not caused by the woman". Furthermore, while his symptoms "might be

similar" if his sternum had indeed fallen, it was "quite clear in this case that you have an ulcer". If his beliefs had been categorically denied by saying "there are no such diseases," he might have continued to worry about sorcery, or at the very least doubted the breadth of biomedicine's knowledge. And to have completely ignored his two explanations would not have resulted in lessened anxiety or positive mental attitude toward his treatment.

Another way to handle the supernatural or bizarre cause issue is to pass part of the buck. This is possible because medical systems which include supernatural cause frequently compartmentalize cure into two parts: removal of the supernatural cause and amelioration of somatic symptoms (the latter, often with medications). This allows a physician to say: "Well, I personally don't know anything about [sorcery; God's punishment; etc.] and I can't deal with it medically. If you think it's caused by it, we can call in a chaplain, or you'll have to go to a special curer to get rid of it. But I *can* cure the *symptoms* you're suffering from."

This approach can create considerable trust in the physician, and significantly ameliorate the image of cocky intolerance that many patients (with strong folk or religious beliefs) see in biomedical practitioners. It should be stressed that many patients have access to alternative healers (folk or otherwise), *do* use them concurrently with biomedical treatment, and frequently give credit for a cure to the alternative mode (cf. Creighton 1977). The more the physician "turns off" the patient by his attitude and intolerance, the more likely that alternative health resources will be utilized in the future.

(2) Folk curers generally accept behavioral and somatic symptoms as naturally co-occurring elements of a syndrome. The stress and anxiety that accompany disease are recognized and often formalized as "official" symptoms of a given ailment. The most heightened forms of anxiety, accompanied by the most alarming behavioral aberrations, frequently point to sorcery — thereby displacing culpability for such behavior to antisocial others. It is not unusual to find a single syndrome (again, most usually sorcery) reflected in symptoms of various extra-somatic systems. A sorcery victim in Bogota, Colombia complained to the curer that he had stomach pain; a snake was in his threat, curling around from behind; his sister was jealous of him; he had bad luck; and there was an owl constantly perched on his chimney. A teenage girl suffering from *duende* (possession by an evil spirit) exhibited amenorrhea, restlessness, catatonia, and typing pornographic statements with the family typewriter. In each case, all symptoms were of equal weight in determining a cause and cure. These are rather extreme cases, yet it is the rare stomach pain, chest congestion, or nose bleed that is not accompanied by some behavioral symptom. The curer may prescribe separate cures (while treating both behavioral and somatic symptoms as part of one syndrome) or treat both with a single act or medication (assuring the patient that all his problems will be reduced). It goes without saying that stigma and guilt of behavioral aberrations are minimized through treatment by a curer (cf. Maclean 1971: 79).

Implications for Biomedical Practitioners

No disease has wholly somatic consequences. Sickness may result in disruption of home life, established habits, interaction patterns, income, sexual behavior, and over all self-image. It may incur the resentment of family and friends called upon to perform unusual services. Or the sick person may impute such resentment even where none is exhibited. Regardless of the severity, illness can and does cause anxiety (thereby becoming a "behavioral" problem) in a society such as ours which places a premium upon youth, beauty, vigor, strength, independence, and winning. The wise physician must recognize our medical system's bias against the inclusion of all but a few standard behavioral symptoms (complaint about pain, inconvenience, quality of hospital service, etc.) as "normal".

Yet, if this is recognized then what? Unfortunately, the problem of how to deal with the "abnormal yet normal" behavioral concomitants of disease is one of the more difficult problems physicians face. Clinicians are quick to call for a psychiatric consult in cases where patients refuse treatment, express the desire to leave the hospital, or act in a "bizarre" manner. The delegation of such problems to psychiatry or the social worker can be a clear signal to the patient that he is suspected of being "emotionally" or "mentally" ill. The vast majority in our society know that "normal people" do *not* have to see such specialists. "Hey, what's going on here? — I'm not crazy!", is a common response to the liaison psychiatrist called in to evaluate the anxious or erractic patient in the cardiac care unit. Consults, therefore, should not be a first resort. A few minutes of sympathetic listening, and even postponement of treatment for a short time, can save anxiety and manpower. If the intern or resident "has no time for such handholding" (a popular and self-perpetuating myth in most teaching hospitals), then a medical student or nurse can spend the time. In most cases, less than five sympathetic minutes are required. Hospital chaplains are usually delighted to be called in for such consults, and are excellent nonstigmatic resources for anxious, non-compliant, frightened patients, or those preparing to leave "against medical advice".

The association of behavioral with somatic symptoms is not merely an "emotional" problem. Many somatic diseases are popularly believed to be linked to certain behavioral or emotional symptoms. Such beliefs can give patients license to behave in ways "appropriate" to the disease. Or — a matter of significance to the taking of the medical history — the presence of physical disease may be deduced by patients from the presence of the supposed accompanying behavioral symptoms. Hypertension provides a good example. Latino migrants to the U.S. (Cohen 1979: 167–168) as well as native middle class anglos (Blumhagen 1980) share a common belief that nervousness and ready loss of temper are symptomatic of hypertension. Cohen has noted that misleading histories can be obtained from Latino patients in response to the question of whether anyone else in the family has had hypertension. Affirmative answers have been given by patients who recall nervous and anger-prone relatives — individuals who were *never* clinically diagnosed as hypertensive (Cohen *ibid*). It is wise for the beginning clinician frequently to ask patients how they know they (or kinfolk) have had such and such disease in the past. Considerable insight can be gained into the manner in which behavior and emotions may be interpreted as symptomatic of physical problems.

(3) Curers in some areas may require the patient to spend time away from home while undergoing treatment, but the majority treat their clientele as outpatients. Many curers also make house calls.

Implications for Biomedical Practitioners

Quite apart from threats to self-image, etc., sickness can be downright inconvenient. Hospitalization can disrupt family operation and create snowballing logistic complications. Lower income patients are especially inconvenienced by hospitalization, insofar as they (a) may hold marginal jobs which offer no sick pay; (b) may have minor children at home with no spouse to care for them; and (c) may live in areas where shopping is not convenient for those who remain to care for the family.

Frequently, the clinician's decision to hospitalize a patient takes no note of the inconvenience of moving out of the home and into an institution at some distance away, while abandoning the family to others. (Sometimes there simply are no "others" — infants may be left in the care of 13 year old siblings, with the hope that neighbors or distant kin will follow through on promises to "look in once in a while".) Anxieties caused by the simple inconvenience of sickness may be quite sufficient to cause patients to leave against medical advice, or give staff a hard time. One way of avoiding or ameliorating this problem is to inquire of all patients, *prior* to admission, about the nature of the inconvenience that will be caused by hospitalization.

Not infrequently, the "need to hospitalize" is based less upon critical medical necessity than the physician's belief that a particular diagnostic or treatment course "would be best" for the patient. "Let's put her in and watch her for a few days" is a common rationale. Often, the decision to hospitalize is based simply upon the physician's estimation that the patient — because of ethnicity, social class, occupation, etc., — would not comply with medical requirements if treated or tested as an outpatient. If hospitalization is definitely required, then it is essential that a social worker be brought into the case immediately, so as to minimize the difficulties caused by abandoning house and family, usually with little notice.

(4) Folk curers tend to accept the patient's view of his own illness. In particular, the curer accepts all of the patient's symptoms at face value, and manifestly bases his diagnosis and treatment upon these. Interestingly, such acceptance of patients' presentation of illness is even more the case in urban milieux where curer and patients are strangers to one another. To a large extent, the patient thus controls his own illness or has a proprietary interest in it. Because urban folk curers tend not to know the patient, and do not represent a clear body of community consensus (cf. Press 1971), they attract and keep their clientele by satisfying idiosyncratic needs. They must compete with each other and with biomedicine, which allows no patient

control over illness. Thus it is unusual that a curer will discount the most bizarre of complaints or most scattered collection of somatic, behavioral, environmental, and cosmological symptoms. Indeed, where possible the curer takes his diagnostic cues from the patient. Knowing this, the patient is free to express those symptoms of most importance to himself, and further, to indicate the kind of diagnosis — and illness — he wants.

Implications for Biomedical Practitioners

We have already discussed the importance of reinforcing the patient's own explanatory model of illness. Modern biomedicine plucks the patient's disease from him and places it in the hands of an impersonal healer with impersonal machinery. Worse yet, biomedicine must fit patient experiences of sickness into its own frame of reference with its own language and with its own parameters of acceptable symptoms, syndromes and cures. In Bogota, Colombia, I found outpatients at a major hospital presenting almost twice as many symptoms to the examining physician as patients of identical social class and migrancy status presented to folk healers (Press 1969). The reason lies with the curer's ready acceptance of the patient's "own" symptoms. The physician, on the other hand, ignores all but those symptoms which reflect the biomedically relevant syndrome he judges to be operating in the particular instance. This is why patients offer more symptoms. They know the physician will dismiss some, and by enumerating more in the first place, they will have more chance that at least a few "of their own" will be accepted. Thus they ensure some "control" over their own illness.

Any disease causes the sufferer to become more aware of his body and his somatic and personal problems. As far as the patient is concerned, all or most symptoms and anxieties he experiences at the moment are part of his present syndrome. Patients may therefore sense and present more symptoms than " necessary". Physicians regularly "sift through" the patient's presented symptoms for the "correct" ones — thereby ignoring or minimizing actually felt symptoms which have already been included by the patient in his own notion of the present syndrome.

When physicians sift through the patient's symptom list, significant "validating symptoms" may be discarded or downplayed. Zola (1966) in studying patients at an eye clinic, noted how Italians view visceral, and Irish view throat-area symptoms as important indicators or validators of illness — regardless of where the majority of other symptoms may be located. I have noted how distress in the "mouth of the stomach" is a ubiquitous symptom among the ill of Bogota, Colombia. Visceral symptoms may be a common Latin American illness validator. I have witnessed an elderly Cuban patient with mild respiratory distress cheerfully respond with "si, doctor", as the attending physician poked vigorously at his abdomen, asking repeatedly if it hurt. The patient obviously felt no such pain. While all presented symptoms need not be given equal weight in diagnosis or treatment planning, all should at least be acknowledged and discussed (it also pays to know the general patient population's repertoire of validating symptoms). The patient should not be left with worrisome "loose symptoms" unrecognized or untreated.

(5) While folk healers may sometimes use unintelligible language calculated to confound (and thus establish awe in) the patient, they almost invariably utilize a common vernacular as well. Explanation of the "pathological manifestation" may be given in biomedical-sounding terms ("duodinal mucosity" is a favorite of one Seville, Spain curer), but etiological explanation is almost invariably linked to the patient's everyday experience and belief system. "You have weak blood" says the curer. Or the patient has worked too hard. His girlfriend is jealous. A dead uncle is displeased with his behavior. His brother envies him. He has eaten something hot when he should have eaten something cold. He has experienced a "shock".

Even where unintelligible or specialized jargon is used, it may seem familiar, or at least endowed with special power. If the patient hears but one mention of Jesus Christ in the midst of the curer's litany, it endows the entire oration with a familiar source of potency. A Bogota curer regularly asked patients to recite responsively such phrases as:

Powerful insignia of the wellspring of the good. In light. In the material of the Hebrew Shade of the light of the Good. In faith . . .

This is unintelligible only in the sense that its manifest function is not explicit. The constituent words themselves are clear and individually strong.

Implications for Biomedical Practitioners

This is not to say that the physician cannot use his jargon. But the biomedical jargon is designed to allow standardized teaching of medicine and standardized communication between medical professionals. It is *not* designed for physician-patient interaction. It serves the physician's ends — not the patient's, and reflects special training, not powers. The physician can — and indeed, should — use the jargon with patients. In this manner he establishes professional legitimacy, if such be his need. But a translation into plain terms is always necessary, and is the more important part of the interaction.

It is difficult to "come down to" the patient's level. Years of specialized training, plus fear of censure by colleagues or supervisors, make plain talk difficult to formulate or express. Brochures made up especially for educating lower-income heart attack victims talk of "high-risk factors" instead of "bad habits". "Menstruation", or even "period" may mean nothing to a black woman who uses the term "monthly". Words such as "congestion", "fetus", "seizure", "anemic", "urinate", or "discharge" seem elemental, yet may be unknown to the patient. It is wise to assume that in any given instance, that patients do *not* understand you — even when (as is most common) they shake their head in assent as you speak and ask if they have understood. Nurses commonly report that patients cannot repeat or even paraphrase the sense of instructions or explanations given by doctors minutes before. It is not merely the words used. Where words contradict long-held beliefs, confusion is likely.

Finally, it is easy to terrify patients with common clinical slang. "Did they take your bloods this morning?" "Did someone come in and take your fetal heart yet?"

(This is a common question to mothers in the labor room.) As a related matter, it is sometimes unclear to patients whether procedures are *passive* (monitoring, testing) or *active* (therapeutic, preventive). One labor room mother asked what would happen to her once the fetal heart and uterine contraction monitors were removed. An electrode had been screwed into her baby's scalp, and a plastic liquid-filled tube had been inserted deep into her uterus (both procedures are common). The wire and tube emerged from her vagina and were attached to a large, complex machine beside her bed. An L.E.D. read-out flickered, a beeping noise stuttered, and a continuous piece of paper emerged from the machine with twin pen tracings. She assumed that the machine was actively doing something *to* her labor and unborn baby. In verbal terms alone, it is easy for a patient — who does not know the word — to assume that to "monitor" a fetal heartbeat means "to make it better". Implying, perhaps, that something is already going wrong.

(6) Curers are usually born in the community and know its mores, history, and scandals. They are aware of past and present threats to its equilibrium, and to specific families. They can thus judge patients' anxieties and problems in historical and social contexts.

Turner (1964) has described the complex and extensive "sociopsy" performed by the Ndembu (Africa) healer, who interviews a number of the patient's kinsmen in an attempt to identify the socio/moral disjuncture that led to illness. Indeed, part of the cure involves orchestrated confrontation between the patient and others with whom he has experienced animosity or distrust. Local curers in village Mexico are usually well aware of intra-familial squabbles which might lead to envy, guilt, and resultant instances and accusations of sorcery. Even where urban curers may not know the patient and his family personally, the bond of shared ethnic identity and knowledge of general ethnic group values can lead curers to anticipate specific kinds of problems or at least be particularly sensitive to their expression by patients. Thus, Mexican-American curers in South Texas or Los Angeles are quick to diagnose illness as stemming from over-eager integration or contact with the Anglo life style (cf. Madsen 1964; Edgerton et al. 1970).

It is important to understand that unlike the biomedical physician, the curer's "license to practice" is tacitly granted by the patient and the local community. He is beholden to no outside authority for permission to practice or for a model of proper practice. Most curers operate in small community contexts where they themselves were born and raised. They have known family and history, and are unlikely (and usually unable) to practice elsewhere. They are thus subject to some degree of control and sanction by the community.

Curers frequently receive their calling via intense and often supernaturally generated personal experience. That these experiences may be wholly fabricated to meet public expectations is immaterial. Most curers cultivate an aura of poverty or public service. Many charge no specific fees, but accept donations instead. They often receive their training in the bosom of the community via apprenticeship with older, known, and respected healers. Or, they learn by themselves, or from a fabled outside healer, or via dreams or possession. Their skills, in other words, are largely self-generated or unrepeatable by others and reflect special abilities, luck, or grace on their parts. Associated with this grace is the notion that not everyone can become a curer simply by study or interest in the profession. The curer's image is definitely one of public service rather than profit-making enterprise.

It is important to recognize that the folk curer's charisma is due at least as much to his personal style (presentation of self, interactional techniques, power-base, reputation, etc.) as to his "science". In addition, folk curers' abilities to generate and manipulate symbols provide a large part of their capacity to heal. It must be stressed again that these symbols are not limited to the "mumbo jumbo" of ritual. Interpersonal management of the patient via intimate knowledge of his desires and value system (and, often, that of his community as well), constitutes symbolic manipulation of the highest order.[2]

Because of their dependence upon personal skills, it is rare that two folk curers exhibit the same diagnostic and curative procedures. I have found this to be the case in small peasant communities as well as in urban settings (see Press 1971; 1975). Indeed, two local curers may differ even in their explanatory models of disease (cf. Kapur 1979: 30). Patients can, and do, shop around for the curer whose style, paradigmatic basis, and explanatory model are most compatible with their needs. In urban settings, particularly, these needs may be multiple and complex, and illness episodes may play a number of different social functions for the sufferer. Folk illnesses may serve as a familiar handle for labeling and responding to sickness in the unfamiliar city. Sorcery beliefs may help to justify failure to achieve economic success. Illnesses identified with the ethnic group can aid in the maintenance of in-group identity and even prevent assimilation (see Press 1978 for a comprehensive discussion of the function of urban folk illness and medicine). Patients often compartmentalize their illnesses and see two or more healers (including MDs) concurrently for different aspects of the same problem (see Press 1969 for additional discussion of this "dual use" phenomenon). Regardless of ethnicity, there is hardly a patient anywhere who has not attempted (and will not continue to utilize) home-medication (herbals, ritual, old prescription drugs, dietary shifts) for the problem presently in the hands of the physician.

Implications for Biomedical Practitioners

Physicians must remember that they are "strangers" to their patients. Neither usually knows anything (certainly little in depth) about the other – the physician's training and life experiences, marital traumas or leisure preferences; the patient's family, community, and social/sub-cultural context. Moreover, the patient is absolutely powerless to control the physician's paradigm or practice. Indeed, the physician himself has little control over these. The doctor and his biomedicine are created, nurtured, and regulated outside the local community and the patient's realm of everyday experience. Standardization of style and science is a conscious goal of both the medical profession and of the gigantic and highly profitable health industry that medicine supports. To a large degree, "all physicians look alike" to the patient, whether the MD be surgeon, internist, endocrinologist, or what have you. As many as 15 years ago, Myerhoff and Larson noted physicians' steady loss of charisma to their amazing and standardized science (Myerhoff and Larson 1965). Their paradigm, identical training, and dependence upon outside-invented and standardized technical wizardry makes physicians largely indistinguishable from one another. The physician's science, not he himself, is the final authority (Myerhoff and Larson 1965: 190). Thereby, the "magic"of the doctor-patient interaction is minimized, along with its important product of symbolic healing.

The dependence of Westerners upon (and worship of) technological sophistication creates a further problem for the physician. This technology, coupled with incomprehensible jargon, extra-community training, astounding equipment, terrifying body-rending techniques, and the locus of healing acts in specialized places, sets the physician and his science apart from everyday life and its uncertainties (both Fabrega [1974] and Foster [1976] provide some excellent discussion on this important difference between biomedicine and non-western medical systems). Modern biomedicine and its practitioners, in other words, should be infallible. Thus, lack of certainty by the physician (i.e., a sincere "I don't know") is more likely to induce stress than to relax the patient through a demonstration that his incredibly trained healer is "just like anyone else" and "only human".[3]

Here, the physician is a clear victim of his science's image and charisma. When uncertain, he can attempt to mitigate stress to the patient by sharing the scientific basis of his uncertainty. This basis almost invariably takes the form of possibilities logically eliminated, with others still pending. Thus, by saying, "Well, we've checked you for (a) and (b) and you don't have these, so now we'll look for (c) and (d) because your symptoms are also associated with these problems" – the patient may feel that his condition is in the *process* of methodical, reductive diagnosis and treatment – not in a blind alley.

In contrast to the folk healer, the physician's image is one of money-making professional as well as healer. The general public is well aware that physicians select their profession as much (or more) for the money as for the cliché-ridden "desire to serve one's fellow man". The physician today who believes that his patients view him as selfless servant of the community's health needs, is severely misled. A deep well of resentment and distrust underlies many patients' attitudes toward the medical profession – even while many of these same patients are totally committed to the biomedical paradigm and its technological wizardry. Indeed, this very commitment underlies the resentment. Modern biomedicine is the ultimate monopolistic "phone company". No competition from alternate therapies or paradigms is allowed. Unable or unwilling to shop around for alternate treatment, the "average" patient is forced into dependence upon the rich physician and his unbending, uncompromising, unintelligible science. This image is all the more common among ethnically divergent patients (but they, at least, may have some access to alternative curing systems should biomedicine fail or admit uncertainty).

Overall, it is most difficult for the physician to solve the problem of image – as omnipotent stranger and paid professional, ruled by his monopolistic science. It is built into the system and its roles. At best one can say that awareness of the problem is at least a tentative step toward its mitigation. The move toward family practice offers a partial solution, although the common belief among medical students that such a practice automatically implies increased personal contact with and intimate knowledge of patients is mistaken. Decentralization of medical practice to local neighborhood health centers is a long way in the future. Indeed, the trend toward group practices concentrated in large "medical arts buildings" (with complex lab facilities, etc.) is actually attracting physicians away from their decentralized neighborhood offices. A few obvious suggestions might help a little. Chrisman notes that "treatments that include recognition of the influence of everyday life will tend to be related to a higher degree of adherence" (Chrisman 1977: 370). This can be done in a variety of ways. Medication regimens can be adjusted to patient work and recreation schedules. Sensitive questioning might reveal that medication taken at certain times and places will enhance the patient's sick role and reduce anxiety over failure to perform to normal standards. Medication taken conspicuously at work, for example, might help reinforce the patient's claim to sickness and reduced performance expectations. Family members can be specified as home treatment-givers if the patient indicates that some family participation in the illness event would be desirable.

Asking friendly, personal questions related to the patient's problem, plus volunteering related personal information in response ("Yeah, my brother had that too, and . . .") can aid in establishing an appearance of susceptibility to common concerns. Sincere encouragement of patients to contact the physician for any question or complication, plus accommodation of treatment scheduling to patient needs, may offer the patient some sense of "control" over his disease and his practitioner. It is easy for the clinical physician to completely terminate contact with the patient once he has written discharge orders. Extra time spent with the patient in discharge-consultation can reveal — and soothe — worries (about returning home as a dependent, ability to care for self, prognosis away from the magical clinical setting, etc.) hitherto unexpressed. If problems surface (even where they are not "logistic" problems of funding, housing, or patient care at home) a social worker should be called in at discharge for additional counseling and expressions of concern for the patient outside the hospital.

Finally, some mitigation of the monopolistic image might be achieved through unfeigned willingness to refer the patient to another physician, or to accept or even encourage some modicum of self remedy or consultation with healers and other types of professionals outside biomedicine. This latter is especially significant where ethnic group patients have access to (and probably utilize) folk curers. Ritual cures (and even herbal ones) will not ordinarily counteract the effects of concurrent biomedical treatment. And it is well known that patients who are actively discouraged by physicians from seeing traditional curers resent this and are quick to attribute cure to the traditional, rather than biomedical treatment. In the long run, this does not promote dependence upon and confidence in biomedical resources.

CONCLUSIONS

In truth, the ideal biomedical health practitioner should be expert in theology, anthropology, psychology and urban studies. This is another way of noting that societal, cultural, ideological and contextual phenomena necessarily express themselves in all aspects of human behavior, and that episodes of disease are not excepted. Of course, no physician, nurse, or other biomedical practitioner can meet these requirements. However, it can be argued that the more aware such practitioners are of the operation of cultural factors in the expression and cure of disease, the more capable they will be of dealing with their culture-bearing patients. It has been suggested that one of the basic problems of biomedical health delivery derives from the nature of biomedicine and its professional organization. It is largely divorced from everyday concerns it is derived from and controlled by scientific, political, and industrial sources outside the local community; it is taught outside the community, and its paradigm allows little or no input from personal symbolic phenomena. Folk medicine and its practitioners are largely the opposite. Some of the basic stylistic and conceptual characteristics of folk healing may be used as a guide to improved management of, and empathy with patients. Most of these characteristics reflect the tacit recognition in folk medical systems of the part disease plays in human social and emotional life. When the disease becomes meaningful for the patient; when the patient believes that he and the healer are in agreement about the kind of disease and its implications; when the patient's anxieties and socio/emotional disjunctures are recognized as legitimate concomitants of disease — then cultural healing can begin, and specific medical treatment itself may be more welcome and effective. Difficult as this may sound, there is truly no alternative. It is to be hoped that eventually, the skills of both social and medical science will be united in the practice of an exceptionally and broadly effective type of medicine.

NOTES

1. Reliance upon curers as biomedical consultants is probably a temporary expedient at best. Native curers are a dwindling group, and are not being replaced by younger recruits (Foster 1976: 18; Press 1973).
2. Even in urban situations, where clients are drawn from diverse societal contexts, folk curers reflect and manage patient symbolic needs. In this case these needs are often highly idiosyncratic rather than community-wide. The curers manage this by following the lead of the patient in diagnosing and assigning cause (Press 1971).
3. In going over files of malpractice suits against one hospital, I have been amazed by the incredible expectations of perfection that patients have of physicians and modern medicine. If the most delicate and dangerous of surgical procedures produces an unanticipated side-effect, patients may respond with great indignation and quick demands for compensation. Such suits will undoubtedly increase in number as biomedicine grows ever more sophisticated.

BIBLIOGRAPHY

Blanchard, E. and L. Young
1974 Clinical Applications of Biofeedback Training: A Review of Evidence. Archives of General Psychiatry 30: 573–589.

Blumhagen, Dan
  1980 Hyper-Tension: A Folk Illness with a Medical Name. Culture, Medicine, and Psychiatry 4: 197–227.
Chrisman, Noel J.
  1977 The Health Seeking Process: An Approach to the Natural History of Illness. Culture, Medicine, and Psychiatry 1: 351–377.
Cohen, Lucy M.
  1979 Culture, Disease and Stress Among Latino Immigrants. RIIES Special Study. Washington, D.C.: Smithsonian Inst.
Creighton, Marie Louise
  1979 Communication Between Peasant and Doctor in Tunisia. Social Science and Medicine 11: 319–324.
Dubos, Rene
  1959 Mirage of Health. New York: Harper and Row.
Edgerton, R., et al.
  1970 Curanderismo in the Metropolis. American Journal of Psychotherapy 24: 124–234.
Fabrega, Horacio Jr.
  1971 Some Features of Zinacantecan Medical Knowledge. Ethnology 10: 1–24.
  1972 The Study of Disease in Relation to Culture. Behavioral Science 17: 183–203.
  1974 Disease and Social Behavior. Cambridge: MIT Press.
Foster, George M.
  1976 Medical Anthropology and International Health Planning. Medical Anthropology Newsletter 7: 12–18.
  1976 Disease Etiologies in Nonwestern Medical Systems. American Anthropologist 78: 773–782.
Freidson, Eliot
  1971 Profession of Medicine. New York: Dodd, Mead.
Illich, Ivan
  1976 Medical Nemesis. Toronto: Bantam Books.
Kamiya, Joe (ed.)
  1976/77 Biofeedback and Self-Control. Chicago: Aldine.
Kapur, R.
  1979 The Role of Traditional Healers in Mental Health Care in Rural India. Social Science and Medicine 13B: 27–31.
Kleinman, Arthur, and L. Sung
  1979 Why Do Indigenous Practitioners Successfully Heal? Social Science and Medicine 13B: 7–26.
Knowles, John H. (ed.)
  1977 Doing Better and Feeling Worse. New York: W. W. Norton.
Logan, Michael
  1973 Humoral Medicine in Guatemala and Peasant Acceptance of Modern Medicine. Human Organization 32: 385–395.
Maclean, Una
  1971 Magical Medicine. Middlesex: Penguin Books.
Madsen, W.
  1964 Value Conflicts and Folk Psychotherapy in South Texas. In Ari Kiev (ed.), Magic, Faith and Healing, Glencoe: The Free Press, pp. 420–440.
Moerman, Daniel
  1979 Anthropology of Symbolic Healing. Current Anthropology 20: 59–66.
Myerhoff, Barbara, and W. Larson
  1965 The Doctor as Culture Hero: The Routinization of Charisma. Human Organization 24: 188–191.

Press, Irwin
    1969 Urban Illness, Physicians, Curers and Dual Use in Bogota. Journal of Health and
          Social Behavior 10: 209–218.
    1971 The Urban Curandero. American Anthropologist 73: 741–756.
    1973 Bureaucracy Versus Folk Medicine: Implications from Seville, Spain. Urban Anthro-
          pology 2: 232–247.
    1975 Tradition and Adaptation: Life in a Modern Yucatan Maya Community. Westport:
          Greenwood Press.
    1978 Urban Folk Medicine: A Functional Overview. American Anthropologist 80: 71–84.
    1980 Problems in the Definition and Classification of Medical Systems. Social Science and
          Medicine 14B: 45–57.
Schensul, Stephen, and M. B. Bymel
    1975 The Role of Applied Research in the Development of Health Services in a Chicano
          Community in Chicago. In S. Ingman and A. Thomas (eds.), Topias and Utopias in
          Health, Mouton: The Hague, pp. 425–443.
Snow, Loudell
    1974 Folk Medical Beliefs and their Implications for Care of Patients. Annals of Internal
          Medicine 81: 82–96.
Sontag, Susan
    1978 Illness as Metaphor. New York: Farrar, Straus, and Giroux.
Stein, Howard
    1979 The Salience of Ethno-Psychology for Medical Education and Practice. Social Science
          and Medicine 13B: 199–210.
Szasz, Thomas
    1962 The Myth of Mental Illness. New York: Harper and Row.
Turner, Victor
    1964 An Ndembu Doctor in Practice. In Ari Kiev (ed.), Magic, Faith and Healing, New
          York: The Free Press.
Waitzkin, Howard
    1979 Medicine, Superstructure and Micropolitics. Social Science and Medicine 13A: 601–
          609.
Weidman, Hazel
    1978 Miami Health Ecology Project Report. Miami: University of Miami.
Zola, Irving K.
    1966 Culture and Symptoms: An Analysis of Patients' Presenting Complaints. American
          Sociological Review 3: 615–630.

SECTION II

CLINICALLY APPLIED ANTHROPOLOGICAL RESEARCH

SECTION II

CLINICALLY APPLIED ANTHROPOLOGICAL RESEARCH

HAZEL HITSON WEIDMAN

RESEARCH STRATEGIES, STRUCTURAL ALTERATIONS AND CLINICALLY APPLIED ANTHROPOLOGY

INTRODUCTION

This chapter describes some of the research, service, and training aspects of clinical anthropology that have evolved over a thirteen year period at the University of Miami School of Medicine in Florida. The author's experience as an anthropologist in a health science setting represents no accidental diversion which led to an unexpected career as a medical anthropologist. It is the logical outgrowth of a graduate training program designed to explore relationships between anthropology and medicine generally, anthropology and psychiatry specifically. This is so despite the fact that at the time of such training in the mid-1950's the field of medical anthropology had not yet emerged fully from its long period of gestation (Wellin 1977). Moreover, the thirteen years in this location constitute only one segment of a longer work history characterized always by an interest in both theroretical and pragmatic linkages between anthropology and medicine. This suggests that if anthropology at the University of Miami-Jackson Memorial Medical Center has had a visible impact upon the structure of some service programs and the functioning of some training programs, it may be due, in part, to the long history of connections between the two fields in the author's training, anthropological orientation, and professional experience.

Clinical anthropology has not yet crystallized fully as a specialty area within the sub-discipline of medical anthropology. Nevertheless, many constituent parts that may be prerequisite to the formation of such a field are beginning to be defined in the literature. There are now sufficient numbers of anthropologists engaged in clinically-related activities that a critical mass may have been reached. Conceivably, this will now allow the development of training programs in clinical anthropology. This chapter describes only what has occured in one health science setting. However, its contribution, together with others in this volume and elsewhere (Shimkin and Golde forthcoming) may be significant in outlining some of the parameters of future training programs in clinical anthropology. Similarly, it may be of value to practitioners and clinical staff in health science settings who wish to learn what their colleagues and counterparts have been doing in their collaborations with anthropologists.

The Problem of Definitions

Currently, there is some confusion about the meaning of the term "clinical anthropology" (Open Forum 1980). Physicians find it especially problematical, because anything "clinical" is linked to clinical practice, i.e., the provision of health care, i.e., therapy. In health science settings, the distinction is made between clinical

N. J. Chrisman and T. W. Maretzki (eds.), Clinically Applied Anthropology, 201–241.
Copyright © 1982 by D. Reidel Publishing Company.

faculty who engage in therapy and non-clinical faculty who do not. The Ph.D.
in anthropology does not certify its bearer as having been trained to practice
therapy. Consequently, the Ph.D. in anthropology does not ensure that its bearer
will have access to credentialing processes within the health science setting. Therefore, from a health science perspective the anthropologist in a clinical setting is
a member of the nonclinical faculty.

From the perspective of medical anthropology, however, "clinical anthropology",
in my opinion, functions at the moment as a useful classificatory device. It helps
to identify a growing field of inquiry and to differentiate from other types of
medical anthropologists, those who are engaged in research, service, and training
capacities in settings designed to provide care to people who are ill or in need of
some type of health professional assistance. Such settings often include programs
to train clinicians in the provision of health services to those who are ill or in
need of health-related support. Clinical anthropology as a substantive field is only
now emerging. Its foundation is being established by the commonalities identifiable in the research approaches, concepts, methods, planning, evaluation, and
teaching strategies employed by anthropologists who work in diverse health science
settings.

Clinical anthropology, when defined as a useful classificatory device, leads to
a further distinction between those anthropologists engaged in clinically-related
professional activities and those anthropologists who, themselves, are therapists.
The former are clinical anthropologists; while the latter are anthropologist clinicians.
Thus, one term, clinical anthropologist, includes all types of medical anthropologists
involved in clinically related arenas; i.e., psychiatric anthropologists, nutritional
anthropologists, pediatric anthropologists, anthropologist clinicians, etc. The label
lumps them together as having something to do with patients, clinics, clinicians, and
the provision of health care. The other term, anthropologist clinician, specifies
that the clinical anthropologist bearing this title is also trained and certified as a
therapist of some sort. When licensed in a particular state, such an individual may
function as a practitioner, whether it be in an institution, a group setting, or in
private practice. Using these distinctions, there are many more clinical anthropologists at the moment than there are anthropologist clinicians. It is likely, however,
that the numbers of anthropologist clinicians will increase in the future.

Entrance into the Field

Anthropologists who enter health science settings do so by invitation. They rarely
walk in and, under the sponsorship of a host institution, create their own positions
by virtue of their grant-winning abilities. Although this model for entrance is, in
fact, a possible one, it does not occur very often. Generally, anthroplogists are
invited in to assist in some way with research projects, service programs, or the
training of health professionals.

More often than might be expected, the charge to the incoming anthropologist
is extremely ambiguous. If research is the focus, it may or may not have been
previously designed and funded. It may be the anthropologist's assignment to

design such projects and develop funding sources to implement them. The areas of research may or may not be specified. This may be left entirely to the anthropologist's discretion. If anthropologists are invited in to plan, monitor, or evaluate service programs, those who provide positions for them may or may not see the full range of contributions which anthropological approaches and perspectives might make and, in effect, may not know how to utilize them properly. If the task for which an anthropologist is invited into a clinical setting is primarily that of teaching, there may be a long period of adjustment and accommodation before the anthropological contribution is viewed as significant and relevant to clinical concerns of the health professionals involved. In brief, although an invitation into a health science institutional structure is proffered and accepted, this does not necessarily mean full acceptance, immediate integration, joyful collaboration and mutually rewarding sets of interactions between clinician and non-clinician participants in the new alliance (Weidman 1976a).

Entrance into the health science field requires all of the standard anthropological sensitivities, approaches, explorations, and accommodations which are utilized ordinarily in any field investigation. It is precisely the trans-disciplinary, trans-system, trans-personal investigative stance of the anthropologist which, in the long run, helps him/her to avoid the two greatest pitfalls awaiting the newcomer to the health science field. One is that he/she becomes something of a threat and too "critical" an observer to be tolerated. In such a case, he/she is soundly rejected as intrusive. The other pitfall is that the anthropologist becomes so supportive and helpful that he/she is increasingly incorporated and ultimately absorbed by a process of co-optation.

The marginal, "alienated" or transcultural investigative posture constitutes the fundamental strength of anthropological contributions in the health science setting. It is essential to anthropology's holism. However, the freedom with which such a posture is put into operation sometimes depends very much on whether or not the anthropologist holds a staff or a line position.

Staff Versus Line Positions

The issue of staff versus line position is a central one not often addressed by administrators on the health sciences side of the anthropology-health science equation or by the directors of medical anthropology training programs on the other side (Weidman 1971). It is important to note, however, that those who enter clinical settings in staff positions have the freedom necessary to become participant observers of every aspect of the organization in which they function. Often they have no authority other than that which comes from their informal influence upon those who hold clearly designated positions within the organization. In contrast, those who accept line positions may have circumscribed authority within a functional division of the organization; however, their investigative freedom as participant observers in the entire social structure may be severely hampered by bounded areas of authority which delineate sub-divisions of the larger system. While the issue of freedom may be crucial in early years or on new assignments in clinical settings, the issue of authority may become central at a later date.[1] Nevertheless, the investigative posture is vital. It underlies all efforts by anthropologists to contribute in meaningful ways to the tasks facing health care delivery and training institutions on the one hand and the literature and theory of medical and general anthropology on the other hand.

The Investigative Posture and Social Change

When anthropologists become involved in clinically related tasks, whether they realize it or not, their overall mission becomes one of social change. For anthropological contributions to be incorporated, there must be some degree of transformation from unicultural to transcultural (or trans-disciplinary or trans-person) perspectives by personnel in the host institution. If there is no movement in this regard, there is little anthropological impact upon either the structure or functioning of service or training programs. Thus, the investigative element that is inherent in anthropological approaches assumes, in such settings, a purposeful character. The investigative posture is not only designed to elicit information for purposes of description or benefit to health professionals; it becomes central, also, in generating strategies for change. When the investigative posture guides behavior enacted from a staff position, the approach, itself, becomes a powerful strategy for change. Anthropological exposure and impact are greatly increased under such circumstances because of the mobility and multiple types of transactions that not only are possible and permitted but are sanctioned.

Both the investigative posture and the transforming mission that have prevailed at the University of Miami-Jackson Memorial Medical Center are reflected in sections to follow. However, a word is in order about the context in which such anthropological applications have been possible.

The Health Science and Community Setting

The University of Miami-Jackson Memorial Medical Center is comprised of the University of Miami School of Medicine and its affiliated hospitals and clinics. Jackson Memorial Hospital (JMH) is the main teaching hospital. It is a publically-supported county facility. As such, it is mandated that JMH be accessible to persons of all groups in Dade County and that it provide them with the best possible care. Such care is given by house officers (residents) who are trained by faculty of the School of Medicine. The School is committed to preparing physicians to practice their specialties in such a way that optimum benefit will accrue to any patient who comes to them for care or for whose care they become responsible.

In the multiethnic receptacle that Dade County has become, particularly over the past two decades, health care increasingly is being offered to patients whose values, experiences, and behaviors may be markedly different from those of the physicians who minister to them. This poses an especially difficult problem for a training institution whose faculty and trainees (the house officers of Jackson Memorial Hospital among others) may be limited by unicultural perspectives. Such single lines of vision restrict their understanding of and teaching about cultural traditions of patients from multiethnic backgrounds or even about the sub-system problems of poor or geriatric patients.

Even though teaching faculty may be aware of cultural factors in health care, the problem persists because they do not have easy access to specific cultural knowledge which might be helpful to them in their interactions with individual patients. Furthermore, the problem is just as great for teaching faculty of diverse ethnic backgrounds as it is for "General American" faculty members by virtue of the fact that all are trained in a unicultural (medically orthodox) mode of thought and action rather than one which is transculturally-oriented.

Given the current picture of a growing awareness of culture-linked problems in both health care delivery and health professional training, it is somewhat shocking to realize that as recently as 1968 ethnicity in Dade County had not yet become a salient issue in health care. Beyond the primarily WASP and secondarily Jewish population base, it was generally known that Bahamians, both black and white, were early settlers to the area and that there were large black populations in three different sections of Greater Miami. It was also recognized that some members of the black communities had moved down from Georgia and North Carolina and that many of these had settled in the rural areas to the southwest. Puerto Ricans were most often identified as being part of the migrant labor population and not inner city dwellers, although this was an inaccurate perception. It was known that Haitians were beginning to appear in small old hotels in the central black section of the city. And the Cuban presence was, of course, beginning to be felt in earnest, not only because of professional and white collar flight from Cuba following Castro's assumption of power in 1959, but also because of the Freedom Flights which began in 1965. Beyond these general understandings of the character of the Dade County community, little was known about cultural, economic, or family configurations in the area from which Jackson Memorial Hospital and its clinics drew the majority of its patients. It was this section of inner-city Miami which entered very early into anthropological activities that had relevance for both service and training programs at the University of Miami-Jackson Memorial Medical Center.

RESEARCH STRATEGIES

At the time of my 1968 appointment in the Department of Psychiatry at the University of Miami, the commitment made was to help transform a conservative, psychopharmacologically and psychoanalytically-oriented system into one that could incorporate a transcultural perspective in its three functions: (a) research, (b) service, and (c) training. The task involved nothing less than systemic change, which, in retrospect, was revolutionary in scope. At the time it seemed a logical undertaking in light of the mutual interest of the author and the departmental chairman in achieving a degree of synthesis of anthropological and psychiatric theory (Weidman and Sussex 1971). The problem, of course, was to translate theoretical knowledge into service and training programs which would reflect that enhanced level of synthesis (Sussex and Weidman 1975).

Research provided a beginning in this enterprise. Over the years and within several departments, research has ranged from large, complex community studies and formal, circumscribed mini-research projects to informal ethnographic investigations. All have been designed to answer specific questions about health care or health professional training. Some of the training-related research initiatives are described in a subsequent section. For present purposes it is important to review one large research effort which led to major structural alterations in mental health services at Jackson Memorial Hospital and is now having further impact in other clinical areas.

The Miami Health Ecology Project was designed to provide basic information about the population to be served by the first community mental health center then being planned for the Miami Area following enactment of Community Mental Health Centers legislation in 1963. The Center was intended to serve an inner-city area adjacent to and surrounding the Medical Center. For a number of reasons which have been outlined elsewhere and need not be reviewed here (Weidman forthcoming; Weidman et al. 1978), this epidemiologically-oriented study was carried out in collaboration with the Department of Pediatrics. In the process, it also became structured as an evaluation study of an ongoing comprehensive health care program in Pediatrics, the service area of which was contained within the boundaries of the proposed community mental health center catchment area. Thus, the Health Ecology Project functioned as both basic and applied research and met the needs of two departments simultaneously. In this context the discussion will center on its contribution to the Department of Psychiatry.

The reader is forewarned that in the sections to follow no attempt is made to convey the substance of project findings. These are available in the Project Report and are presented in part in other publications. (Weidman 1979; Weidman forthcoming; Weidman et al. 1978). Instead, there is an attempt to make explicit for the reader some of the conceptualizing and change-related strategies inherent in anthropological contributions to the health science setting in Miami.

THE HEALTH ECOLOGY PROJECT

The Health Ecology Project of the University of Miami was supported by the Commonwealth Fund in 1971. It was a comprehensive, comparative study that investigated health problems, health beliefs and health practices in five predominant ethnic groups in a low-income inner-city section of Miami. The groups are: Bahamian, Haitian, Southern Black, Cuban, and Puerto Rican. Several innovative features of the study are highlighted here. In addition, central areas of inquiry are outlined, and general types of findings are described that contributed importantly to the planning of the previously-mentioned community mental health program.

Innovative Features

The importance of the Health Ecology Project mapping effort cannot be over-emphasized. At the time the study was initiated, lack of accurate information about the people in the area left no alternative but to take to the streets, making observations and talking to local residents. A large amount of supplementary environmental information was also accumulated, coded, and translated onto a base map with overlays. These provided a rich source of information and displayed in an easily assimilated manner not only the predominant population clusters but the organization of health care in relation to community characteristics and cultural groups. The series included the following:

(1) Base map showing neighborhood gathering places, such as food stores, restaurants, laundromats, coffee windows, bars, pool halls, and theaters.
(2) Overlay showing cultural territories (geographic boundaries of ethnic enclaves), industrialized areas and bus transportation routes.
(3) Overlay showing location of orthodox medical and dental facilities, displayed according to specialty categories.
(4) Overlay showing churches and observable non-orthodox healing resources, such as religious article stores, occultists, and naturopaths.
(5) Overlay showing census tracts and block groupings to allow the plotting of various kinds of census data against the full backdrop of neighborhood, cultural, and health-related information shown by means of the first 4 base map/ overlay combinations.

Later, additional maps were prepared to show the distribution and location of traditional healers identified for each group on the basis of field investigations.

The full set of maps allowed visualization of a large amount of complex material. When used in lectures, the series functioned as an extremely important heuristic device in community agencies, the medical center, and the College of Arts and Sciences classroom settings.

By design, and for various reasons described in the project report, research assistants were mature women who had already raised or were still raising their families. They were representatives of the ethnic groups under study and were untrained researchers when they joined the project. Although there is nothing exceptional about the use of "indigenous" workers in various community health programs, there may be uniqueness in the amount of formal interviewing and writing of ethnographic reports which was required of them, including interviews with traditional healers.

A combined anthropological/sociological approach was utilized. Ethnographic data, recorded at the time of or immediately following a questionnaire interview, provided, during the period of data analysis, the means of monitoring the accuracy of certain types of survey responses. Ethnographic materials also allowed the comparison of *emic* (cultural within) and *etic* (orthodox from without) data in an unusually effective way.

The combined basic/applied characteristics of the research project were somewhat unusual. The size and scope of the project, its urban emphasis, and its focus upon ethnicity were exceptional in the health field at the time of its inception and during its implementation. The project's importance for planning and evaluating service programs and for the training of health professionals is noteworthy. Also, the entire research effort, undertaken from within a health science setting, functioned as a more influential strategy for change than might have been the case had it been conducted in another context.

Areas of Inquiry

The investigation was guided by the *health culture* concept. This concept refers in a holistic way to "all of the phenomena associated with the maintenence of well-being and problems of sickness with which people cope in traditional ways within their own social networks and institutional structures" (Weidman et al. 1978). To fully grasp the importance of the health culture concept, two major analytic approaches are utilized: one emphasizing a cognitive dimension; the other stressing social system or social organizational components. The *cognitive* dimension includes world view, values and beliefs, conceptual guidelines for health action and the symbolic structure of therapeutic rituals. One must look into theories of illness prevention, health maintenance, views of bodily functioning, etiology, diagnosis, treatment and cure in order to understand the cognitive aspects of the health culture concept.

In contrast, the *social system* characteristics of a health culture relate to its organization as a health care delivery system. One must become familiar with the structure and functioning of organized sets of health/illness related roles and behaviors in order to understand the operation of a health care system — a system that is primarily reparative or therapeutic in nature and only secondarily preventive.

Overall, a particular health culture functions as an integral and essential part of the cultural tradition of an ethnic group, regardless of whether or not that group may have left its country of origin many years previously. Consequently, the concept of health culture is inextricably linked to that of culture in this theoretical orientation.[2]

With the health culture concept as its organizing principle, the Health Ecology Project, among other things,

(1) assessed in five ethnic groups the patterning of symptoms and conditions revealed first by *etic* (orthodox) categories and instruments and then by *emic* (cultural within) categories of illness;

(2) determined some of the symptoms which, *emically*, combined into meaning clusters to allow beginning self diagnosis of a condition (syndrome/illness);

(3) probed underlying *emic* perceptions of bodily functioning which are relevant to etiological views and illness processes;

(4) inquired into patterns of self-care designed to alleviate symptoms and cure conditions and examined beliefs about the maintenance of well-being;

(5) explored patterns of utilization of both orthodox and traditional systems of care;

(6) examined the roles of healers predominant in various traditional health care systems, including patient/healer interaction, contexts of curing, forms of

payment, referral networks, recruitment, training, and relationships to orthodox providers of care;

(7) traced, by inference, etiological theories, therapeutic practices, and medicinal preferences of traditional healers on the basis of patient reports and healer self-reports;

(8) compared the value orientation profile of project sample members with that previously established for representatives of the dominant cultural system (Kluckhohn and Strodtbeck 1961);

(9) compared aspects of world view and values in traditional and orthodox health cultural systems.

General Findings

Health Ecology Project findings demonstrated the fact of cultural differences in the manner in which aches and pains and other ailments are defined as symptoms about which any individual might be concerned. In each group there were patterned ways of describing complaints and presenting them to health professionals when something was sufficiently wrong that professional care was sought.

In each of the five ethnic groups studied, conditions (syndromes) were identified by symptom clusters organized in ways that were not identical with criteria used in establishing diagnoses according to orthodox medical categories. Falling-out, a condition extensively described and discussed in a previous publication is a case in point (Weidman 1979).

Project findings also indicated that the process of linking certain sets of symptoms together and identifying them as a particular syndrome with its own label is based in each group upon patterned perceptions of bodily functioning that sometimes differ markedly from orthodox views on such matters. Project data revealed within each group widespread use of home remedies that were consonant with traditional views about bodily functioning and causes of illness. Results also documented the utilization of traditional healers; sometimes in place of orthodox health care; sometimes in conjunction with it.

Within each group striking incompatibilities of orthodox and traditional views existed on the topic of physical/spiritual and natural/unnatural illness distinctions. "Spiritual" and/or "unnatural" illnesses were perceived to be magically or supernaturally caused and consequently fell, utlimately, outisde the realm of authority of orthodox health care. The research also established the presence of many types of traditional healers in the various communities within the study area. It further demonstrated the central role of such healers in offering treatment for "spiritual" or "unnatural" (magically or supernaturally caused) conditions.

In brief, Project findings documented the presence in Miami of viable health cultural traditions that were influencing health/illness behavior within each of the groups studied. These results have served to eliminate from this setting one of the common responses anthropologists often receive when they introduce exotic ethnographic data to emphasize theoretical points they wish to make. The response often takes the form of, "That's very interesting, but it doesn't happen here", or

"We don't have to worry about that here". In Miami, this is no longer an acceptable way to avoid having to deal with matters some health professionals might wish to disregard. The data exist. They are drawn from local communities. They are current. They are convincing. They have direct relevance to health care.

Concepts as Strategies for Change

The concepts of *culture* and *health culture*, which guided the Health Ecology Project are considered, in their own right, to be important factors in initiating change in a health science setting. Two additional change-oriented concepts began to be used in a similar way as preliminary findings emerged from the project's substantial pilot study, completed early in 1972. As project discoveries about cultural differences were made available to health professionals, I began to introduce the concept of *co-cultures* into teaching sessions. This was a calculated move, designed to encourage perceptual shifts on the part of clinicians from a unicultural to a transcultural vantage point. Although the health culture concept allows recognition that the conceptual system of an ethnic patient is just as deep-rooted and integral to his sense of well-being as is that of the clinician, it does not require an immediate and automatic assumption of a transcultural posture in order to grasp its full significance for health care. The co-culture concept is far more efficient in this regard. The author introduced this term as a way acknowledging the equivalent function of health cultural traditions for both ethnic patients and orthodox health professionals.

When a person uses the term, co-cultures, he assumes a perceptual set that automatically juxtaposes cultural systems. Juxtaposition in turn provides the basis for comparison of congruent and non-congruent elements in them. In reality, this is nothing more than the classical anthropological investigative stance. In clinical teaching, however, it is far more important to focus upon the traditions themselves, or upon the bearers of cultural traditions, rather than upon the perspective that allows the simultaneous assessment of similarities and differences between the patient's health cultural views and those of the health care provider. Nevertheless, the anthropological posture is assumed automatically with adoption of the co-culture concept. There is no way to use the term without recognizing that more than one cultural system is included as a referent. Furthermore, the word implies co-equal status for the health cultural traditions which guide and support the various coping and health-related behaviors of those who participate in them. Consequently, the term encourages a non-judgmental stance.

Although greater equity is posited by means of the co-culture concept, there is no way to escape the fact that each orthodox practitioner carries the medical, social, and legal responsibility for improving, to as great an extent as possible, the health status of each patient who comes for care. Similarly, there is no way to escape the fact that if the patient refuses to accept or is unable to comprehend and comply with orthodox interventions, the practitioner may be rendered powerless to meet his responsibilities in this regard. It is easy to argue, then, that the clinician is placed in a stronger position to achieve the outcome desired by recognizing that co-cultures may be involved in every clinicial transaction. Such recognition allows for the possibility of culture brokerage if negotiations should be necessary to ensure not only compliance but also appropriate utilization of health care facilities.

In summary, by moving from the concept of *culture*, to that of *health culture*, and then to the *co-culture* concept. in conversations and teaching sessions, an attempt is made to generate in clinicians a perceptual shift from a unicultural to a transcultural position. It is the latter stance which makes it possible to engage in *culture brokerage*, another key term that I introduced into the health science setting in Miami in the early 1970's.

Culture brokerage relates to the process of establishing meaningful, strategic, or significant linkages between separate cultural or sub-cultural systems (Weidman 1973, 1975, 1976b). The person who engages in such mediating processes functions as a culture broker, in a role to be discussed in greater detail below. In the context of clinical activities, culture brokerage encourages behavior by health professionals which, theoretically, should lead to greater success for the clinician and a better outcome for the patient. In order for the health practitioner to negotiate between divergent health cultural beliefs and practices, it is necessary to determine the nature of the beliefs and concerns that guide the patient's behavior. Only then can areas of difference or incompatibility be determined. And only after these are identified can mediation be attempted. In the process, however, the following changes in clinicial transactions are likely to occur:

(1) a greater understanding of the person who presents with specific complaints;
(2) an enhanced response to points of concern tied to the patient's symbolic system as well as to those related to the practitioner's diagnostic system;
(3) the development of more meaningful connections between the requirements of orthodox clinical reality and requirements of the patient's own clinical reality;[3]
(4) the establishment of a foundation whereby the orthodox rationale for intervention may be incorporated more easily into the patient's repertoire of health-related understandings; and
(5) a more humanistic interactive process which tends to establish a stronger affective bond between the patient and the health professional.

Thus, culture brokerage joined the concepts of culture, health culture, and co-culture as strategies designed to alter perceptions and elicit changed behavior in clinical areas of a health science institution. Their use was supported by a wealth of empirical data accumulated over a five year period in the local communities from which many University of Miami-Jackson Memorial Medical Center patients are drawn. These anthropological concepts assumed even greater importance in planning for the community mental health program which would serve a geographical area extending beyond but including the study area of the Health Ecology Project.

STRUCTURAL ALTERATIONS IN THE ORGANIZATION OF HEALTH CARE

We, in the Department of Psychiatry, wished to design a community mental health program that would avoid the high drop-out rates and patterns of underutilization so often associated with such programs in low-income or multiethnic areas. Consequently, we stressed responsiveness to the needs of the people for whom care would be provided. Since we knew a great deal about such people and their needs, it was a relatively simply matter to design an appropriate program.

The following characteristics prevailed in the area: social positions near the bottom of the social stratification system; marginal subsistence; deleterious environmental conditions; overcrowding; poor housing; lack of private transportation; poor public transportation; language differences; illegal alien status for some; distrust of both formal institutions and "other" ethnic groups; lack of awareness of available social services; high rates of crime, etc. (Weidman et al. 1978). These were acknowledged.

We also acknowledged the presence of cognitive systems and perceptions that diverged in many ways from those of orthodox providers of mental health care. We took into consideration differences in world view and value orientation; diverse health-related beliefs and behaviors; varying perceptions of bodily functioning and views about causes of mental illness; different paradigms for interaction with healers; differing views about action required for cure of ultimate causes of illness, misfortune, etc. We also respected the documented presence of traditional healers and patterns of utilization which led easily, and often simultaneously, to both traditional healers and orthodox practitioners. Given these circumstances, the planned program incorporated a number of strategies for innovation.

First, the decision was made not to rent or erect a mental health center building to which patients would be expected to come for care. Instead, the plan was to deploy Bahamian, Haitian, American Black, Cuban, Puerto Rican, and geriatric teams out into the areas where these groups were known to reside. Second, priorities were established which focused primarily upon prevention and then on culturally-appropriate care if there should be breakdown of some sort. Third, Jackson Memorial Hospital facilities, to which the community mental health program was linked, would function to provide back-up services only. Fourth, because of the emphasis on prevention and culturally sensitive care, six key positions would be established for social scientists (preferably anthropologists) of the same ethnic background as the population served. Fifth, the social scientists in these key positions would be called "culture brokers". Sixth, in responding to the needs of individuals in the respective communities, culture brokers would engage in brokerage of two types: (a) that between the community and the dominant social and political system on the one hand; (b) that between traditional and orthodox health cultures on the other hand.

The planned program was funded in 1974 for an eight-year period. Until March of 1981, when it assumed independent status, this community mental health service component of Jackson Memorial Hospital achieved national recognition for being truly responsive to the needs of the diverse ethnic groups and a large number of elderly within its federally designated service boundaries. Internal evaluation has shown it to be efficacious in reducing the number of hospital admissions

RESEARCH STRATEGIES 213

for patients from the area served (continuation grant of CCMHC 1977). The August, 1975 issue of *Psychiatric Annals* is devoted in its entirety to a description of the program shortly after its inauguration. A more recent description is imminent (Lefley and Bestman in press), and a more detailed description of its origins and inauguration is contained within the *Miami Health Ecology Project Report*, Volume I (Weidman et al. 1978).

The formalization of a professional culture broker position has set some potent forces for change in motion. It is this formalization which makes a crucial difference between the Miami program and others (such as the Cornell Navajo project [Adair and Deuschle 1970]) which have had people functioning in similar roles but not formally trained as social scientists (anthropologists) or formally identified as "brokers" carrying training responsibilities along with service ones.

There is also a fundamental difference in the way the culture broker concept has been defined in Miami and the way it has been described in the anthropological literature on social change. In this literature the culture broker concept has applied primarily to mediators between units bound by asymmetrical relationships, such as those between superordinate (national) and subordinate (local) systems (Geertz 1960; Wolf 1956). The label has been used descriptively and after the fact; i.e., after a successful mediating or brokerage role had been achieved. In contrast, the concept, as I translated it into the health field has stressed coordinate status for the two systems involved in any clinical transaction (Weidman 1973, 1975, 1976b). Furthermore, through the creation of a position in a service program and by assigning preliminary role requirements to it, a purposive cast has been given the concept which was not present before. Asymmetry in the culture broker role does still exist in the brokerage responsibilities between various communities (local) and the broader social and political system (metropolitan); while symmetry prevails in brokerage between health cultural traditions.

With respect to traditional healers in particular, it is noteworthy that networks in each of the ethnic communities easily allow the collaboration of traditional healers and orthodox practitioners when an individual's mental health problem requires such collaboration. Furthermore, it is the transcultural perspective supporting this program and the brokerage elements within it which makes such linkages not only acceptable but, for certain numbers of patients, essential.

In both types of "linking" responsibilities inherent in the culture broker role-set and in the research and training aspects of the role as well, the goal is systemic change that will benefit the community and the individuals living in it. Thus, change is sanctioned in the role requirements initially set forth for the culture broker position (Weidman 1973; Weidman et al. 1978). Furthermore, additional role attributes (rights and responsibilities) are being explored and developed in the separate communities and with the elderly (Sussex and Weidman 1975; Weidman 1975). In this regard, it should be noted that the incorporation of culture broker positions and the persons who fill such positions constitutes a most significant alteration in the structure of such an organizational system as does the multiethnic model itself.

In summary, it may be acknowledged that anthropological theoretical orientations, research, and conceptualization contributed to the design of a large service program in a health science context in a multicultural setting. Anthropologically-oriented positions were created and incorporated as integral and essential parts of a clinical program. Culture brokerage at many levels became a major characteristic of the role-set of these "non-clinicians" (on the health science side) whom we (on the anthropological side) would now consider to be clinical anthropologists. The mandate to innovate has generated emergent mental health strategies which vary from group to group but contribute toward raised health levels for the low income populations being served.

The significance of this large mental health program within the context of this chapter is that it introduced structural alterations in the health care delivery system. Furthermore, the new service organization continues to strengthen and encourage a transcultural perspective on the part of clinicians involved in the provision of mental health care and the training of mental health professionals. Community/hospital relationships first established by Health Ecology Project research assistants have been reinforced and augmented by the community mental health service which grew out of it. The community mental health program now offers an unusually supportive context in which our current training and research strategies in primary care are being implemented. We are assured community contacts and ethnic group assistance in the field activities associated with the conduct of various explorations in ambulatory care.

CLINICALLY RELEVANT ANTHROPOLOGY

During the years of successful implementation of the community mental health program there was, in other sections of the medical center, a growing awareness of the need for cultural expertise. Anthropological attention was increasingly directed to cultural issues in health care in other departments, and in mid-1979 a strategy was devised to increase the efficacy of ambulatory care for patients of multiethnic background. I initiated the shift which was sanctioned by the chairman of the department of psychiatry, the medical school dean, who is the University's Vice President for Medical Affairs, and the associate dean who functions as Assistant Vice President for Medical Affairs. A training proposal was developed, and financial support was provided by the Community Hospital Education Council of Florida. Anthropologist colleague, Clarissa S. Scott, joined in this undertaking on a part-time basis as the training activity began.

The Training Facility

The training facility is the Ambulatory Care Center (ACC) of Jackson Memorial Hospital, which is centrally located in the medical center. This is a five-story structure which has sixteen teaching/service-unit modules, conference areas and classrooms as well as laboratory and radiology units, medical records, central supply, pharmacy, and administrative offices. It houses the ambulatory care·clinics of the four departments in which the training occurs.

The Task

The task is to explore ways in which cultural factors affecting health care might be introduced into the training programs of residents in Pediatrics, Internal Medicine, Family Medicine, and Obstetrics-Gynecology. Such explorations are intended to lay the foundation for extensive programs in the future. The purpose is to help prepare primary care physicians to practice their specialities in such a way that patients who come to them for help will benefit to the fullest extent possible. Part of helping physicians in training to gain the means of ensuring optimum benefit for their patients involves the development of strategies to increase patient compliance so that hospitalizations may be reduced and health levels raised. Thus, our immediate goals are twofold:

(1) to provide resident physicians in four medical specialities of the Ambulatory Care Center with information and experience that will allow them to acquire specific cultural knowledge and to incorporate, overall, a transcultural perspective in their approach to, interaction with, and treatment of multiethnic clinic populations; and

(2) to teach residents to work with the patient's beliefs and perceptions as a baseline in helping patients understand and learn the orthodox medical views supporting the care that they receive.

Early on, it was decided to focus upon second-year residents for two reasons: first, to ensure reinforcement of cultural awareness as second year residents became third year residents; second, to encourage dissemination of newly acquired expertise to others in the training hierarchy as third and second year residents supervised first year residents and medical students who followed them. However, it will be seen that the training efforts have spilled over into other areas. The anthropologists are very much "trainees" as well as "trainers". Also included in this "trainee" category are clinical faculty, teaching fellows, nursing faculty, staff nurses, health educators, nutritionists, and social workers. In one context or another, we have been engaged with representatives of each of these groups in matters related to training and patient care. In addition, patients themselves are considered "trainees" because of their need to comprehend the meaning and nature of the health care offered them. The preliminary steps taken to launch this pilot training project were sufficiently cumbersome that they need to be touched upon here.

ACCESS TO CLINICAL AREAS

Access to clinical areas and activities constitute no problem for a staff anthropologist in a home department. In four unfamiliar departments, however, access to clincial areas must be assured by a series of meetings with hospital, nursing, and medical school health professionals at various levels of administrative responsibility. The legitimizing process undertaken in Miami is as follows: first, the Assistant Vice President for Medical Affairs called a meeting of departmental chairmen and other persons involved in training programs. Following that, individual meetings were held with the following persons:

(a) The chairman of each of the four clinical departments.
(b) The medical director of the Ambulatory Care Center.
(c) The administrator of the Ambulatory Care Center.
(d) The nursing director of the Ambulatory Care Center.
(e) Training Directors in each of the four departments.
(f) Teaching faculty in each of the four clinical areas in the Ambulatory Care Center.
(g) Supervising and head nurses in each of the four clinical areas.

Medical directors and teaching faculty of each clinical area then introduced the anthropologists (Weidman and Scott) to residents, nurses, aides, etc., either in the patient-care areas or during regularly scheduled staff conferences. Individual introductions were made to selected residents with whom the author worked directly in each service unit of the four medical specialities. The same processes occurred during rotation through each unit. While Weidman rotated, Scott concentrated on patient interviews.

At the end of two years of half-time involvement in these explorations, there is no question but that the role definition achieved is one of "teaching faculty" and "member of the health care team". Nevertheless, initial perceptions included the following characterizations:

(a) The new person in the clinic is the equivalent of a graduate student engaged in doctoral dissertation research.
(b) The new person in the clinic is a non-physician clinical researcher.
(c) The new person is a medically-informed observer.
(d) The new person is a specialist from a different department.

While none of these perceptions prohibited freedom of action, the characterizations of (a) and (b) may have been slightly more inhibiting than the other perceptions. Over the months, however, as cultural information began to make a difference in outcome or in the understanding of specific problems in health care, these views changed first to a definition something like: "helpful members of the faculty who are not too much in the way in our busy clinics" to, finally, "teaching faculty and collaborative members of the health care team". The point to be made is that when there are no precedents for clinical anthropologist roles in ambulatory care, they must evolve in much the same way they do when anthropologists enter foreign villages.

Participant Observation

The anthropological method of participant observation is central in this pilot effort. The process of rotation through each of the four units and the joining of residents on their assignments, during ward rounds, at case conferences, and in examining rooms has allowed an understanding of the broader context in which residency training in ambulatory care occurs. This type of participation provided, in a relatively brief period, knowledge of the following:

(a) the system of services provided by JMH and each of the four university departments;
(b) the structure of the training program in each of the four departments;
(c) the organization of the ambulatory care units of the four medical specialities; i.e., the manner of assigning nurses, assigning patients to residents, and patterns of processing patients;
(d) the schedules for various types of clinics in the primary care units of each of the four medical specialities; i.e., the date and location of general and specialty clinics;
(e) the assignment schedule for residents rotating through the various clinical areas;
(f) the schedule and location of case conferences and lectures attended by residents in each of the four medical specialities;
(g) the structure of the medical chart, the location therein of laboratory reports, progress notes, referrals and consultation notes;
(h) the meaning of medical symbols, notations, and abbreviations that are part of the medical record of each patient seen in the Ambulatory Care Center;
(i) the computerized system of record keeping and scheduling of patient appointments.

Interviewing

Patient interviews are conducted quietly in waiting rooms, in separate interviewing rooms, by telephone, during pre-arranged home visits, and in a collaborative way with both residents and teaching faculty. Interviews are initiated by anthropologists or they are held at the request of physicians. In those instances when cultural information seems especially important for a positive therapeutic result, the matter is pursued further with both the attending physician and the resident responsible for a particular patient's care.

Record Review

In an effort to identify general areas of poor compliance which might be explored for the impact of beliefs and traditions different from those of the orthodox health care system, a series of record reviews has been undertaken. In each of the four clinical areas of the Ambulatory Care Center (ACC), all patient records have been reviewed for anywhere from two-week periods to a full month. With the cooperation of nursing service and clinical staff, second sheets of the computerized medical record were collected for review. Ordinarily discarded as redundant, these carbons were maintained in the clinical areas and were destroyed in the usual manner upon completion of the inquiry into *recorded* problems of compliance.

For those who wander into clinical areas with a desire not to disrupt the flow of clinic activities and yet to gain a general impression of patterned problems of medical management, this is a productive, initial step to take. For example, in the

Pediatric specialty clinics *recorded* evidence of poor or non-compliance clustered around the medical management of asthma, cardiac conditions, and epilepsy. And in the continuing care clinic of Pediatrics, nutritional problems were pronounced, with frequent notations by resident physicians that there was poor compliance in such matters. Some mothers of infants were offering solid food at much too early an age; while some mothers of toddlers were providing far too much milk in the diet and not enough solid food in the form of vegetables and meats. For older children in the continuing care unit of Pediatrics dietary control again emerged as an important area of poor or non-compliance in the medical management of both obesity and juvenile diabetes.

Other interesting findings have emerged from such reviews. For example, a survey in the Internal Medicine Unit of the ACC revealed that for those patient records showing poor compliance with *diet* and poor compliance with *medication* for the conditions of hypertension and adult-onset diabetes, Blacks were over-represented in relation to their percentage of the clinic population during the period in which the record survey was conducted. Since most of the patients visiting the ACC clinics are indigent, and many live in comparable inner-city neighborhoods, this raises the possibility that cultural factors may be at work. Identification of such patterning opens the door for more focused inquiry and more focused teaching around general problems of compliance in each of the four medical specialities.

While record reviews in each of the clinical units of the ACC have helped to surface general areas in which cultural factors might be contributing significantly to problems of poor compliance, the anthropological technique of contextualization has led to the recognition of structural or organizational impediments which may also interfere with a better outcome of health care.

CONTEXTUALIZATION

Contextualization is the process of understanding every component of a unit in which health care is provided and then tracing a patient's movement through that system, into the home and community and back again for the next visit. By proceeding in this fashion with patients from diverse ethnic groups whose health conditions and compliance problems seem identical, it is possible to identify significant weaknesses in the network of care as well as ethnic differences in attempts to manage particular conditions. In other words, contextualization is useful in pinpointing structural weaknesses in the health care delivery system and also in identifying specific points at which cultural factors may be inhibiting a favorable outcome of medical intervention.

The process of contextualization in the Internal Medicine unit of the Ambulatory Care Center produced important information relating to issues of compliance with both diabetic and hypertensive regimens. On the one hand the information suggested a weakness in the health care system which might be remedied by a medication "hot line". This would insure immediate access to medical advice at the time questions regarding medication arose. Thus, regardless of the patient's ethnic background, compliance might be improved by prompt answers to questions about stopping medication, stretching it over a longer period of time than was intended, increasing or decreasing it, changing medication, or renewing prescriptions, etc.

On the other hand, when patients of the same ethnic background offered information that began to reveal patterned responses to questions about the management of diabetes or hypertension, then impediments other than social organizational ones appeared to be at work. Examples are provided by several Hispanic diabetic patient comments to the effect that one might become "dependent" upon insulin if it is taken too regularly and for too long a period; or, to the effect that "once you start taking insulin, the eyes go bad". Examples from several Black hypertensive patients include statements such as the following: "I don't need medicine if I stay calm"; or "I use other things to cool the blood and bring it down"; or "If I don't have a headache, I know my blood pressure isn't high enough to need medicine." With patterned responses like these, the problems of compliance surely involve more than weaknesses in the structure of the health care system. The process of contextualization allows both types of information to be elicited and provides guidelines for more intensive inquiry into *emic* views about managing chronic conditions. It also provides important information to be utilized in clinical teaching.

A second example of contextualization recently described in another context relates to problems in nutritional counseling in Pediatrics (Weidman forthcoming). Several structural features in the pediatric continuing care clinic functioned to minimize the chances that a mother whose infant or child required dietary management would have the necessary guidance and reinforcement from the nutritionist. By correcting these weaknesses in the functioning of the system, both health care providers and the mothers of children had a better opportunity to achieve their common goal, which was, of course, better health for the child involved. Strengthening the system ensured that mothers and the nutritionist would meet. This allowed the next, and much more difficult step to be taken: i.e., an attempted mediation between medical prescriptions about diet and traditional prescriptions guided by ethnic food preferences, ideals of healthy infant weight, and other rules about good health. The anthropological contribution at the point of mediation is also substantial and frequently leads to additional research and the development of new teaching strategies.

TEACHING STRATEGIES

Clinical Instruction

When any of the investigative techniques of participant observation, interviewing, record review, or contextualization leads us to patients whose cultural beliefs appear to be important inhibiting factors in compliance or outcome, the matter is discussed with either the resident physician involved or the attending physician. If the resident is one with whom there has been no prior contact or working relationship, the matter is first discussed with the attending physician in the area through which the resident involved is rotating. The diagnostic and therapeutic issues are discussed with the attending, who is a member of the teaching faculty. Then, the attending physician, the resident physician, and the anthropologist(s) meet together in the patient care area to develop ways of negotiating between the orthodox and the traditional cultural approaches to the patient's care. The meeting is long enough to communicate the essential aspects of the problem but brief enough that it does not unduly interrupt the resident's pace of work or the flow of patients through the clinic.

In the eyes of the resident, the anthropological contribution is sanctioned automatically by the engagement of the attending physician in the process. Furthermore, it is non-threatening, because it is directed toward therapeutic efficacy with a specific patient. Under these circumstances the introduction and use of cultural information is usually very well received. It is the resident who implements the strategy in interactions with the patient in the examining room. Thus, the experience is his/hers alone. As such, it provides the basis for subsequent explorations and learning.

One dramatic instance recently described in another context reflects the transformation which may occur when cultural factors are taken into account in health care (Weidman forthcoming). The case is one in which the doctor was approached by a patient with many reservations about orthodox health care because of prior unfortunate experiences. Initially, the patient was perceived by the doctor to be "schizophrenic" because of his "flat affect" and his experience of hearing voices in the night. Following use of the teaching technique outlined above, the interactive pattern changed to one of great warmth between doctor and patient following a series of negotiations between orthodox views and traditional cultural interpretations of the symptoms presented. The physician achieved the therapeutic goals he had set forth, and the patient was content that all of his concerns had been addressed and that he was feeling better. The diagnosis of schizophrenia was revised.

In addition to one-to-one teaching in the clinics with second and third year residents, our work is also having an impact on a wider audience via other mechanisms of instruction. Some of these are reviewed below.

Participation in Staff Meetings

When any of our informal investigations reveal patterns of structural weakness in the health care system or patterning of any sort that might warrant further discussion and inquiry, a place is requested on the agenda of a forthcoming staff meeting in whichever clinical area is involved. For example, one of our record reviews in Pediatrics suggested the over-representation of Black children suffering from iron-deficiency anemia and an over-representation of Hispanic children considered to be obese. This has become a focus of further inquiry and health educational concern in the Pediatric unit involved. In addition, the structural weaknesses regarding nutritional counseling, mentioned above, were resolved as a consequence of discussion during a staff meeting.

Videotaping

On many occasions Dr. Scott's interviews in the home have been so revealing of cultural beliefs regarding home management of health problems that videotapes have been made on subsequent visits. These are made with the patient's consent for use in medical teaching. The tapings are financed by funds for medical student instruction, and the tapes are used in the first year Introduction to Medicine course. They are also utilized in one and two-day workshops on the transcultural perspective in health care to be discussed below. Additional tapes have been requested for use in teaching medical students on their Liaison Psychiatry rotations. These resources are available for use in other health professional training contexts as well.

Case Conferences

We have explored with great success the use of the case conference method of instruction. For example, with the support of the chairman of the Department of Family Medicine and the training director of this department, three dramatic cases have been presented in which cultural factors played a crucial role in the successful treatments of patients. The physicians involved were at different levels of training and responsibility, one a member of the teaching faculty, one a second year resident, and one an intern. Each presented the medical facts, the puzzling aspects of symptoms, diagnosis, and therapy, the manner in which cultural information was utilized, the importance of that information, and the successful outcome that occurred as a result of taking both traditional and orthodox views into consideration. The anthropologist (Weidman) then elaborated upon the cultural aspects of the case, including discussions of world view, health culture, perceptions of bodily functioning, etc. In each instance the entire presentation and the lively discussion which followed were tape recorded. The tapes are being transcribed, edited, and submitted for publication in the *Journal of Family Practice* as Grand Rounds presentations. The clinicians carry senior authorship responsibilities in this undertaking, thereby gaining additional experience in presenting the approach to their peers. These strategies generate far more interest and personal investment in such matters than might be the case otherwise.

Team Teaching

One teaching effort which is becoming more structured in the Department of Family Medicine involves the use of videotapes of resident-patient interactions. We have found that this allows a multi-layered teaching/learning format which can have a broad ripple effect. For example, when a patient's visit with a resident is videotaped (with the patient's written permission), the tape is utilized to assess various parameters of interaction such as: interviewing skills, interpersonal behavior, patient education about medical conditions, prescription instructions, counseling in primary care, etc. It is also possible during such analyses, to introduce cultural information which benefits not only the resident, but also the member of the teaching faculty and any teaching fellows who may be present. As the anthropologist contributes insights and cultural data to the critique of the interaction, the physicians present are able to absorb cultural information linked specifically to the patient's concerns in relation to medical diagnosis and management. Similarly, as the attending faculty member and the teaching fellow comment and advise the resident, the anthropologist is able to understand points of particular medical and interactional concern. Everyone benefits, including, ultimately, current and future patients.

Faculty Development Seminars

When videotapes of patient-resident interaction in the Family Medicine Clinic are especially good teaching tapes, they are also used occasionally in Faculty Development Seminars. Six to eight Family Medicine faculty members (not always the same ones) meet weekly for inservice sessions designed to strengthen their teaching ability. After viewing a segment of a videotape of resident-patient interaction, the tape is stopped, and faculty engage in role-playing. One faculty member acts as "resident"; while, first a physician and then an anthropologist take turns guiding the "resident" to a more skillful interactive approach prior to sending him/her "back into the examining room" with the patient.

The role-playing exercises are followed by comment and advice from other faculty members present. Such sessions contribute to more efficacious teaching methods on the part of all faculty and frequently function, as well, to underscore the importance of cultural factors in health care. We have found, for example, that at times cultural views are clearly expressed by the patient who appears on the videotape. Medical faculty, however, may be unaware of their full meaning and uncertain about utilizing such information in their analyses of the "resident's" performance. The Faculty Development Seminar use of videotapes and role-playing allows a greater understanding and internalization of the cultural issues involved. Unquestionably, this will, in time, influence all levels of residency-training in Family Medicine as more members of the faculty become at ease with a cultural component in their teaching and in family practice. The value to the anthropologist participant in such faculty development seminars is just as great. In no other context is it possible to practice clinical teaching, a mode of instruction to which anthropologists ordinarily are not exposed.

Workshops

One teaching strategy which we would not have predicted would be very popular is that of the one-day workshop. We have found it to be a very productive teaching mode. The workshop format first emerged in response to a request from nursing faculty at Jackson Memorial School of Nursing for an intensive staff development seminar on cultural issues in nursing. It was designed as an all-day workship and offered continuing education credit, with learning objectives clearly specified. It included discussions of the concepts of culture and health culture, the use of natural therapeutic remedies and the use of spiritual therapeutic measures by Black American patients. It also described Haitian health care in Haiti and the United

States and Cuban health care in Cuba and the United States. Videotaped interviews with Black and Hispanic patients were used to maintain a clinical focus, and attention was given to techniques for eliciting cultural information. A fieldwork assignment was made, during which the ethnographic approach and beginning transcultural skills were to be put to use with any patient who may have been defined as a "problem" patient. A second half-day meeting followed completion of the field assignments. During this session, selected case studies prepared by nursing faculty were analyzed and discussed to further clarify processes which were operating in their interviews with "problem" patients and to reinforce the transcultural (trans-person) posture.

Although this workshop was developed for nursing faculty specifically, it now constitutes a basic training format which can be offered in any clinical area for any group of health professionals. It is currently being modified to accommodate three additional requests. One comes from the Department of Family Medicine, one from Pediatrics, and one from the Veterans Administration Hospital, which is an affiliated teaching hospital of the University of Miami School of Medicine.

Family Medicine

In collaboration with the Department of Family Medicine, a two-day workshop is being planned for October of this academic year (1981). It is designed to acquaint first and second year residents with problems of rendering care to a multiethnic clinic population. A general orientation with study groups will constitute the first day; while focused attention on diabetes, hypertension, and other major illness categories (including *emic* "unnatural" illnesses) will be the work of the second day. Both anthropologists and Family Medicine teaching faculty will participate in study group discussions and in case presentations as a way of reinforcing the collaboration required in bringing physicians in training to the transcultural perspective in the provision of health care.

Pediatrics

In Pediatrics, the impact of the Haitian migration to South Florida is being felt in many ways. One of the most striking patterned problems, however, reveals itself in the number of Haitian babies hospitalized with severe dehydration and other complications from prolonged diarrhea. They are far sicker than any other group of children hospitalized for such conditions and often must remain in the hospital for extended periods of time. Two requests have come from Pediatrics for assistance with this problem: one from the clinical director of the continuing care clinic of the Ambulatory Care Center; the other from Pediatric nurse educators. Informal research on this problem (to be discussed below) will culminate in a workshop with Pediatric health educators; while a special seminar on this topic will be held for pediatric faculty and staff in the Ambulatory Care Center.

Veterans Administration Hospital Nursing Staff

A third use of the workship format is scheduled as this manuscript goes to press. It is to be held at the Veterans Administration (V.A.) Hospital adjacent to Jackson Memorial Hospital in the medical complex. This workshop, like that of the Jackson Memorial Hospital School of Nursing, also provides continuing education credit for V.A. nursing staff. Inasmuch as there is an unusually rich mix of nurses of diverse ethnic origin in the V.A. hospital, some will participate as panelists and others will function as study group participants with specific tasks. Commentary, overviews, and cultural analyses will be provided by anthropologists (Weidman and Scott).

It should be noted that the emergence of training workshops as a viable teaching strategy comes as a suprise to us. We would not have predicted that such large blocks of time would be made available for teaching about cultural factors in health care. This suggests that the problems involved in the management of patients from multiethnic backgrounds are of such magnitude in Miami that a transcultural approach is becoming a prerequisite to genuine communication between health professional and patient. We would add that it may be a prerequisite, also, for higher rates of compliance with medical regimen and ultimately for improved outcome of care.

CURRICULUM DESIGN

To date, anthropological explorations in clinical realms have not led to major involvement in curriculum design; however, some contributions have been made to curriculum planning in the Department of Medicine. As of July 1, 1980, this department initiated a primary care track as part of its General Internal Medicine Training Program. Within this track a curriculum is being developed that deals with practical patient problems that are outside the realm of standard internal medicine residencies. Some of the components of this track (but not all) are as follows:

(a) Emphasis on prevention and maintenance outside the hospital.
(b) A shift from episodic care to continuity of care (outpatient and hospital).
(c) Multidisciplinary teaching, including, among others, psychiatrists and anthropologists.
(d) Patient education and health promotion.
(e) Community preceptorships in private offices of Department of Medicine attending physicians.
(f) Cost containment and cost effective medical practices.
(g) Comparative evaluations of primary care trainees and standard internal medicine residents re: patient emergency room use and hospital admissions, cost containment, etc.

Clinical training remains at the heart of the program, with each resident consulting the attending physician on each patient visit. But, also being built into the curriculum are weekly clinical conferences, primary care seminars, a journal club, a research seminar, a lecture series on non-internal medicine clinical topics, a mini-course on Epidemiology and Public Health, and research activities with Department of Medicine and primary care physicians.

It is significant that anthropological perspectives and cultural factors in health care are becoming an integral part of this primary care track. The expectation is that within five years or so this track will attract approximately 50—70% of the Internal Medicine house officers, thereby changing considerably the type of internist graduated from this Department of Medicine. We anticipate that there will be increasing participation by anthropologists in curriculum design and evaluations as this program evolves. There is no guarantee on this point; however, the program directors and anthropologists are already working closely together in various research and training activities in the Internal Medicine clinical areas.

FORMAL RESEARCH PROJECTS

As the point is made in both small and large ways that culture counts in health care, there has been more openness from clinicians and at the same time a more critical attitude which is leading to mini-studies on specific problems. The reasoning seems to be as follows:

Yes, I can see that in this case cultural beliefs made a difference in compliance and in outcome, but how general is this? How do we know that this patient is not atypical for his cultural group? How do we know where we need to develop more structured training around some of our major problems in health care?

The answer has been that it might be worthwhile to examine such questions systematically. Consequently, we have embarked upon formal mini-research projects in Internal Medicine, Pediatrics, and Family Medicine.

Internal Medicine

In Internal Medicine, an anthropologist, an internist, a nurse clinical educator, and a clinical pharmacist have embarked upon a carefully controlled study to determine the value of using cultural knowledge to promote compliance with the hypertensive regimen. In broad outline the plan is to compare the conventional patient educational approach (which will include helping the patient to tailor medication-taking to his or her daily living pattern) with one that acknowledges and incorporates the patient's health cultural beliefs and behaviors into the teaching session. The goals are to increase patient compliance with anti-hypertensive medication and improve blood pressure control.

Pediatrics

One of our previously mentioned observations from record review in the Pediatric continuing care clinic is that obese Hispanic children were over-represented in the patient population of this unit during a month long review of all clinic records. This observation, among others, has led to the design of a comparative study to examine the influence of mothers' cultural ideals of healthy infant weight and related feeding practices on obesity.

Family Medicine

The value of a circumscribed training module oriented to the medical management of diabetes is currently being assessed in Family Medicine. Using a control group for comparison, the module requires three sessions and involves residents at each level of training (PGY1, PGY2, and PGY3)[4] who are following insulin-dependent, adult-onset diabetic patients in the Ambulatory Care Center. This module builds upon the doctoral dissertation research of Dr. Clarissa Scott (1980) who, earlier in her career, functioned as Field Coordinator for the Miami Health Ecology Project. It is specifically addressed to utilizing the patient's *emic* views to increase the patient's orthodox understanding of the illness. The evaluation design includes periodic measures of compliance and degrees of control of the patient's condition. It also includes both patient and resident self-reports of satisfaction with the management of the illness at specified intervals.

We consider small, circumscribed formally structured research projects of this type to be important teaching strategies for the following reasons, some of which warrant careful research in their own right.

(1) The research questions are being asked about cultural factors in health care, compliance, health education, and outcome.
(2) The research designs are sound; therefore, the questions asked may be answered in unequivocal terms.
(3) Empirical data from such studies serve to erase any lingering questions about the importance or lack thereof of cultural beliefs in matters of compliance, the success of health education, etc.
(4) Empirical data influence decisions about curriculum.
(5) Empirical data from sound research provide substantive materials to utilize in teaching.
(6) When integrated into training programs, empirical data regarding local patient populations and specific techniques of medical management reinforce other efforts designed to achieve both the short-term and long-range goals of our work.
(7) Empirical data are persuasive in influencing health-professional and patient interactions. Both patients and health professionals benefit from the use of such data.
(8) Medical students who become involved as research assistants during work-study periods learn from such projects and are possibly influenced in their care of patients by such participation.
(9) Research efforts of this sort bring multidisciplinary persons from faculty, staff, and trainee populations together in ways which encourage cooperation and collaboration; thus, more integrated ways of working together emerge in many different contexts.

INFORMAL STUDIES

Informal ethnographic inquiries constitute a continuing aspect of anthropological

activity in clinical settings. In Miami these are carried out in and around more
structured responsibilities, but they have direct implications for patient care as
well as medical education. Several examples follow:

Internal Medicine

In Internal Medicine we are being drawn into an analysis of problems faced by
health care providers as they attempt to treat high rates of tuberculosis, particularly
among Haitian refugees who continue to arrive in boats of all sizes upon the shores
of South Florida. The problem is not restricted to this group of newcomers to
Dade County, but within the Haitian community the tuberculosis rate appears to
be 10 to 15 times higher than the base rate for the county as a whole. Major areas
of concern center on the apparent inability of many such refugees to identify initial
symptoms of tuberculosis and to seek care during the early stages of the illness.
We know from both Wiese's studies (1971, 1974) and the Health Ecology Project
(Weidman et al. 1978), that symptoms orthodox physicians associate with early,
intermediate, and advanced stages of tuberculosis tend to be defined by Haitians
as four separate illness categories or "disease" entities. We are finding, also, that
there is a great confusion in the minds of many Haitian patients about early releases
from the hospital (with continuing medication and follow-up in ambulatory care
clinics) when the patient still "feels sick". The reverse problem also is common.
Many Haitian patients question the need to continue medication for months
after they again "feel well". Once released from the hospital, medication ordinarily
is required daily for an additional 15 months. Health professionals find, however,
that frequently it is discontinued almost immediately. Moreover, many patients
very quickly are lost to follow-up. There are many reasons for such behavior,
but aside from "feeling well" and, therefore, seeing no need to take medicine,
two extremely salient ones are: (a) the need to be unencumbered in the quest for
employment and (b) the fear of being jailed or deported, because "They won't
let you stay if you are sick". This informal ethnographic inquiry is ongoing.

Pediatrics

In Pediatrics we are accumulating ethnographic data which will be incorporated
into the above-mentioned forthcoming workshop with health educators and a
special seminar for Pediatric faculty, residents, and staff to be held during the
academic year. The focus of this special inquiry is on problems of managing diarrhea in Haitian babies.
     The extreme morbidity of Haitian babies hospitalized with severe dehydration
and other complications from prolonged diarrhea constitutes a puzzling problem
to pediatricians at Jackson Memorial Hospital. The management of Haitian babies
with diarrhea presents a challenge in ambulatory care settings as well. We have
learned, for example, that when home remedies fail to help their children, Haitian
mothers usually first seek help from private physicians or community clinics. In
these settings the physicians instruct the mothers to stop their traditional practices
designed to cure diarrhea, but they do not. The children are then hospitalized,

both out of necessity and also as a strategy by local physicians to block the continued use of traditional practices which are harmful to the children.

We do not yet have all the answers we need to begin cultural negotiations around the management of diarrhea in Haitian babies; however, we do have some insights into the problem. We know from our prior research, for example, that a form of milk of magnesia, *magnesie en boule*, a "cold" remedy, is given for "hot" diarrhea (with fever) and, also, that "hot" substances are given to counteract "cold" diarrhea (without fever) (Weidman et al. 1978). Such practices support the hypothesis of the clinical director of the pediatric continuing care clinic that mothers of Haitian children with diarrhea are giving them some hypertonic substance or substances which heighten their morbidity rather than alleviating it. Additional factors which appear to be relevant in this regard are as follows: [5]

(a) Haitian mothers must work; therefore, they do not nurse their infants in Miami.
(b) "Formula" is a new idea to them. They do not understand the need to refrigerate formula (and may have no refrigerator).
(c) Under conditions of poverty and crowding in which many Haitian refugee families live, sterilization of formula bottles is essential but little understood by Haitian mothers.
(d) Undiluted evaporated milk is often given as a substitute for formula.
(e) Adult table food, which contains large amounts of fat, is fed to Haitian babies beginning at the age of three or four months.
(f) Haitian mothers reject instructions to give their infants with diarrhea only Pedialyte (an oral electrolyte solution) for a certain period of time. They see it to be "just water" and say that their babies will die without food.
(g) Milk is not perceived to be a "food"; so in the event Haitian mothers attempt to follow medical instructions to eliminate food for a certain period of time, this does not pertain to milk. When they give their infants milk, they are not "feeding" them; they are offering them something to drink.
(h) "Something to drink" often includes goats milk from the Hispanic community, which is seen as providing more "strength" than other forms of milk.
(i) Honey is defined as a "hot" food which provides strength to infants and may be added to liquid substances, including formula and milk.

Almost all of these behaviors may be viewed by pediatricians as actually or potentially harmful to Haitian babies. The investigation is continuing, however. As we feel more secure in identifying the predominant cultural patterns and home remedies that are used in an attempt to "bind" the digestive process and cure diarrhea but which in effect exacerbate the condition in Haitian infants and small children, processes of training and cultural negotiation will begin. The crucial question is whether or not brokerage between belief systems and an acceptable process of education about orthodox views will be possible. Certainly, cultural accommodations are required if compliance and an improved outcome are to be achieved.

Gynecology

A number of areas of non-compliance have emerged in Gynecology which warrant attention; however, none seems more problematic than the management of pelvic inflammatory disease, which includes an array of conditions which need not be reviewed here. Within this broad category none seems more entrenched and fraught with difficulties than the management of salpingitis (inflammation of the Fallopian tubes) among Black patients particularly. Gonorrhea accounts for many cases of salpingitis, but we have found confusion in the minds of many such patients about the etiology of "pus tubes", as this condition is called within the Black community. There is confusion, as well, about the meaning and purpose of therapy, and about the frequent recurrence of the condition. In order to sort out some of the areas of non-compliance and the reasons for them, we have embarked upon an informal ethnographic inquiry.

Patients with salpingitis are interviewed in the Gynecology unit of the Ambulatory Care Center prior to or following their scheduled appointments. Information gathered to date corresponds extremely well with community data collected previously through the Health Ecology Project. Presenting symptoms include severe, contraction-like pains in the abdomen. They are episodic and may be associated with nausea, and an array of other symptoms. Many Black women in the community and in the clinic see the condition as caused by contamination ("dirt" of some sort which has "poisoned them" and led to a generalized "blood" problem). They frequently comment that they "don't understand" what the doctor is saying about the problem and what the treatment is supposed to achieve. "They give me shots and pills, but it comes back." Some believe that because of the number of symptoms they have (fever, weight loss, pain, lack of energy, etc.) that "something more" must be wrong. The feeling is that this is not a localized problem; that it is more extensive than the doctor suggests. Sometimes the thought is expressed that there is need for "something to pull the poison out": Importantly, in the case of "pus tubes" home remedies are considered to be ineffective. It is recognized that penicillin and pain pills are necessary. The feeling is, however, that these do not go far enough to effect a cure; therefore, the condition recurs.

Health professionals, on the other hand, see the condition as recurring because of poor hygiene, an active sex life, multiple sex partners and, in the case of gonnorhea, contact with a specific bacterium. A "cure" would require greater cleanliness, possibly reduced sexual activity and greater restrictions on the number of sex partners involved in order to reduce the chances of being reinfected. While this is so on the one hand, some Black patients with whom we have spoken see no relation between "pus tubes" and sexual activity *per se*. They see "dirt" as one of the primary causes, but it may come from the air, a toilet seat, a douche bag, or, possibly a dirty penis. "Dirt", of course, sometimes has magical connotations, and the extent to which spiritual or supernatural activity may be perceived as part of the problem of recurrent salpingitis remains to be clarified.

It is apparent from our work to date that sexual behavior within a large segment of the Black community served by JMH, is defined as "good" and "desirable" and necessary for health. The consequences of abstinence or reduced sexual contact are always negative ones, such as headaches, nervousness, and, ultimately, mental illness. Thus, the orthodox provider of care says that salpingitis recurs beccause of poor hygiene, frequent sexual encounters and numerous sexual partners; while the Black patient with "pus tubes" tends to see the problem as recurring because the health care provider has not given the proper treatment to clean the body or the blood. There are other problems of compliance related to examination of sexual partners, but these will not be reviewed here. Medical advice to reduce the frequency of sexual activity or to limit it to a single partner would be intrusive. Advice to have sexual partners examined and treated is rarely followed. Another type of advice to prevent recurrences of salpingitis might be to encourage the use of condoms and to reduce stress levels, advice which would have little meaning to many patients.

This informal ethnographic inquiry is reaching the point that a strategy session will be held in the near future to discuss our findings with the Gynecology clinical director. Next steps could lead in two directions: (a) toward a more controlled, comparative study among patients of different ethnic background (with residents participating) and/or (b) toward a full staff conference (including residents) to discuss not only our findings but also health education strategies that might be used with patients suffering from chronic salpingitis.

MEDICAL STUDENT INVOLVEMENT

One of the advantages of the clinically-linked mini-research projects mentioned above is that medical students have an opportunity to participate as research assistants while on two-month work-study stipends during summer months. Some students engage in administering questionnaires, conducting patient interviews, monitoring compliance by means of pill counts, prescription renewals, and insulin measurements, etc. Others investigate various aspects of medical management problems for particular conditions. They explore issues of (a) diagnosis, (b) therapy, (c) patient compliance, (d) patient definitions of the illness, (e) patient beliefs about its proper management, and (f) life circumstances and events which also influence compliance and outcome. Thus, some students learn from more formal research endeavors; while others learn the process of ethnographic research by means of contextualization and ethnic group comparison.

Arrangements are made with the clinical directors of the medical speciality areas in which the various health problems are explored, to have the students participate in a formal discussion of the work completed. At the end of the two-month work-study period, the student is allowed to prepare and present at a full staff conference a formal paper reporting his/her findings and making recommendations about strategies that might be employed in (a) increasing compliance and (b) educating the patient about the orthodox medical beliefs and practices underlying the treatment received. Implicit in this process are some important teaching elements which, hopefully, will not be lost on faculty, staff, and residents.

Other medical students are supervised according to individual needs and specific requests. For example, a third year medical student has requested supervised reading in medical anthropology along with his required work in the coming year. He had an interest in the field of anthropology during his undergraduate work and now sees the relevance of this to his career as a future physician. His intent is to follow such reading with fieldwork during his fourth year when time will be available to him for this.

At the request of the Department of Family Medicine, supervision is also being provided to two medical students who will participate in a clinical clerkship in Brazil during the coming summer. They will have contact with a number of Indian tribes in the Amazon Basin and need guidance to appropriate medical anthropological literature which will help them know how to elicit cultural information and to begin to utilize a transcultural perspective in their clinical work.

PATIENT EDUCATION

As the point has been made that culture can be important in health care, it has become much easier for us to collaborate with health professionals in exploring new ways of explaining orthodox views and orthodox therapeutic efforts to patients. During discussions with clinicians about specific problems of patient comprehension and compliance, practitioners make medical information explicit for the benefit of the anthropologist. The anthropologist, in turn, makes cultural information explicit for the benefit of the health professional. Then, together, strategies are developed to help orthodox care to become meaningful to the patient in terms of his own understandings. When the discrepancy between the two is not too great, the patient may be brought to a fuller comprehension of the orthodox position, first by contrasting that position with the patient's views; second by showing in what way the patient's understanding makes sense but is not quite correct under the circumstances involved; and third by consistant and repeated clarification of the orthodox position on each visit. When the discrepancy between the two belief systems is extensive, however, special effort is directed to helping the patient to receive three messages:

(1) That the Health professional *understands* the patient's views of his/her health problem, its etiology, and what might be perceived to be appropriate therapy;
(2) That the health professional *respects* these views by addressing in a professional manner each of the patient's concerns about symptoms and reassuring the patient that, in this instance the problem is different;
(3) That the health professional *cares* about the patient by explaining fully what the problem is (in his/her opinion); what the prescribed therapy is designed to do, and what positive, beneficial signs the patient might look for to know that the treatment is working.

The transcultural perspective is implicit in dealing with both narrow and large

differences in belief systems. It should be noted, however, that in order to trans-
mit the type of messages outlined above, practitioner-patient interaction may be
altered markedly from that usually in existence in clinic settings where cultural
differences are not taken into account. The interaction is altered in a direction
compatible with the achievement of goals set forth at the beginning of this section.

Inasmuch as the argument is for a more relativistic, transcultural perspective
in health care, it may seem paradoxical that there is equal concern about transmission of the orthodox view to patients of multicultural background whose health
cultural traditions, we say, are deserving of attention and respect. Our position on
this point is that the potential strengths of orthodox medicine cannot be realized
without a fair degree of compliance with prescribed therapies. Also, we accept a
great deal of evidence that eclectic absorbtion of health related beliefs and therapies
is a continuing process inherent in the evolution of all health cultural traditions.
The process, however, occurs in individuals who are the bearers of those traditions.
Consequently, the view is held that the more meaningful linkages there are between
orthodox and traditional approaches, the better chance there will be for increased
compliance and raised health levels.

This is a very different hypothesis from that which has been explored in the
literature to date; namely, that compliance will improve when patients are taught
medically accurate details about their conditions. Repeated studies have disproved
this hypothesis (Haynes et al. 1979; Sackett and Haynes 1976). However, investigations have not yet carefully examined the hypothesis that compliance and outcome
will improve when orthodox medical knowledge is transmitted to the patient in
relationship to his/her own understandings of the illness process.[6] If this hypothesis,
also, is disproved following similar studies by many investigators, then it may be
wise to recognize that the high value placed upon health education within the
dominant culture and the orthodox health institution is unsupported by social
facts in the field of health care.

Until such time as we may know the answer to this second type of question, we
shall proceed on the following assumptions: (1) that health beliefs and practices
are absorbed by the patient in an eclectic fashion, (2) that compliance and outcome
will improve through orthodox health education that is meaningfully linked to
the patient's belief system, and (3) that the more coherent the segments are that
are transmitted by health professionals and absorbed by patients, the greater
the congruence there will be in the long run between the clinical reality of patients
and the clinical reality of health professionals. Such congruence requires, of course,
the transmission of coherent segments of traditional health cultural beliefs to
the orthodox health professional in order for the question to be properly examined.

In brief, from a transcultural, investigative posture of anthropology there is no
conflict between support of relativism on the one hand and orthodox therapeutic
regimens on the other. One (relativism) may work with the other (unicultural
strategies) to achieve the common goal of both the health professional and the
patient; namely, an improved state of well-being.

In the long-run, the provision of health care may be made easier for both patients and practitioners because bridges between traditional and orthodox views are being forged in the process. It is possible, in fact, that the primary value of the negotiating mode of interaction, is nothing more than a way to improve communication and rapport between patient and practitioner. Each begins to listen to the other. Thus, a two-way teaching-learning process of the sort described, may function to allow a more humanistic orientation to prevail throughout the entire set of interactions. Compliance is likely to be improved on these grounds alone. Consequently, improved health status may be linked to greater compliance based upon an enhanced trust and faith in the practitioner *because* of the relativistic posture of the clinician.

Whatever future experience may prove, the difficult task of orthodox health education for patients of multiethnic background is discussed in the context of every consultation, every case presentation, every seminar, and every workshop in which we participate. In addition, it is the challenge of patient compliance and patient education which has led to both formal and informal research strategies described above. In Internal Medicine the issue is that of compliance with the hypertension regimen. In Pediatrics, the two areas in which we are working relate to diarrhea in Haitian babies and obesity in children, particularly Hispanic ones. In Gynecology the problem is that of pelvic inflammatory disease generally and salpingitis, specifically, for Black patients in particular. And the teaching strategy undertaken in Family Medicine relates to compliance with the diabetes regimen.

Health education for patients from multiethnic backgrounds is an integral component of our research and training activities with health professionals, whether these be medical and nursing faculty, residents, staff nurses, or medical students. The fact that we increasingly are able to work collaboratively with practitioners on particular management problems suggests a fairly high level of integration achieved to date by means of these explorations.

CONSULTATION AND THE CREDENTIALING PROCESS

As word spreads that cultural factors may have an important bearing on outcome of health care, there are increasing numbers of requests for anthropological consultation. These are both individual in nature and group related. Individual requests tend to be for patients whose diagnostic picture is confused and who are not responding to orthodox therapy. Two cases of this type have been described recently (Weidman forthcoming). Examples of requests for group consultation and assistance include those from JMH health educators: one group working with diabetic patients; another working with mothers of Haitian infants. Another request has come from a pediatric social service unit focusing on teenage preganancies.

While group consultations about programs create no problems regarding rights and obligations of anthropologists in clinical settings, the matter of individual patient consultation does raise extremely important questions. For example, although the medical chart clearly specifies sections for physician notes in contrast to notes by others, does an anthropologist, untrained in patient evaluation, patient care, or even input into patient care have the right to write in the chart?

As a faculty member in a clinical department, there is no question about the right (or the responsibility) to respond to a consultation request from a physician for an anthropological opinion about a patient. An anthropological assessment is made and outlined in the chart. Advice is proferred in writing therein about actions which might be helpful in patient care. It then becomes the responsibility of the patient's physician to either write orders acting on that advice or to disregard it. If the anthropologist were not to use the chart in this way, cultural information of value to many persons involved in the patient's care would be lost. Also, as Kaufman has stressed, consultation notes which reflect an anthropological perspective and include cultural content, condensed though it may be, function importantly in staff and house-officer education as well as in patient care.[7]

Nevertheless, the medical record is a medico-legal document, and anyone who writes in the chart is subject to subpoena for court appearances in the event of malpractice litigation. If an anthropologist has gone through the institutional credentialing process and functions according to a list of privileges approved by a series of formal hospital committees and governing bodies, then such a person would be covered by the same institutional malpractice insurance provided other credentialed health professionals. If such a person has not gone through such a credentialing process, however, or has overstepped the privileges listed and authorized, then he/she may become personally liable for his/her own legal defense and payment of any damages that might be required by a court.

In Miami, more frequent consultation requests and increased collaboration with physicians in patient care has led the author to the point of initiating a request for formal credentials and delineation of privileges. The application will be submitted to the Credentials Committee of Jackson Memorial Hospital, to the Joint Conference Committee of hospital and medical school representatives, and to the Public Health Trust which governs JMH hospitals and clinics. It may be some time before this process is completed. It is mentioned here as an issue with which increasing numbers of anthropologists will have to deal as they become more fully engaged in clinical action.

CONSULTATIONS WITH TRADITIONAL HEALERS

The distinction made by many Black patients between "natural" and "unnatural" illnesses and by many Hispanic patients between "physical" and "spiritual" illnesses limits the extent to which the orthodox health care system has meaning for them. As long as a particular health problem is viewed as a "natural" or a "physical" illness, it is possible to attempt to develop meaningful linkages between orthodox and traditional health belief systems. Once an illness is defined by the patient as an "unnatural" or "spiritual" one, however, the orthodox system becomes somewhat less relevant. It has no standard therapies for "supernaturally caused" illnesses; therefore, the brokerage task assumes different characteristics.

"Unnatural" or "spiritual" problems that orthodox practitioners would consider to be psychiatric in nature ordinarily are treated in traditional health cultural systems by traditional healers. The cosmology which defines such conditions and delineates the therapy appropriate to treating them is so alien to orthodox psychiatric approaches that, generally, there is no point in requesting psychiatric consultation or suggesting referral to a psychiatrist.[8]

We have found it necessary, in such cases, to request consultation from reputable traditional healers. These are persons with whom we established relationships as part of our prior Health Ecology Project research. Such relationships have been maintained within the framework of the multiethnic community mental health program described above. At times patients are referred to such persons; at other times the healer is called to the clinic.

Often traditional healer consultations include therapeutic actions which prove extremely beneficial to patients suffering from "supernaturally-caused" disorders (Weidman forthcoming). Dramatic improvements in patients' conditions have occurred in remarkably short periods of time as a consequence of such contact. Continuing care by the healer in conjunction with ongoing care by orthodox practitioners is left to the discretion of the patient. In some instances we know that contact with the traditional healer has continued. In other instances a single visit has been sufficient to transform a situation from one in which the patient fails to respond to orthodox interventions to one in which the patient responds remarkably well. It is significant that the patient ordinarily continues under the care of the orthodox physician while accepting welcome assistance, also, from the traditional healer.

On the basis of current patterns, we find that in Family Medicine alone, we may expect four to six patients in any two-week period to be candidates for consultation with a traditional healer. Frequently, the patients so afflicted are indigent, with no financial means of access to such persons. Consequently, consultation fees become the key to improved health status for a certain percentage of the patient populations with which we work.

We have been in an unusually strong position to meet needs of this type in our clinical activities because of the structure of our community mental health program. The Cuban and Haitian unit directors are anthropologists whose ethnic backgrounds match those of the communities they serve. Each has an extensive community network that includes traditional healers whose work they know well. There is another resource in the director of the Bahamian unit who is not a social scientist. He is a Bahamian ordained minister and spiritual healer who grew up in the Bahamas. In his capacity as a salaried member of an orthodox but innovative health care system, he has functioned as a consultant to medical practitioners. In his capacity as a Bahamian traditional healer he has also, at the request of orthodox practitioners, provided therapy to patients in both hospital and clinic settings. He has done so without remuneration despite the fact that some of the traditional remedies he uses contain very expensive ingredients.

Referral networks which include traditional healers in Bahamian, Haitian,

American Black, Cuban and Puerto Rican neighborhoods are beginning to be so well established that, in a sense, they represent an expanded component of the orthodox health care system. As such, they require the same types of fee for service arrangements that would be expected for any consultation request to an orthodox specialist. Inasmuch as third party payments do not include the services of a traditional healer in the state of Florida, and county funds are not available for such purposes, funding must come from other sources. We are currently exploring ways in which such traditional healer consultants to indigent patients may be reimbursed according to standard fee schedules prevailing in the area.

Requests for consultation from traditional healers, like those for consultation from anthropologists, raise some important medico-legal issues. Consultation is one thing; therapy — and *unorthodox* therapy at that — is quite a different matter. Consultation advice may always be accepted or rejected by the attending physician. If, however, a recommendation for traditional therapy is acted upon, that order enters the record under the physician's signature as the medically responsible person. Therefore, in a litigious society prudence suggests that an added step be taken prior to the writing of such an order. That step would entail full discussion with the patient, and a request for a signed informed consent form indicating his/her desire to be treated on the premises by a traditional healer with the orthodox practitioner present or not as desired. Such an informed consent form becomes part of the medical record and is obtained prior to the writing of an order by the attending physician for traditional therapy.

Hospital risk management offices are only now coming to terms with some of the medico-legal questions raised by these recent alterations in the structure of orthodox health care. Each question satisfactorily answered represents an accommodation to shifting patterns of health care based upon the incorporation of a transcultural perspective. And each accommodation is designed to increase responsiveness to patient needs and concerns while increasing the efficacy of the care provided. Whether or not a genuine transformation is underway remains to be seen. It is exciting, nevertheless, to witness here and there the impact of anthropological contributions in a health science setting which benefit both patients and providers of health care.

COST EFFECTIVENESS

Cost effectiveness is very much a theoretical and pragmatic issue in the evaluation of uniculturally versus transculturally oriented service programs. In a training institution such as that of the University of Miami School of Medicine, service programs rest first upon the vision and experience of its clinical faculty. They rest secondly upon the house officers of the university's teaching hospitals and clinics; i.e., the resident physicians who are being trained by faculty of the School of Medicine. With greater experience in our training and research strategies, we anticipate that there will be a solid core of clinical faculty and a group of third year residents with whom it will be possible to embark on a study of cost effectiveness of the two modes of health care delivery.

There has been dramatic evidence from our own experience in Miami that cultural responsiveness in health care is cost effective (Lefley and Bestman in press; Rubin and Jones 1979; Weidman forthcoming). There are also increasing numbers of cases being reported by other investigators that are in line with our findings (Eisenberg and Kleinman 1981). Consequently, until a systematic study is feasible, we shall proceed with every exploratory approach and investigative technique that we can devise to achieve the goals toward which our efforts are guided. Until proved wrong, we shall assume that transculturally oriented health care is more cost effective than uniculturally oriented care.

In summary of this section on clinically relevant anthropology, the description of our work demonstrates the extent to which the initial focus upon ambulatory care residency training in four clinical departments has been broadened. We have responded to many requests outside this training arena. Collaboration has been undertaken with health professionals in whatever ways seemed important and meaningful to them. In addition we have contextualized, conceptualized, strategized, and initiated processes designed to encourage movement from a unicultural to a transcultural perspective.

The beauty of this exploratory project is that it allows us to be responsive to the needs of both providers and consumers of health care. In the process gradual changes are occurring in the structure of training programs and service systems. In the long run such structural alterations provide the means of answering unequivocally some of the questions prevailing in the current literature. For example, one key question is whether or not outcome is favorably affected by taking cultural beliefs and practices into consideration when orthodox care is provided. Our work and that of others suggests that it is. A second question is whether or not traditional healers affect outcome in a way orthodox healers cannot. We have striking evidence that they can. A third question is whether or not traditional healers legitimately can become part of the structure of orthodox medicine, either by incorporation or by referral networks. We are currently engaged in such a legitimizing process in Miami. Nevertheless, systematic investigations are needed to examine these and many other central questions to ensure that we are not lured on only by anecdotal material. It is entirely possible that formal inquiries into such matters will be feasible in Miami in the not too distant future.

During the two years in which this pilot study in ambulatory care training has proceeded, Clarissa Scott and I unquestionably have come to be perceived (a) as members of the teaching faculty for residents in ambulatory care, (b) as contributors to the health care of ambulatory patients of multiethnic background, and (c) as collaborators in health education for such patients. We anticipate that an additional two years will see many of our emergent strategies crystallize and become formal aspects of residency training in the four medical specialties in which we function as well as in other areas of the medical center.

Implications for Training in Clinical Anthropology

There are implications in our work for training in Clinical Anthropology. As formalization occurs, the dimensions of our clinically-related activities will become more sharply etched. At that time the incipient training possibilities in clinical anthropology that are unfolding may materialize into a full-blown program. For example, Dr. Irwin Press of Notre Dame, a professor of anthropology and academically-based medical anthropologist, spent a sabbatical year with us. The year (1980–1981) was designed to give him clincial experience which is not available to him in his home institution. In addition, persons who hold Ph.D.'s in anthropology, some already specialized in medical anthrpology, are beginning to request post-doctoral training in clinical anthropology to be carried out in this health science setting. Furthermore, we have been receiving requests recently for experience in transcultural nursing, from faculty of the University of Miami School of Nursing, located on the Coral Gables campus. This school of nursing, under the leadership of Dean Evelyn Barritt, recently has adopted transcultural nursing as its guiding orientation and educational mission. Nursing faculty without prior experience in translating the transcultural perspective into patient care are feeling the need to "learn by doing" in the hospitals and clinics of Jackson Memorial Hospital.

Formal Assignments and Committee Responsibilities

As in any institution of higher learning there are formal demands upon anthropologists in health science settings which sometimes place them in influential positions in the organization. One of these in a school of medicine is the curriculum committee of the Medical School Council. I presently sit on such a committee in Miami and, therefore, am in a position to add formal weight to medical student education which is in line with changes occuring at the residency-training level.

Scott is in an even more direct position to influence the character of medical education in the preclinical years. She functions as coordinator of the Department of Psychiatry's behavioral science teaching for the freshman and sophomore Introduction to Medicine course. She also carries co-coordinating responsibilities for the entire medical student pre-clinical curriculum. In each capacity, she has the opportunity and the responsibility to help prepare effective behavioral science teaching content and devise behavioral science teaching strategies for medical students. In Miami this realistically includes a strong anthropological component; thus reinforcing and preparing students for many of the anthropological contributions occuring in other contexts.

CONCLUSIONS

This chapter has reviewed some of the strategies I have employed in attempting to better integrate the respective contributions of anthropology and medicine to health care in a multiethnic setting. Much of my work has been considered exploratory. Nevertheless, it has opened the door for colleagues to follow and become involved in clinically related activities in a way that might not have been possible without such incursions into clinical realms.

Although clinical anthropology is not yet fully formed as a specialty area within the sub-discipline of medical anthropology, there is clearly need to prepare anthropologists to function in ways similar to those outlined here and in other chapters in this volume. On the health science side there is receptivity to and need for anthropologists to be so engaged. Unfortunately, there is currently precious little training for clinical anthropologists which will prepare them to work with clinicians of various types.

If we were to formalize into a training program some of the aspects of our work in Miami, the syllabus would include many of the topics which have been touched upon herein. The sub-headings utilized above have not been designed specifically for such purposes; nevertheless, they serve as guidelines to parameters which might be incorporated into training programs for clinical anthropologists. For example, methodological approaches could include: participant observation, record review, contextualization, formal research design, and ethnographic inquiry. Similarly, the social mechanisms which allow theoretical and substantive material to be introduced could include one-to-one teaching, team teaching, staff conferences, case presentations, seminars, workshops, and consultations.

Additionally, although the processes of planning, implementing and administering various research strategies have not been made explicit, they represent training issues, nevertheless. The use of research strategies in clinical settings suggests the need for training in research design, proposal writing, implementation and administration of grant support, acquaintance with computer technology and computer use, as well as techniques for indexing, recalling, and analyzing ethnographic and life history materials.

Thus, whether the reader's interests lie on the professional side or the academic side of anthropology in health science settings, this chapter may be of some value in sorting out various dimensions of work that are currently operational in the field of clinical anthropology.

NOTES

1. In Miami some of the greatest points of tension over the years have been related to the timing of shifts from staff to line positions and vice versa as change strategies have dictated. Anthropological views have frequently but not always been decisive in this regard. In several instances it has been possible to maintain the staff position despite various types of pressure to accept line positions of considerable responsibility and authority. At another time, when a strategic shift to a fairly central line position seemed (and has proved to be) crucial for continued anthropological/psychiatric program development, multiple organizational and administrative constraints prevented it.
2. Following Harris (1971), we have consistently used the definition of culture as "The learned pattern of thought and behavior characteristic of a population or society . . . a society's repertory of behavioral, cognitive, and emotional patterns."

3. Kleinman et al. (1978) have directed attention to the concept of *clinical reality* as a useful, relativistic term.
4. Shorthand for postgraduate years 1, 2, and 3, referring to first, second, and third year residencies.
5. We are indebted to Claude Charles, M.A., for his assistance in our explorations of this problem. Mr. Charles functions as Haitian Culture Broker in the community mental health program which grew out of the Health Ecology Project.
6. This is the intent of our formal research on compliance with the hypertensive regimen which is being conducted with faculty in the Department of Internal Medicine and JMH clinical staff.
7. Lorraine Kaufman (1981) made this point during a workshop on Training Issues in Clinical Anthropology, held during the Annual Meeting of the Society for Applied Anthropology, Edinburgh, Scotland, April 11–17. It might be added here that consultation note writing is a skill which must be developed to be effective. It should, by all means, become an integral part of a clinical anthropologist's training.
8. Snow includes a summary of successful attempts by orthodox practitioners to deal with the issue of "unnatural" illness in health science settings. See Snow (1978). As more persons with joint degrees in medicine and anthropology apply integrated approaches to patient care, it is likely that there will be an increase in reported instances of orthodox success with patients whose illnesses are believed to be magically caused. The question in our mind is whether or not joint degrees are necessary. Is it possible that adoption of a trans-cultural view in health care will have the same impact without masters or doctoral level training in anthropology?

REFERENCES

Adair, John and Kurt Deuschle
    1970 *The People's Health*. New York: Appleton-Century-Crofts.
Continuation Grant
    1977 Continuation Grant of the Comprehensive Community Mental Health Center of the Mental Health Division of Jackson Memorial Hospital and the University of Miami, Department of Psychiatry, 12–19–77.
Eisenberg, Leon and Arthur Kleinman (eds.)
    1981 The Relevance of Social Science for Medicine. Dordrecht, Holland: D. Reidel Publ. Co.
Geertz, Clifford
    1960 The Javanese Kijaji: The Changing Role of a Cultural Broker. Comparative Studies in Society and History 2: 2: 228–249.
Haynes, R. B., et al.
    1979 Compliance in Health Care. Baltimore: The Johns Hopkins University Press.
Harris, Marvin
    1971 Culture, Man and Nature. New York: Thomas Y. Crowell, p. 624.
Kleinman, A., L. Eisenberg, and B. Good
    1978 Culture, Illness and Care. Annals of Internal Medicine 88: 2: 251–258.
Kluckhohn, Florence R. and Fred L. Strodtbeck
    1961 Variations in Value Orientations. New York: Row, Peterson and Co.
Lefley, Harriet P., and E. W. Bestman
    in press Community Mental Health and Minorities: A Multi-Ethnic Approach. *In* S. Sue and T. Moore (eds.), Community Mental Health in a Pluralistic Society. New York: Human Services Press.
Open Forum: Clinical Anthropology
    1980 Medical Anthropology Newsletter 12: 1: 1980, and Open Forum: Clinical Anthropology (continued) Medical Anthropology Newsletter 12: 3: 1980.

Rubin, Jeffrey C. and Judy Jones
   1979 Falling-Out: A Clinical Study. Social Science and Medicine 13B: 2: 117–127.
Sackett, D. L. and R. B. Haynes
   1976 Compliance with Therapeutic Regimens. Baltimore: The Johns Hopkins University
         Press.
Scott, Clarissa S.
   1980 The Influence of Patient Beliefs on Compliance to Therapy for Diabetes Mellitus.
         Unpublished doctoral dissertation, University of Miami.
Shimkin, Demitri and Peggy Golde (eds.)
   forthcoming Anthropology and Health Services in American Society. In preparation for
         University of Illinois Press, Urbana, Illinois.
Snow, Loudell
   1978 Sorcerers, Saints and Charlatans: Black Folk Healers in Urban America. Culture,
         Medicine and Psychiatry 2: 69–106.
Sussex, James N. and Hazel H. Weidman
   1975 Toward Responsiveness in Mental Health Care. Psychiatric Annals, 5: 8: 8–16.
Weidman, Hazel H.
   1971 Difficulties of Synthesis: Conceptual Blocks and Administrative Hang-ups. Paper
         presented at the 30th Annual Meeting of the Society for Applied Anthropology,
         Miami, Florida, April 14–18, as part of a symposium entitled, "How Goes the Holy
         Trinity? An Appraisal of Psychiatric Anthropology in Five Medical Settings Today."
   1973 Implications of the Culture Broker Concept for the Delivery of Health Care. Paper
         presented during the Annual Meeting of the Southern Anthropological Society,
         Wrightsville Beach, North Carolina, March 8–11.
   1975 Concepts as Strategies for Change. Psychiatric Annals 5: 8: 17–19.
   1976a In Praise of the Double Bind Inherent in Anthropological Application. In Michael
         V. Angrosino (ed.), Do Applied Anthropologists Apply Anthropology?, Athens:
         University of Georgia Press, pp. 105–117.
   1976b On Getting from "Here" to "There." Guest Editorial, Medical Anthropology News-
         letter 8: 1: 2–7.
   1979 Falling-Out: A Diagnostic and Treatment Problem Viewed from a Transcultural
         Perspective. Social Science and Medicine 13B: 2: 95–112.
   forthcoming Research, Service and Training Aspects of Clinical Anthropology: An Institu-
         tional Overview. In Demitri Shimkin and Peggy Golde (eds.), Anthropology and
         Health Services in American Society. In preparation for the University of Illinois
         Press, Urbana, Illinois.
Weidman, Hazel H. and James N. Sussex
   1971 Cultural Values and Ego-Functioning in Relation to the Atypical Culture-Bound
         Reactive Syndromes. International Journal of Social Psychiatry 17: 2: 83–100.
Weidman, Hazel H., et al.
   1978 Miami Health Ecology Project Report, Volume I, University of Miami offprint.
Wellin, Edward
   1977 Theoretical Orientations in Medical Anthropology: Continuity and Change Over
         the Past Half-Century. In David Landy (ed.), Culture, Disease, and Healing, New
         York: MacMillan, pp. 47–58.
Wiese, H. Jean
   1971 The Interaction of Western and Indigenous Medicine in Haiti in Regard to Tuber-
         culosis. Unpublished doctoral dissertation. University of North Caroline at Chapel
         Hill.
   1974 Tuberculosis in Rural Haiti. Social Science and Medicine 8: 6: 359–362.
Wolf, Eric R.
   1956 Aspects of Group Relations in a Complex Society: Mexico. American Anthropologist
         58: 1065–1078.

ATWOOD D. GAINES

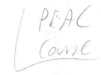

KNOWLEDGE AND PRACTICE: ANTHROPOLOGICAL IDEAS AND PSYCHIATRIC PRACTICE

INTRODUCTION

In the practice of clinical psychiatry, an essential feature of praxis is the accumulation of knowledge about patients through the interpretation of their presentations, both aural and behavioral. It is upon the knowledge base derived from a variety of sources, embodied and disembodied (e.g., written records) that diagnostic, managerial and dispositional decisions are based. Because the confrontation of individual patients, prospective patients and physicians (and physicians in training) may be seen as a fundamentally hermeneutic interaction, it can be suggested that biomedical clinical "knowledge" is but interpretation, interpretation of symbols and signs in terms of particular, and particularistic interpretive schemata (see Good and Good 1981).

Because interaction in clinical settings is an essentially interpretive process, it is of considerable importance for the improvement of clinical praxis to evaluate interpretive frameworks such as social-cultural anthropology, which may have demonstrative impact upon clinical interpretive processes and hence on the construction of clinical reality. Toward this end, this chapter addresses the problem of knowledge and praxis in clinical psychiatric settings, including emergency room consultations and open and closed wards in a public non-profit hospital. It will be demonstrated here that social-cultural anthropology,[1] as a body of theory, a stock of knowledge and a set of methods, can make contributions to clinical interpretations and thus to clinical psychiatric practice.

The Construction of Clinical Reality

Research on psychiatric practice has long noted that exogenous factors can influence clinical assessments. Researchers focusing upon the social class of patients and practitioners have pointed to the impact of such status differences upon clinical interpretations and dispositions (Brill and Storrow 1960; Derogatis et al. 1971; Myers and Schaffer 1958). Differences in ethnic group membership between healer and patient have also been seen as contributory to problems of clinical interpretation (Katz, Cole and Lowery 1969; Dorfman and Kliner 1962).

It is now well known that different ethnic groups perceive psychiatric symptoms differently (e.g., Sanborn and Katz 1977; Katz, Sanborn and Gudeman 1969; Katz, Cole and Lowery 1969; Marsella 1980; Gaines 1980; Good and Good 1981; Kleinman 1977, 1980; Kiev 1968; Reynolds 1978). As well, illness experiences vary radically across cultures (Good 1977; Marsella 1980; Zborowski 1978; Kleinman 1977, 1980). The members of various cultural groups may be said to perceive different illness realities based upon their divergent Explanatory Models (EM's,

N. J. Chrisman and T. W. Maretzki (eds.), Clinically Applied Anthropology, 243–273.
Copyright © 1982 by D. Reidel Publishing Company.

Kleinman 1975, 1977, 1980). We also find differences in EM's in various sectors of the same health care system (cf. Freidson 1970; Kleinman 1980; Twaddle 1974) and, importantly, among individual professional healers (cf. Abrams and Meador 1976; Gaines 1979, 1982; Light 1976). Actors' varying explanations in the clinical setting influence interactions and interpretations occurring in that context.

The catalogue of exogenous factors affecting diagnosis, and hence, patient management, has also been shown to include practice orientations of Western psychiatric professionals (Duehn and Mayadas 1967), cumbersome or limiting diagnostic nomenclatures (Gaines 1979, 1982) as well as various sorts of errors, intentional and unintentional (Morrison and Flanagan 1978). The demonstrated impact upon clinical interpretations and patient management of such exogenous factors throws into relief the fact that from the physician's (or the patient's) point of view, the clinical encounter is not a mere decoding of clear signs of distress which leads directly to the invocation of particular diagnostic labels and the assignment of therapeutic regimes.

The critical problem which must be addressed, then, is the interpretive, or hermeneutic nature of the medical encounter. The medical encounter is but a species of social encounter or interaction. In all such interactions, meanings are brought to and exchanged by actors through the employment, patterned and idiosyncratic, of various symbolic forms. Patient and healer, as the actors in the medical encounter, should be seen as engaged in the interpretation of the context of the encounter (as symbolic itself) and of the symbolic forms manipulated by the other during the encounter. Symbols may be seen as embodiments of meaning and are such things as words, acts, events and or gestures (cf. Geertz 1973). Participants' understandings of a given encounter are grounded in preexisting definitions of the medical or psychiatric encounter as a species of encounter and are also derived from the exchange of meaningful elements in the encounter itself. (Depending upon the experience of a given individual, the medical or psychiatric encounter may be seen as either a new form of interaction or as a repetition of a previously known form of encounter. Hence we cannot suggest that reality is created anew in each encounter.)

When we consider that encounters in medical and psychiatric contexts are interpretive, we are led to a concentration on meaning and understanding. What meanings do certain behaviors have? What do we understand the presentation of particular behaviors to mean? What are the meanings of patients' social or physical characteristics? In the meaning-centered approach to medical interactions recently elaborated and clarified by Byron and Mary Jo DelVecchio Good (1981), we see that the critical psychological mode of experiencing is "verstehen", (to understand), rather than "wissen" (to know) or "erklaren" (to explain). As they have written, "all illness episodes should be seen as fundamentally semantic" (i.e., meaningful) and all clinical transactions between patient and healer "should be seen as fundamentally hermeneutic" (Good and Good 1981: 4).

We may see that clinical reality is in fact constructed and that the construction is the result of hermeneutic processes that elucidate meaningful (to a given context) elements. Clinical reality for patient and healer is a construct or constructs (as they often differ, cf. Kleinman 1980), created by interpretation. As such, alterations of the knowledge base concerning a given patient, or the provision of new vantage points from which to view him/her, can all contribute to different and fuller interpretations of patients and their presenting complaints. So, as we alter the hermeneutics, the interpretive processes of the clinical encounter, so too we alter the nature of clinical reality which is thereby constructed.

In this paper, interest will focus upon clinical psychiatric interpretations and the impact upon them of social-cultural anthropology theory, knowledge and methods. Having set this formidable task, it will be necessary to leave aside from our consideration the important issues of the fundamentally semantic nature of medical and psychiatric illness episodes to focus only upon the construction of clinical reality by psychiatrists. Although this paper assumes a meaning-centered approach to psychiatric illness, we focus only upon healers' interpretations of patients' semantic illness realities.

Setting

The data presented here were collected during research on psychiatry in a large 600 bed general hospital which I will call Kahala-Kokua General Hospital.[2] The hospital is located on the island of Oahu amidst the marvelous cultural diversity of Hawaii. Psychiatric attendings and residents discussed here are affiliated with the medical school of a local university which provides psychiatric personnel to Kahala-Kokua. Residents usually spend a year-long rotation in the hospital providing in-patient and out-patient services, consultation liaison work or other tasks on the different psychiatric services. Kahala-Kokua Hospital is one of serveral hospitals which provide emergency psychiatric care to the approximately 800,000 people of the island.

In addition to emergency and out-patient services, Kahala-Kokua General also maintains an in-patient mental health facility. From 15 to 18 of the beds are apportioned to the closed section of the ward. Patients were seen in the open and closed wards of the facility as well as in the emergency room.[3]

In the following, we will consider cases that demonstrate that the construction of clinical reality is altered by the introduction of aspects of anthropological science. The cases show that aspects of anthropological science can provide the basis for the deconstruction and subsequent reconstruction of clinical psychiatric reality. Cases will be presented and the contributions of anthropology to the construction of new clinical realities analyzed. Contributions of anthropological theory, method and/or knowledge will be assessed case by case. This means of presentation saves both time and space as the consideration of the same cases under different rubrics would require some repetition of identifying information. As well, the use of cases allows for the demonstration of the efficacy of applying different aspects of anthropological science to the same case. By utilizing a case approach, it will be seen that various components of the science may be simultaneously relevant to the reconstruction of clinical reality.

The cases chosen for presentation here were selected to highlight issues that I think are especially significant in that they present at least a glimpse of the major issues of the construction of clinical reality where anthropological science may be able to make a contribution.

THE CASES

Case 1

A 26 year-old male was admitted to the psychiatric unit of Kahala-Kokua General Hospital. The patient's diagnosis upon admission was "schizophrenic". (The diagnostic nomenclature in use by the attendings and residents in this study is that of DSM II. Although drafts of DSM III were available in the department, there had not been any systematic attempts as yet to switch to the new nomenclature or nosology). The patient, unemployed for some time, was the son of a Japanese father and an Okinawan mother. He had been born in another city on another island in Hawaii. The patient was admitted after being found wandering about near Waikiki and was without permanent residence or means of support.

Upon admission, the patient gave his name as "Bob Edlax". While his given name seems to have been correct, the family name he gave was an enigmatic fabrication. It was some time before the meaning of his pseudonym could be unraveled through the use of some ethnographic knowledge of American popular culture.[4] In addition to the problem of his family name, Bob presented clinicians with a problem regarding his self-definition of ethnic identity. Bob claimed that he was white. This problem of social classification of self and other will serve as a focal point for the examination of folk theories regarding racial and ethnic identity held by clinical professionals involved with the case. These folk theories were part of the clinical assessment of Bob Edlax.

I was made aware of Bob by a level two resident (second year of a four year residency program) who suggested that Bob might be of interest to me. It was then known among the residents among whom I worked that I had some interest and research experience in the field of ethnicity. This was one reason it was suggested that I might want to meet Bob Edlax. The resident's suggestion came on the second day of Bob's stay in the hospital. Neither the resident nor the attendings (or the ward staff for that matter) had any doubt whatsoever about the "character of danger" manifested by Bob. It was certain that he was schizophrenic. And, one of the definite symptoms of that condition was the frequently verbalized ethnic self-ascription of "white". It seemed fairly obvious that a claim of Anglo ethnicity by a man that was clearly phenotypically Asian constituted yet another symptom of the disorder that afflicted the patient. But was this claim really another symptom of schizophrenia?

When I was told about Bob's belief that he was a "Haole" (local Hawaiian term which originally meant "foreigner" but which now refers to whites only), it occured to me that the assertion was not wholly inconceivable. I met Bob on Kahuna, the open psychiatric ward of Kahala-Kokua Hospital. I was accompanied by Dr. Unger, the level 2 resident who had first told me of Bob, and Dr. Hanneman who was Bob's attending and an extraordinarily sensitive clinician.

During that first encounter, Bob often and firmly asserted that he was "Haole". As he said, "I'm Haole, not Asian. I hate those Asian bastards. I like those people" (he then pointed to a female Haole ward clerk). On subsequent days, Bob was to get into difficulty for verbally and possibly physically abusing other patients who were Asian. These hapless people, not knowing of Bob's existential position, would make 'mistakes' such as sitting next to or speaking to him. Bob interpreted such acts as declarations by these Asian others that he too was Asian and that they were claiming him as one of their own, an identity he vehemently denied. We might note here that in assuming a white identity, Bob seemed also to have incorporated racist attitudes toward Asians which he viewed as part of white identity. Bob did have a refined notion, a specific kind of white identity in mind.

Not only did Bob see himself as a Haole or white, but as a special sort of white, a "new creature" as he explains in this exchange with a medical student. The exchange had been taped the morning I met Bob. I was able to view the tape the evening of the day I first encountered him.

Medical Student: What is your ancestry?
Bob: Ancestry is, huh, oriental's blood; along a Japanese father and an Oki (derogatory slang term for Okinawan) mother.
MS: How do you view yourself?
B: As a new creature.
MS: As a new creature? Could you tell me about that?
B: You, have you ever looked at the back of the pyramid, at the eye?
MS: Huh?
B: (On the back of the) dollar bill, I mean.
MS: Oh. Yes.
B: You'll see the Virgin Mary was really an Egyptian god, Orsiris. When they came to the planet, they started sucking the humanoid out of the modern man and putting the space creature, the new creature, into it. Once Jim died, he left his legacy for his brothers to follow 'cause he knew they would have a hard time doing that. He had no brothers, I don't know ... he had friends but he left it for the new creatures, where race does not mean anything, just peace and brotherhood among nations of the world. People like (the Joneses) and many prominent families, perhaps in the US of A, who disagree with the ways of Rock'n Roll. Once we start realizing who these children are, you know, what's gonna happen? It's going to be anarchy.
MS: These new creatures of yours, they're involved with Rock'n Roll?
B: Yea. Rock'n Roll to the world, yeah. Food, Jesus, Krshna, maybe even Krshna will be included.

This portion of the interview gives us a view of the major elements of Bob's cognitive world; severe problems over personal identity, popular music culture ("Jim" refers to Jim Morrison who died in Paris in 1974 and who was the lead singer of the Doors, a famous Rock group of the late sixties and early seventies), pop culture (Eastern religion), sustenance (here in the form of food, elsewhere in conversations including the interview from which the above was excerpted, it is garbage or manure), money and spiritual/new creatures. In terms of anthropological theory, I will focus on the problem of race.

Bob, as we have seen, denied being Asian. He claimed instead that he was Haole or white or Anglo, the term he would employ changed from time to time, day to day. Attending health professionals attributed this "nonsensical" claim to his illness. In fact, Bob showed more anthropological understanding of the cultural construction of ethnic categories than did the people who were trying to help him. Of course, this is a case of being right for some of the wrong reasons.

As has been shown in anthropological research, ethnic distinctions are made on the basis of subjective criteria without regard for putative objective criteria (Barth 1969). Further, research has shown that there are not, in fact, any biologically distinct races of man (Washburn 1972). Bob had recognized that "in common sense terms ... , the idea of race is built not simply on the notion of likeness but also on the idea of consanguinity. A race is a group of individuals who share certain characteristics by virtue of their common ancestry" (Stocking 1968: 164). However, after "physical anthropologists subjected these characteristics to more and more careful measurement (during the last half of the 19th century), the racial 'likeness' became a statistical rather than an individual phenomenon, and common ancestry became almost a gratuitous assumption" (Stocking 1968: 165).

Also, as Montagu has noted,

Most readers will be aware that the social (sometimes called the "sociological") concept of race, the doctrine, to put it briefly, that there exist superior and inferior races, has long been unacceptable to anthropologists. What most readers may not be aware of is the fact that the *biological concept of race* has become unacceptable to a growing number of biologists on the one hand and to an equally increasing number of physical anthropologists on the other (1970: xi).

(The original statement appeared in 1964.) Of course, Franz Boas, the father of American Anthropology, showed us at the turn of the century that 'race,' language and culture were independent of one another.

A biological conception of race implies that human populations are distinct in terms of certain measurements, but these measurements produce indications that there is a great deal of overlap among supposedly dissimilar groups. Hence, "mankind cannot be subdivided into one group with zero per cent and one group with 100% frequencies for any one character" (Hiernaux 1970: 36). It has been clearly recognized that any system of racial classification, whether it contains seven, nine or however many 'races' must be based upon arbitrary criteria (Montagu 1970; Hiernaux 1970; Stocking 1968; Washburn 1972). As Hiernaux asks, "If any racial classification is arbitary, for what purpose can it be of any use?" (Hiernaux 1970: 40). The concept of race, therefore, is seen as useless and misleading as a scientific concept (Washburn 1972; Montagu 1970; Hiernaux 1970). The concept of race must be regarded as a folk theory, a cultural form of social classification (cf. Gaines n.d.). As much is indicated in UNESCO's 1950, 1964 and 1967 formal statements on the scientific basis of the concept of race made over the last 30 years (cf. 1969), i.e., there is no such basis.

Thus, Bob evidenced a more scientifically modern conception of culture as the molder of behavior in the face of his contemporaries' clearly 19th century notions of the "three races" (white, black, yellow). Recognizing this understanding allows us to see a critical area of his problem, that of self-identity which was intimately bound up with American notions of racial identity. (Blu [1980] indicates that the racial ideology is giving way to an ethnic ideology and shows this is 'what is happening to the notion of race', a question posed by Handlin [1957] and Stocking [1968]).

Bob was trying to say (unsuccessfully) that, "while I may look Asian, I am culturally Anglo". How do we know this was what Bob was trying to say? After listening to Bob, I formulated and asked him directly if this is what he meant by his assertion that he was white. As I posed the question, Bob leaned forward with much interest. When I finished, he smiled and enthusiastically responded, "Yes! That's it! That's it exactly!"

Now we can see that Bob's self identification is not, as was thought initially, a schizophrenic symptom. Treating it as such also fails to center upon the patient's central problem, self identity. Because he felt he was Anglo, obviously he had greatly ambivalent feelings toward his parents. It is not surprising that he sometimes denied that they were his parents. While he no doubt cared for them, he also felt hatred and contempt for them because they had given him the physical appearance which made it difficult if not impossible for him to be accepted as a member of the Anglo ethnic group. So it is not surprising that he would doubt his parentage from time to time.

I do not here suggest some vaguely Langian idea that the madman is really an architect of a logical new reality in response to illogical external pressures and that the mental patient is the one who is 'really' in touch with reality. Rather, it is shown here that a patient exhibiting schizophrenic symptoms is demonstrated to be less out of touch with reality than initially would appear to be the case.

In other respects, Bob's case presents us with a chance to see the use of ethnographic knowledge in a clinical situation. That is, the anthropologist was able to gain some rapport with the patient because of some ethnographic knowledge of pop culture which paralleled his own. The author could make sense of the patient's statements where often others could not. In the exchange with the medical student above, Bob's statements made virtually no sense. First, let us clarify some of Bob's statements from the first excerpt and then provide a second excerpt which highlights the patient's focus on a specific cultural domain.

In the first excerpt, Bob talked of "new creatures", among whom he counted himself, and linked these creatures to Rock and Roll. We can see that his identity as a new creature in part refers to his freedom from traditional social classifications which made him Asian. He sees himself as a member of an Anglo subculture, Rock and Roll, the members of which are above such invidious distinctions. He thus equates Rock and Roll with the formulation of a world culture and a decline in racial notions of social classification. This identification of music and social change is not, of course, unique to Bob; Bob has in fact internalized a major message of the 1960's-cultural upheaval as social change, freedom and justice through music (and other art forms). Two further things are important.

First, Bob sees new creatures as being in the vangaurd of change. This makes sense of his other statements that Asians were "stuck, rigid, traditional". "They don't understand Rock and Roll." For Bob, he could not be Asian *and* be progressive or revolutionary. This negation leads to a desire to deny his parents explicitly or implicitly ("I am a new creature", i.e., not the son of a Japanese man and an Okinawan woman). Second, new creatures must of necessity be involved with the revolutionary agent, the music. As a consequence of this last belief, he talked in seeming riddles using song and album titles, song lyrics and the names of record labels and Rock stars. So most of his discourse would be comprehended by another member of the subculture or, as in this case, a student of that subculture. Bob's concentration on a single subcultural domain appears again more clearly in the second excerpt below. While schizophrenic symptomatology is readily observable, Bob's utterances are clearly less than totally random. Making some sense of his speech requires knowledge of the domain in which he speaks, as we will see when we analyze this next bit of conversation with Bob.

MS: You said sometimes you feel you're being controlled by others. How?
B: Yes. When I get in contact with the new creatures, the immortals to be more exact.
MS: How can you tell you're coming into contact . . . ?
B: I feel peace, content, well being, happiness in my inner soul, way down inside, and I feel content.
MS: Have you come in contact with new creatures recently?
B: Yes. Mike Snow.
MS: Who is he?
B: Rock'n Roll musician (a personal acquaintance, not a major Rock figure), vocalist, child of God, flower child, latter-day flower child. We'll record on Swan Song. Bet on contract approval by the Corporation.
MS: And you're a rock star or musician?
B: Yes, musician. Everybody is a star, but you have to prove that yourself before they can reap the cake, that was left out in the rain. But we know who we are and we're going to to try to make it on Swan Song. (Bob begins to doze off here but continues) Try to understand it. Not all love is in vain. It's not a homosexual relationship either. [(aside) Don't know where that word came from. It's in the media all the time.] It's really more like aspiring towards a cheapened communion between brother and sister. My sister is an Indian girl (gives name) who I look forward to seeing, loving and taking away to Hollywood, once I find her.

And later in the same interview, Bob says:

B: Music is my only friend, (well) not really, (it is) one of my friends.
MS: What other friends do you (have)?
B: Freaks. Not really, children who grew up in the world until they got burned. Can't explain revolutionary philosophy from the Sixties. Can't explain . . . unless you grew up and listened to records then. (I have) a guardian angel, French. Came to take care of me;

compassion and pity for a lesser man. She's been through so much burn. Helped me to take the burn off, to have more rational and compatible behavior for Americans.

When the medical student gave Bob a proverb to interpret, he answered it in a way consistent with his focus on Rock;

MS: Can you tell me what the proverb, "A rolling stone gathers no moss" means?
B: (without hesitation) No sticky connections, no shady connections. It's a groove, but no connections. Shady groove but no shady connections. No sticky fingers, there might be some sticky fingers but there is nothing sticky about it.

Using these excerpts, I hope to point out briefly the utility of ethnographic knowledge when used to interpret patients' utterances and for the understanding of those utterances by their placement in a subcultural context. Although ethnographic knowledge is the immediate key to unraveling the patient's discourse, it should be kept in mind that the anthropological assumption that there *would* be a key and that discourse would be patterned according to *some* cultural context is the necessary starting point for understanding.

Bob's statements about control and contact evidence classic schizophrenic symptomatology. However, he seems not to receive any sort of orders or criticism from these contacts as is often the case with this disorder. Bob talks of certain social categories, e.g., "child of God, flower child, latter-day flower child". In this he is referring to significant social categories of the Sixties' scene. The phrase, "latter-day" indicates Bob's awareness that the Sixties have indeed passed. (We should note that the "Sixties" actually refers to the time between 1963–4 and 1972–3.) He refers specifically to that time in American history when Rock'n Roll matured into Rock and became the dominant form of musical entertainment (recorded and live). Bob, in his discourse, is faithful to Rock music. We see virtually no references to such musical forms as Rhythm and Blues, Country and Western, Jazz, Opera, Classical or any of the more recent musical developments which include Reggae, Disco, Punk, New Wave (i.e., American Punk), Country Rock or Folk. He does make reference to the Blues, however, because the Blues serves as the basis for Rock but not the other forms of popular music. Thus, all Rock musicians are also Blues musicians and employ the Blues musical scale. Fifties' Rock'n Roll does not nor do new forms such as Punk.

So it is that the Rock world with which Bob identifies is that of the Beatles, the Rolling Stones, Cream, Led Zeppelin, the Who, Sly and the Family Stone, Ten Years After, the Doors, the Jimi Hendrix Experience, the Jefferson Airplane and so forth; "Heavy" or "Super" groups all. In the first excerpt, Bob referred to Jim Morrison of the Doors as well as some of the secular and religious themes current in the Sixties. In the second excerpt he actually focuses almost exclusively on the subcultural domain of Rock.

First, the "immortals" to which Bob refers are the legends of Rock who have gone on to that Great-Concert-in-the-Sky. These include Morrison as well as Janice Joplin, Jimi Hendrix, Duane Allman (Allman Brothers' Band), Brian Jones (the

Rolling Stones), John Bonham (Led Zeppelin), Keith Moon (the Who) and most recently and tragically, the brillian lyricist John Lennon.

The name, "Swan Song" is that of a relatively new record label (ca. 1975). Its first and still major artist is a group led by Briton Paul Rogers called "Bad Company". The group represents the remnants of a late-Sixties' group with a substantial cult following called, "Free". [Perhaps Bob was attracted to this label because of its home base, Los Angeles, and more importantly because 'Bad Company' is the type of company he feels his parents and disapproving others think that he keeps (e.g., freaks, flower children, burn-outs, etc.)].

Bob then goes on to make the statement that, "everybody is a star". This is the title of a famous song by Sly and the Family Stone and refers to the Sixties' notion of the inherent value in everyone. The next statement he makes, "before they can reap the cake, that was left out in the rain" is a direct quote from the psychedelic song written by Jim Webb entitled "MacArthur Park". This use of a line from a song actually appears earlier in this excerpt. When Bob said he felt content and well being, "way down inside", he was using a line from Led Zeppelin's song, "Whole Lotta Love". He does this again later in the excerpt when he repeats the phrase, "Can't explain . . . ". This is a reference to one of the Who's early hits which carries this title.

After Bob used the line from "MacArthur Park", he began to doze off. As he does, he provides us with a marvelous example of a relaxed ego allowing repressed material to enter consciousness (though it was clear that Bob did not need to be drowsy to allow such material to gain access to consciousness; periodically, Bob would say his father wanted to have sex with him or that he wanted, or was afraid of, having sex with his father. He said the same of his mother, and expressed fears of homosexual interest other males had in him.) After saying, "Try to understand it. Not all love is in vain", he regains full consciousness. He then negates the relationship between himself and his friends who are going to make it on Swan Song by saying, "It's not a homosexual relationship either. (In an aside) Don't know where that word came from", and so forth.

Even in these statements, Bob draws from the Rock idiom. He makes use of "Love in Vain", an old (ca. 1930) slow blues written by Robert Johnson, the legendary Bluesman, and made popular with Rock audiences at about the turn of the decade (1970) by the Rolling Stones. In an apparent attempt to further deny any homosexual feelings toward his musician friends, Bob begins to talk of a women he once met.

Bob's use of the kinship terms "brother and sister" derives from the rhetoric of the 60's. In that rhetoric (and the world view it expressed), a cue is taken from Black culture wherein unrelated individuals are referred to by kinship terms. The usage is logical in the context of the rhetoric of the "love generation" the members of which are of one generation (conceptually) and are all children "of love", "of Peace", "of God", or "of Rock'n Roll". As members of the same generation and offspring of one or another entity (Rock'n Roll, love), members are obviously, if only symbolically, siblings. Hence, depending on gender, everyone is a 'brother' or a 'sister'. His Indian sister is a woman he met whom he felt was compatible with the goals of Rock (peace, love, krshna). He also mentions a French guardian angel.

The angel was a real person, an older woman who was a friend of the family and with whom Bob communicated from time to time while he was a patient. Here as elsewhere, Bob would characterize the relationship as more than friendship, perhaps for the same reason he brought up the Indian woman in this excerpt after mentioning his relationship with Mike Snow.

The interpretation of the proverb that Bob offered finds him thinking concretely about rolling stones. However, Bob is thinking not about just any rolling stones, but about *the* Rolling Stones. Bob's interpretation is in fact a string of references to recordings of the Rolling Stones'. His statement, "no sticky connections" refers to the Stones' 60's hit, "Connection", and to the title of one of their most successful albums, "Sticky Fingers". "No shady connections" again makes reference to the song "Connection" but also to another album title and another song. The album is entitled "Made in the Shade" and the song is "Standing in the Shadows". Bob goes on to state in different combinations these titles but adds the slang term "groove", which, while used in the '60's, is older and is a term for good music. He is also, no doubt, making a pun on 'shady grove'.

In this first case we have seen a schizophrenic with severe problems in social self identity and sexual identity but we are here concerned only with the former. Bob had clearly cathected Rock music and Sixties' culture as the essential elements of white identity. Having internalized these over the years (he was an ardent follower of the alternative life styles of the Sixties and early on had dissociated himself from Asians), he was disturbed about his rejection as a viable white ethnic because of his Asian appearance. His identity as a new creature was supposed to leave his old racial identity behind but others, because of their own racial theories, would not allow him to alter his identity.

In this case we have used anthropological theory and ethnographic knowledge of popular culture to show not that a patient was improperly labeled as schizophrenic, but rather to highlight elements that were used to diagnose his condition and to signify a particular level of distress (severe). These elements were misinterpreted by clinicians. Hence, while Bob was certainly ill, and schizophrenia was the nature of the illness, he was perhaps not as ill as his physicians were led to believe by virtue of their folk definition of racial identity. This case shows how clinical reality is created according to psychiatric interpretive schema which in this instance were also folk cultural theories (cf. Gaines 1982). This reality was reconstructed through the application of anthropological theory and knowledge.

The next case will highlight the efficacy of cultural anthropological methodology in the case of a manic in-patient who posed some management problems for the staff of the closed ward unit of Kahala-Kokua's psychiatric facility.

Case 2

A 35 year-old Jewish male, Max Huhn, was admitted to Kahala-Kokua's locked psychiatric ward after being brought to emergency by the local police. Max had been picked up at the local airport where he had gotten into difficulty with the management of a few retail outlets there. Max was diagnosed upon admission as "manic-depressive, manic". After several days on the locked ward, he continued to give considerable trouble to both patients and staff. Max was being maintained (that is, it was hoped that he would be soon maintained) with a combination of antipsychotics and lithium. Despite heavy doses of both, Max remained easily rouseable and combative. He was abusive to other patients, ward staff and psychiatric care team members. I first talked with Max in the company of his care team. Max was asked about his background and refused to give any information. He was asked about his present condition and he began to shout, "There's nothing wrong with me. I'll sue you. I'm being kept here for no reason." Max was a very angry man. He insulted everyone, called them "asses", "turkeys" and other less flattering names.

It was difficult for attendings or residents to get much out of Max. He would shortly end any interaction with insults and by angrily leaving the interviews (which were conducted on the ward at one or another of the tables situated there in the ward's lounge area). One important feature of interaction I had noticed among psychiatrists and their patients which I felt bore directly on the problem of Max's reluctant communication was the nonreciprocal nature of interaction. To illustrate, on one occasion I observed a 30 year-old schizophrenic Japanese male patient, an ethnic local, who had made a drawing of a woman. A female attending physician asked him about it, inquiring if he was, or had been, married. The patient looked at the psychiatrist and asked pointedly, "Are you married?" The female psychiatrist responded, "We're here to talk about you. Whether I'm married or not is unimportant. Let's talk about you". The patient smirked; then in a begrudging and curt manner, he answered further questions, offering nothing more than the required responses.

The point here has to do with methods in anthropology. That is, just as society may be seen as a system of exchange, and even predicted thereon (Mauss 1970), so too interactions may be seen as based upon reciprocity. One technique in the conduct of participant observation, the principal method of social-cultural anthropology, is the conversion of field encounters into conversations rather than formal unidirectional interviews. Since an exchange involves a two-way conversation, an informant's response may be more positive when he realizes the flow of information is two-way. In contrast, sociological research often employs an extractive process whereby respondents are administered questionnaires that control and artificially narrow the interchange. So it goes in psychiatry, too, that a patient may wish to engage in natural conversation, only to have this desire frustrated.

It was clear that Max took questions to be invasive. When he angrily asked his interrogator the same question as was put to him, he received no reply. So, Max would not answer questions put to him by people who failed to reciprocate with him and who he felt were falsely imprisoning him. Also, we should keep in mind some background material. Max, of course, was seen as a manic-depressive in a manic phase. It could be pieced together that there had been some earlier episodes similar to the present one. During this manic phase, Max had taken his savings from his bank in the midwest and bought a plane ticket to Hawaii.

It is in Hawaii that Max comes under the aegis of public authority, first the police and then psychiatry. Upon his arrival in Hawaii, Max had begun to spend large sums of money; just how much was unknown. Once on the ward, aside from the verbal abuse he heaped upon staff persons, Max maintained what Goffman would call an occult involvement; he constantly carried a bag around the ward. Periodically, he would leave the bag unattended and pretend to take no notice of it. Actually he would maintain a watchful eye on it. He would not relinquish possession of it to staff, nor would he divulge to anyone the contents of the bag despite repeated queries by staff members.

In the view of Max's team care group (the team consisted of an attending, a resident, a medical student, and from time to time, an anthropologist), he was "a very sick man". One indication of the severity of his condition was his total denial of his illness. He refused to acknowledge that anything was amiss. Further, in addition to his apparent lack of insight, Max was uncooperative, secretive, combative and insulting. All were seen as by psychiatric staff persons as indicative of his very serious mental condition.

It should be noted that there are two different issues related to communication in this case. The first problem is that of the non-reciprocal nature of interaction between physicians and patients. The second issue is the problem of the abuse which Max heaped upon staff members. With this background, we can look at what transpired when Max was approached and related to in a different interactional mode, one that takes reciprocity as the basis for social interaction and that is employed in the course of social-cultural anthropological research.

We shall see that by placing Max in an interactional mode which he apparently felt was appropriate, we discover that his denials of recognition of his problem and situation were expressions of his displeasure with his treatment. That is, in a single interview with me Max discussed all of the issues that had been problematic in his relationship with his caretakers. As may be seen below, communication with Max was facilitated by reframing the interactional mode from extractive to reciprocal, thereby allowing self-disclosure[5] on the part of both interlocutors. I should mention that Max remained somewhat surly throughout the conversation, but he was at least communicative.

Anthropologist: Excuse me, Max. Would you mind if I sat down here and talked with you for a
        while?
Max: I don't care what you do.
A: Thanks. Max, I was wondering if you were married. If you are, your wife might like to know
        you're here.
M: Are you married?
A: Not any more. I got divorced about eight years ago. What about you?
M: I was married, too.
A: But not any more?
M: No.

A: Did you come to Hawaii to see her or your kids? (It was not known whether Max had any children at this point).

M: No. They're on the mainland.

A: Your kids too?

M: Yeah. Do you have any kids?

A: Yes. A son. He's getting up there in years, he's nearly eleven.

M: Oh yeah. (Max then took out his wallet and extracted several pictures of children, one male and one female. He placed these on the table without making a comment. Max had been secretive about his wallet, refusing to give it up or allow any one to see it.)

A: Oh, those are good-looking kids. (The children, about seven to ten years of age seemed part Asian. I suspected but never confirmed that Max's wife was from Hawaii and that he had been there before.)

M: Yeah.

A: Was it rough ending the marriage?

M: Yeah.

A: Were you ever sick before your marriage broke up?

M: No. It started after it broke up.

A: So you've had these problems only since the marriage ended? (I repeated this question to make sure he was recognizing his present condition as an illness or at least a problem).

M: Yeah. I was O.K. before that.

A: Why do you think that is?

M: Hmm. (I) don't know. Couldn't take it I guess.

A: What about coming here. What brought you here?

M: What brought you here?

A: A job.

M: Oh. I just came.

A: To do what?

M: I don't know.

A: Did you bring anything besides the bag?

M: Hmm.

A: Is the bag important?

M: No. Just what's in it.

A: What do you have in it?

M: Gold, money.

A: What do you mean?

M: (Max then bent down and opened the bag and gave me a glimpse. There were indeed gold coins. In the brief look that I got, they seemed to be commemorative coins in sets of two and three. I saw some gold chains as well.)

A: That looks important all right.

M: (Max then began to pull slips of paper out of his wallet, which he had left in view during our talk. The slips of paper were receipts for purchases. He had a great many. I quickly glanced through them noting that all were dated in the last several days before his admission and some were for very expensive items. I could not figure the value but was aided by one last slip that Max handed me. It was his tally of how much he had spent. The tallies came to something like $6,000.00. It was these purchases that he had in his bag.)

A: Well, Max. This is valuable stuff. It might be a good idea to keep it locked up until you're ready to go home, don't you think?

M: No. I don't trust them. If I give it to them they'll steal it and I can't do it.

A: Do what?

M: I figure that if I keep it, it's O.K. If someone around here takes some of it while I have it, I can sue the hospital.

A: Is that why you sometimes leave the bag alone?

M: (smiles, for the first time) Yeah.

Max and I talked a bit longer but important elements of the case can be seen in the above. Clearly, Max does recognize that he is ill. Also, right or wrong, he has a theory, an EM (Kleinman 1980) of the etiology of his illness and knows its history. The lack of recognition of his illness and its history led the team care members to see Max as very sick, which he was, but not so sick that he lacked cognizance of his illness. As well, he divulged his secrets to me without a great deal of resistance. He would periodically test my intentions, my stake in the interaction, and my view of him as an interactant by asking me the same question I asked of him. The lesson here is that Max, as well as many other patients, did not like to be *talked to* or have information *extracted from* him. He wanted to be *talked with* and considered an equal in the interaction. Subsequently, team care members *did* recognize and said that their view of Max's condition needed rethinking in light of the display of insight reported above.

A second problem was alluded to earlier with regard to communications with Max. That is, while he insulted people regularly, the only response from ward and attending staff was a mild "that's not appropriate". However, the ward philosophy, which was frequently articulated, stated that "patients should be treated as normal individuals". This was honored in the breach. If the ward personnel did in fact feel that this was the appropriate tack, perhaps other behaviors were called for with reference to Max. Fortuitously, a medical student working on the ward approached me with a pertinent observation.

The medical student, "Jack", on his psychiatric rotation, was a part of the team which was caring for Max. Jack wanted to talk with someone about what he felt was "inappropriate" behavior on the part of the ward and attending staff. He chose me to talk to about his feelings. Jack felt that Max should not be allowed to go about insulting people. He personally did not like it and felt it was inappropriate for staff to tolerate such rude behavior. I agreed with Jack and suggested that one might see it from a subcultural point of view. That is, that the 'subculture of psychiatry' as premised upon the WASP culture of the wider society tended to be nonconfrontational and ill-equipped to handle displays of strong emotion. Jack, a Japanese-American, agreed but said this particular inability was not shared by him. (In late 1979, I had the opportunity to observe a psychiatric ward in Northern California where all ward staff persons were Black. The ward staff evidenced not the least hesitation in physically or verbally correcting patient behavior which they found inappropriate. In one instance, a Anglo patient, who had just arrived on the ward for evaluation, began to tell a ward clerk how patients should be treated. The Black ward clerk instantly became angry and said, "Don't tell me how to run my ward. You hear me, mother-fucker?" Startled, the patient went on to say that he was "only trying to be helpful". The ward clerk then said, "I don't need your help, turkey. Now hit the door", i.e., leave the ward. The patient did not understand the clerk but the clerk quickly explained, "Get the fuck out, fool. Hit the door!" The clerk thereupon took the arm of the patient and dragged him to the door, unlocked it, and pushed the patient out. The other clerks did not stir or take any note of the scene. Other patients were treated firmly and with dispatch if they acted in a way contrary to the needs of their ward staff.)

ATWOOD D. GAINES

I asked Jack what he felt should be done. He said, "I think I should go over to him (to Max) and tell him that I don't like being insulted and that I'm not going to allow him to continue to do it." Jack had noted the discrepancy between the ward philosophy and the actual practices by saying, "If we're supposed to treat them (the patients) as normal (individuals), then they should be told when they're doing something wrong the same way they would be if they were outside". I agreed and told him that his idea was a good one.

Jack did inform Max of his dislike of Max's behavior and made it clear that while Max might be angry about his treatment and enforced stay in the hospital, he (Jack) was angry about the way Max treated him. The outcome of this interaction was that for several days Max was indeed much better behaved toward others, especially Jack.

This last aspect of the problem which Max presented may be seen as soluble through the application of a theoretical distinction drawn in social-cultural anthropology; that is, the distinction drawn between the real and the ideal levels of culture. All cultures and subcultures have ideals, notions of the proper order of things, and of right and proper behavior. Often, these ideals are mistaken for accurate representations of reality by informant and anthropologist.

Too, it is often the case that social actors will wear what may be termed "masks" as they portray to an external observer the ideal forms of behavior associated with their group or subculture. In this way informants conceal behavior which might be damaging to their image (cf. Berreman 1972) and thereby manage the impressions they make upon others. In our case here, there was a clear disjuncture between the stated normative rule concerning the treatment of patients and the sanctions which were invoked in response to violations of stated rules of conduct. This disjuncture was noted by the anthropologist and the medical student.

For the anthropologist, the observation derived from a normal comparative research procedure wherein normative statements are checked against actual behavior. Comparisons of behavior with idealized abstract statements about behavior should be made to assess the distinction between the real and the ideal. In addition, norms or values or 'rules' of behavior given in the abstract should be compared with behavior in actual contexts rather than seen as abstract, disembodied, trans-contextual rules.

In this next case, we will see the use of ethnographic knowledge about a particular social category or identity and that identity's characterological concomitants which allows for the deconstruction of a clinical reality, "schizoid", developed during a case conference.

Case 3

During a departmental case conference in the department of psychiatry at a university in the local area, an interview was presented on video tape. The subject was a young Chicano male who appeared to be in his early twenties or very late teens. The subject was being interviewed by a psychiatrist. The information provided the audience, which consisted of attendings and residents from this and another psychiatry department, made no mention of the person being a patient nor was mention made of any disorder. The tape was being presented to interested parties for their comments and assessment.

The young man talked of the difficulties of life, "the Man", who made life difficult for him and others. He talked in a slow, accented, inarticulate manner and remained slouched deep down in his chair. "Carlos", as we will call him, wore a sweater and a knit cap; the latter he wore pulled down, covering his ears. Given the climate in Hawaii, it was not the most appropriate attire, especially since he was indoors.

Carlos was extremely vague in his responses. "Did you go to school?", his interrogater asked him. "Yeah. Did that. (It was) a trip. Hey. Sociology, man. It's the Man, keeps you down. Little man can't do nothing. Hey, I know". After listening to the tape, a discussion followed in which the possibility of a psychotic disorder was developed.

Several faculty members thought the individual was probably "schizoid" based upon a number of factors. The factors that were mentioned by faculty in support of their suspicion that Carlos was schizoid included the vagueness of his responses, his very low key attitude with almost flat affect, his inappropriate manner of dress and his static, very slouched, posture. When several other members of the group began to be persuaded that some schizoid symptomatology was present, I offered some ethnographic information which served to deconstruct this clinical reality which was yet in the process of construction.

At this point in the discussion it seemed appropriate to point out that Carlos was a "low rider", a member of a major social category in California and the American Southwest, though certainly a novelty in Hawaii. I also suggested that Carlos was, it seemed, a quite normal low rider; for Carlos's dress, including the knit cap pulled over his ears, was more or less a low rider uniform. Sometimes the sweater might be exchanged for a white or black tee shirt, but otherwise Carlos was in uniform. I mentioned that there were perhaps several hundred thousand such low riders in California alone.

Generally Latinos, low riders are a very large social category and social identity which comprises men (primarily) and women of all ages whose most prized possession is their cars. These are lavishly painted in all sorts of colors, and have additional chrome pipes (usually non-functional) added to them. The interiors of the cars are expensively redone in leather, velvet and other materials. The major preoccupation of low riders (when not working to support their cars) is showing off themselves and their cars by "cruising" along certain well-known thoroughfares. Making an impression is very important; the performance of the cars, speed, etc. is not. The appellation, "low rider", derives from the fact that the springs are cut from the undercarriage of the cars and the shock absorbers removed. The cars then ride only inches from the ground and often cannot go up driveways or over bumps in the road higher than a few inches.

So it is that in many areas, urban and rural alike, one can see hundreds, if not thousands of low riders who sit, dress and talk exactly like Carlos[6]. But in Hawaii, people of Carlos' social identity, a subcultural identity of a wider Hispanic cultural tradition, are very rare. I saw but one other member of this subculture during my year in Hawaii. That was a female who was brought to the emergency room unconscious. She said she had been kidnapped by a man who had promised her a job if she went with him to Hawaii. She was from San Jose and had left a two year old child whom the patient 'thought' was in the care of her sister.

The faculty members and residents present at the case conference, with one important exception, as I will note below, were not aware of the existence of low riders or their characteristics and, I believe, were still somewhat skeptical after my discussion. However, my interpretation, which deconstructed a budding clinical reality, soon received support from a level two resident in the department in which the case conference was taking place. After my discussion, the resident said, "I'm from Los Angeles, and there are thousands of guys like him (like Carlos) there. (I think) Dr. Gaines is right. He's just a low rider. I don't think there is anything wrong with him".

We see in this example that some knowledge of a social identity with which professionals in this Pacific setting had little experience altered clinical judgments about an individual. The change is from a view of the individual as evidencing a particular form of pathology to a view of the person as a normal member of a rather large subculture. I must admit that not all faculty members were completely convinced. I suspect that some might have surmised that *all* low riders must be schizoid if Carlos is typical of them.

In the next case, I will present an example of a failure in the reconstruction of clinical reality. Yet the failure points up the influence of exogenous factors on the construction of clinical reality and also the potential contribution of anthropological theory and knowledge for the construction of more viable clinical realities that can assist in making differential diagnoses. We will see here that subcultural professional demands can sometimes supersede those of the clinic as the source of psychiatric/medical clinical constructions.

Case 4

A 29 year-old Portugese-German male was the subject of rounds on a psychiatric in-patient service in a hospital affiliated with Kahala-Kokua's psychiatric training program. One of the residents caring for the patient had suggested to faculty that the patient would be interesting enough to warrant the attention of a professor from the East who was then visiting the department. Dr. Seldon, as we will call him, was widely known for his rare combination of psychoanalytic therapeutic expertise and practical and theoretical knowledge of psychopharmacology. I attended the rounds with residents and Dr. Seldon to observe it as a subcultural event of the profession, as I often did, but also as a special variety of that event, that with a well-known visiting psychiatrist (who was willing to look into a case for pedagogical as well as therapeutic reasons).

The patient, "Roger", was brought into a room by a resident. In the room, where Dr. Seldon would interview the patient, were residents, one attending, the author and Dr. Seldon. The patient was locally born and raised by a Portugese Catholic mother and a southern German Catholic father. The patient's major complaint was described by the resident as depression. Roger did a lot of crying, both in the hospital and before coming in. Remarkably, the patient was a functioning entertainer. He regularly performed on stage in clubs in the tourist areas of Honolulu. After performances, he, as he said, "sort of collapsed". He spent most of the time between performances in bed, often crying. The resident who was organizing the rounds said that the patient had been a veritable mass of sobbing protoplasm until shortly prior to the interview.

In contrast to this picture, Roger remained attentive throughout the interview and responded rapidly to questions, elaborating on the answers. He clearly enjoyed the attention the interview provided and no doubt construed it as a performance.

During the interview, the patient took great pains to explain what a failure he was. He said he had never done well in school and, in fact, was always at the bottom of his class. He said he had never been successful at anything in his life. It was striking that he sought to convince us of his inability to perform in life. But the performance was laced with some levity; he would use humor to convince us of his ineptitude.

Dr. Seldon: How did you do in school?
Roger: I didn't (smiles). I was always last in my class(es). I couldn't win for losing. I stayed at the bottom of the barrel. I was always stupid.

The patient appeared well-kept. He was a decent-looking man without any apparent infirmities and appeared in moderately good physical condition. In short, he did not appear to be the stupid clod he wished others to believe he was. The patient spoke clearly to the group and in Standard English. This is a bit of ethnographic information which has some importance in this context. I mentioned above that the patient was born and raised in the urban Honolulu area of Oahu. The circumstances of the patient's upbringing were rather modest; this is again an important piece of information.

After talking with the patient for some time, during which a fairly full history was taken, the patient was excused and Dr. Seldon set about analyzing the case. From the history and symptomatology, Dr. Seldon quickly ruled out drug abuse. In the analyses of aspects of the case it was apparent that Dr. Seldon's method was educational. But, as well, the rounds provided a time for Dr. Seldon to bring to bear his expertise to clarify a puzzle facing residents at the host institution.

Residents had suggested that the patient was suffering from some form of depression which did not have any precipitating crises. They could offer no real explanation for the patient's inconsistent behavior. I believe it was the inconsistencies of the patient's behavior and his occupation as club singer which led Dr. Seldon to wisely consider and reject drug abuse (including alcoholism) at the outset. Dr. Seldon then suggested that other psychogenic disorders might be kept in mind as possible explanations of Roger's behavior, though all of those mentioned was termed only 'slight' possibilities which nonetheless should not be overlooked.

Though many of the explanations centered on psychogenic disorders, no striking
data were gleaned from the patient's life history.

His background seemed perfectly ordinary, including graduating on time from
both junior and senior high school. Dr. Seldon, taking into consideration the
patient's reported poor performance in school, then suggested that the patient "just
might have some borderline mental retardation". For several reasons, including the
bits of ethnographic data mentioned above, I objected to this interpretation, and
suggested that this was unlikely in this case. Dr. Seldon replied that an auxiliary
group (in California) had recently shown that as many as 30—40 per cent of (California) school children evidenced some learning disability due to at least some
minimal retardation. I suggested that perhaps that high figure had more to do
with the number of ethnic minorities in California schools than with problems of
retardation. Dr. Seldon said he felt comfortable with their figures and we went on
with the consideration of Roger's case.

I later realized that my behavior was not 'appropriate' for several reasons. First,
as I became more knowledgeable of the subculture of psychiatry, it was clear that
the suggestion advanced by Dr. Seldon was not meant to be the "answer" to the
puzzle with which Roger presented us. Rather, the suggestion was meant to provide
a fresh perspective from which to view a troublesome problem. Residents were
centering on only one explanatory model, that of psychogenic depression. The
visiting professor wanted to provide a new domain, another model for consideration
by the group just as a possibility. My objections tended to make the diagnosis more
concrete than it really was, short-circuting its negotiation.

So although my disagreement may have had some basis in clinical reality, it
detracted from residents' interaction with Dr. Seldon and obstructed his attempt
to provide the possibility of an organic basis for a problem which had been viewed
only in the light of psychogenic etiologies. Later, I was rightly chided for "detracting
from the residents' time with Dr. Seldon". So, as is often the case in the early
stages of anthropological fieldwork, the anthropologist, like a naive child, does
sometimes get underfoot. So it was in this case. But, I would like point out the
potential benefit that the application of anthropological science to this case might
have had.

First, Roger's concern to convince us of his failing appeared to me to be merely
an example of what I have found is a common form of discourse in the Mediterranean Culture Area and in the daughter cultures of that area; i.e., the Latin and
Islamic traditions. I refer to this form of discourse as *the rhetoric of complaint*.
The source of this rhetoric is a cultural tradition that extolls suffering as a virtue.
Suffering is seen as ennobling. Those who do not suffer, or who do not bear their
suffering well, are not viable, worthy individuals. So it is in the Great Traditions
of the Mediterranean that people normally employ this mode of discourse as the
means of managing an impression of themselves as good, true folk and ultimately
as saintly, for we note that all saints suffered. The rhetoric of complaint, then,
is simply a mode of discourse, a means of presentation of the self, and is not
necessarily a faithful rendering of social reality or personal history.

In this chapter, we have already seen this rhetoric at work in the case of Carlos the low rider. Carlos talked of 'the Man' who kept people like him down. He also mentioned 'forces' and 'they' who were unknown adversaries. (These ideas were seen by some faculty members as a bit paranoid). For both Roger and Carlos, there is a desire to portray the self as a victim of some one or some thing (e.g., of "the Man" or of stupidity). Both use a mode of presentation which carries the meta-communication that the speaker has suffered and/or is suffering: and that by virtue of that suffering, they should be seen as good and decent people at the mercy of outside forces over which they have little or no control.

The internal inconsistencies of Roger's story show us the "painting of a por-trait" style of self presentation (cf. Lee 1959 on the presentation of the Greek self). In this style, the portraits convey great meaning, but are not always accurate renderings of personal past or present. Elsewhere, I have argued that there are two distinct cultural traditions in the West, the Northern European Protestant and the Mediterranean Culture Areas, each exhibiting broadly similar characteristics internally but striking contrasts when compared (1982). Each cultural tradition has a particular worldview and conception of person. The two conceptions of person which I discussed are the "indexical" and the "referential". The former is that found in the Mediterranean while the latter is that of the Northern European Pro-testant Area. The rhetoric of complaint outlined here is the mode of presentation of the indexical self where self is created, as a portrait, for a given encounter, thereby indexing that encounter. The indexical self is created as a marker of a given encounter. The self portrayed changes from time to time, encounter to encounter, in contrast to the referential self (Gaines 1982). The referential self is a stable self such that discourse about self refers, more or less completely depending upon the interaction, to an historical self factually described. (Of course, the facts are but interpretations). Thus, as is true of Celtic areas (which, excepting the Scots, are Latin as well), the people of the Latin tradition tell stories, they don't give facts.

It appears in our case that Dr. Seldon accepted Roger's rhetoric and used it as a basis for the construction of an alternative clinical reality. However, it is noteworthy that while Roger said that he was always a failure and always at the bottom of his class(es), he managed to graduate on time from both junior and senior high school in a state where many locals do not complete their secondary education. It seems plausible to suggest that someone with the difficulties described by Roger might have failed a grade or two and/or failed to complete his secondary education. There is another point, relating to Roger's use of Standard English, to be considered as well.

Roger must be regarded as a "local". This is an term used by people of the island to refer people who are locally born and reared. The term does not separate many ostensibly distinct "racial" or ethnic identities from one another. Thus, the term lumps together local 'Japanese', 'Hawaiian', 'Portugese', 'Chinese' and 'Korean' individuals. "Local" identity is an amalgamation of these identities into an emergent identity that is distinct from any one of the contributing cultural groups. One of the features of the local identity is "Da Kine Talk". This is the name of the local dialect which is spoken by most people who are local born and raised, regardless of their original language. (Exceptions are some "kama'ina's", native born whites of high social standing, or others of comparable social standing who associate little with the local people. However, many of these people can 'put on' the dialect if they so desire.)

Since Roger was born and raised locally in a middle- to lower middle-class family in Honolulu of the 1940's and 1950's — i.e., a far less urban area than it is today; and given the circumstances of Roger's rearing, it might be suggested that Roger was possessed of an above average level of intelligence and may have been a rather diligent student. This is suggested by the fact that Roger acquired communicative competence in Standard English while those around him did not. This view of Roger is quite different than that suggested by Dr. Seldon.

In this case, some ethnographic knowledge could have been marshalled to rule out particular diagnostic entities advanced to explain the case. Both ethnographic knowledge and theory of the presentation of self were potentially capable of transforming clinical reality. However, subcultural concerns of this specialty of biomedicine relating to the nature of visitors' rounds took precedence in the consideration of a confusing case.[7] Status and pedagogical considerations influenced the construction of clinical reality. The hermeneutic nature of the clinical encounter is highlighted here in a manner different from that of the other cases. Also highlighted in this case is the need for caution and the construction of appropriate means for cross-disciplinary communication in clinical contexts.

The next case I will present concerns anthropological knowledge and anthropological method and how these two aspects of anthropological science contributed to the deconstruction of one clinical reality, "chronic schizophrenia", and the construction of a new clinical entity, "mental retardation". On this occasion, the construction of a new clinical reality led to a change in the disposition of the case.

Case 5

A 41 year-old Hawaiian-Portugese-Chinese ("local") female appeared in the emergency room of Kahala-Kokua one summer evening. The woman was brown-skinned and heavy set with short black hair with streaks of gray. She was casually dressed in an aloha shirt, shorts and slippers (called zori or thongs by tourists). The woman, "Alice", seemed very anxious. She also behaved in a peculiar manner. Alice had been seen first by a social worker who worked as part of the emergency room team. The social worker, after talking with Alice was at a loss as to what to do. The resident-on-call and I talked with the social worker about her.

Social Worker: We're undecided about what to do. She's been here and State (the State hospital). I spoke with her mother (by phone), who sounds crazy and (with) her brother, who sounds crazy, too. She's on Thorazine, 200 mg. I don't think she needs to be hospitalized, but I don't know what to do about her. She constantly talks about her appearance.
Resident: What does she want?

SW: Can't tell. She changes. She came in because (she said) she was beaten by her father-in-law. (As it turned out, Alice was struck by her step-father after she had hit him).
Res: We have only one or two beds. (i.e., there were only two beds at most for a female which were free at that time for psychiatric patients).
SW: You don't want to use one for her.

The resident, the social worker and I went to interview Alice after her records arrived.

Res: Where do you stay?
Alice: Home.
Res: Where is that?
Alice: (very loudly, like a child reciting an important dictate of a parent) *1–2–4–7–6* Ulupaula Street, Kaneohe, Hawaii.
Res: Who do you live with?
Alice: My mother and step-father.
Res: Why did you come here?
Alice: My brother and sister-in-law brought me. (Delivered in a wide-eyed deliberate manner as if she had to work very hard to get it right, as with her address given above).
Res: Why did they bring you?
Alice: I hit my step-father with a plate (delivered like a knowingly naughty, but nonetheless triumphant little girl). He punch me! Hit me. Bruise my back (clumsily turns to show us where on her back she was hit).
Res: Why did you hit him?
Alice: He was vulgar.

And so the interview went. Alice answered questions in the same childish manner throughout. She spoke in a loud voice with some slurring of speech (and in the local dialect which I have not tried to render here; e.g., "My brother and sister-in-law brought me" actually was more like "Mah brudda an' seesta-en-law braw' me"). She was perfectly oriented, though anxious. Her manner struck me as a "cloak of competence" as anthropologist Robert Edgerton (1971) called it. The cloak is the mantle of adequacy which Edgerton found that retarded persons developed in order that they might avoid being stigmatized as incompetents. So after talking with Alice for over an hour, we asked that Alice leave the room. We explained to her that we were going to discuss her case and then we would call her back and talk with her again and that she could wait in the other room. While we told her this she became anxious simply because she couldn't follow what was being said to her so rapidly. We discussed her case when she did leave.

Res: What do you think?
Anth: Mental retardation.
Res: Right, she's not schizophrenic.
SW: Is she diagnosed as schizophrenic on the record? (i.e., she *is* diagnosed . . .).
Res: (Yes) "Chronic Schizophrenia" each time in the records is what it says. (The file on Alice was huge. She had been at Kahala-Kokua a number of times and at the State institution a number of times. She had been periodically institutionalized since she was 16 years old).
SW: It's hard on one impression . . .

Res: Maybe I'm too sure . . . .
Anth: I'm very sure, too. She's not schizophrenic at all.
Res: No, she's not. Maybe thorazine is stopping her thoughts; but if she is schizophrenic,
       she's not at all decompensated.

We conferred for a while longer on what to do, deciding to call her relatives
again. I wanted especially to talk with Alice's mother who might be able to tell us
more about her. Alice's brother was located but he would not come for her. When
we told her that her brother would not come for her, Alice became somewhat
frightened and angry raising her voice and saying, "Don't lie", "Don't lie". We
assured her that we were not lying. I asked her if she had been hearing voices.
"No", she said. I asked had she ever heard voices and she said, "No. I'm not crazy!
I'm just dirty. My mother didn't give me a bath."

Anth: Does your mother usually give you baths?
Alice: Yes.
Anth. Why?
Alice: 'Cause it gets hot and I need one.
Anth: Well, we have a room for you if you would like to stay here tonight.
Alice: No, I want to go home.
Res: You don't want to come into the hospital overnight?
Alice: No. I won't (stands up and gives us a childish, but serious scowl).
Res: If you won't come into the hospital, there is nothing we can do for you. You just have
       to leave if you don't come in.
Alice: Then I'll leave; walk home Pali (mountain pass to the other side of the island where she
       lived).
Res: You won't come into the hospital?
Alice: I won't stay hospital (local dialect often drops prepositions and articles).
Res: Then you can leave. (Alice walked out).

The resident felt that Alice was not ill enough to be hospitalized but felt he
would give her a room based upon her limited capacities due to the now recognized
mental deficiency, a condition which nowhere appeared in her voluminous records.
The excerpt above in which her new diagnosis is discussed indicates that the resident
was not anxious to advance a new clinical reality. I very much felt as though I
needed to act as an advocate for the patient, the new diagnosis, and as a support
for the resident's view, which paralleled my own because clinical reality is, as noted
in the discussion of Case 4, resistant to change for other reasons than in the presentation or interpretation of symptoms. I suggested that if we considered the patient
retarded, then she could not be kept in the hospital if she were unwilling to stay.
This suggestion resulted in the discussion above which ended in Alice's departure
from the hospital.

Shortly after Alice's departure, her mother called the hospital (she had been
contacted earlier by the social-worker and refused to pick up Alice). She was irate
because we had let Alice leave the hospital. The resident asked me to speak to
Alice's mother when we were informed she had called and was then on the phone.

Mother: She crazy. Everybody can see that. What kind docta's you got there, let somebody
        crazy go? Where she go?

Anth: Home.
Mother: How she get home?
Anth: The bus, I assume.
Mother: There's no bus this time night. How she get home? Why you let her go?

After Alice's mother had vented her anger, I got her to talk about Alice and discovered some previously unreported medical history which seemed to confirm the contention regarding Alice's retardation.

Mother: I'll sue Kahala (if) something happen to her.
Anth: Well, Mrs. Sousa, we can't commit her involuntarily. She is not sick enough to commit. She has to be dangerous to herself or to other people. The quarrel she had at home isn't enough to say that. We asked her to stay but she did not want to. So, we have to let her go because she is not sick enough for us to be allowed to keep her against her will. Alice was not confused; she knew the day, month, year, where she was, how she got here. In other words, she was not confused or disoriented.
Mother: But she crazy. She went Maui one time and came back. Took the bus home and didn't remember nothing. She don't know where she is or what she do. She forget. I know, I take care of her.
Anth: Yes. Well, you have 41 years experience with her and we have only an hour's (experience), but with Maui, she knew how to get there and back didn't she? But when she was here, she was oriented and not confused. Anyway, how long has she been like this?
Mother: Since she was four years old.
Anth: And what happened to Alice when she was four?
Mother: She got sick. She had a fever and slept for days and vomited and shook. But we lived way out, no doctas, long time ago. But later see docta and he say nothing wrong 'cause she look normal. But there was something wrong, they just didn't understand mental illness then. She never was same after that ... Then she went into hospital (the State hospital) first time when she was 16.
Anth: I see. Since then, since four, she's had this problem, she's been like this?
Mother: Yea, she crazy.

Alice's mother and I talked a few minutes more. I tried to suggest that Alice was not mentally ill, but had sustained some brain damage during that episode when she was four. The difference between schizophrenia and retardation from an illness was lost on her, however. In her classification, they were one and the same thing, "crazy". After finishing my conversation with Alice's mother, I told the resident of my findings on the illness episode in Alice's fourth year. He looked at the social worker who, along with the other medical staff members of the emergency room, was quite sure that Alice was schizophrenic and said, "See? I told you". He (and I) clearly felt vindicated.

SUMMARY AND CONCLUSION

In this chapter the value and utility of social and cultural anthropological knowledge, method, and theory for clinical psychiatric practice have been explored. I have suggested that anthropology does have "special methodology and special results as a consequence which do make a difference" (Maretzki 1976: 83) in the construction of clinical reality and hence in the practice of clinical psychiatry. I have not focused here on dyadic therapeutic encounters because of the limits of my own experience and, hence, the data I might offer. It seems obviously, however, that issues would be raised in therapeutic contexts that could well be approached by psychiatrists with anthropological tools.

We have considered the specific nature of the differences which the application of anthropological theory, method, and knowledge made or might have made in five clinical encounters. Each of the five cases illustrated the application of at least two of the components of social-cultural anthropology. In Case 1, social-cultural theory concerning social classification and ethnographic knowledge of popular music and the Rock subculture of Anglo culture were shown to disentangle the seeming total disorder of the utterances of a young schizophrenic man. It was also suggested that Bob's condition was not as indicative of total decompensation as clinicians had thought because of their construction of a clinical reality in part based upon their folk notions of racial identity. Of course, clinicians share these beliefs with the bulk of the members of the wider society, so this is not a case where professional medicine holds a belief at variance with lay persons.

Case 2 was an example of the utility of anthropological method in clinical contexts. The procedure of comparing stated norms, rules or behavioral descriptions to actual behavior in various contexts was shown to be efficacious in improving patient management. As well, the use of reciprocity in interaction, a methodological tack stemming from a theory of society as reciprocal exchange, was demonstrated to be an effective means for improving communication between patient and other which allowed for clarification of the patient's self-awareness and self-assessment. Barriers to communication can cloud perception by clinicians of patients' levels of self-awareness thereby obscuring diagnostically significant levels of patients' insights into their own conditions and situations.

The utility of anthropological knowledge about social categories was highlighted in the third case. Knowledge about "low riders" as a social category and knowledge of subculturally normal modes of presentation — verbal and behavioral — were shown to provide for a reconstruction of clinical reality in the sense that apparent clinical symptoms were shown to be subculturally patterned behaviors.

In Case 4, we saw an example of anthropological naïveté which, combined with extra-clinical, professional subcultural pedagogical considerations, resulted in failure to incorporate ethnographic and theoretical material into the construction of a more appropriate clinical reality. The case, in a different way than the others, makes the point that clinical reality is a hermeneutic construct and as such is potentially alterable by the appropriate introduction of anthropological insights.

The final case considered in this chapter was that of Alice who, for a quarter of a century, seems to have been misdiagnosed. Here anthropological theory, method and knowledge assisted in the transformation of one clinical reality, "chronic schizophrenia", into another, "mental retardation".

The emphasis in this paper has been on a semantic or meaning-centered view of clinical reality. This approach contrasts with the empiricist and physicalist approaches dominant in psychiatry and other branches of Western biomedicine. A meaning-centered approach suggests that empiricist and physicalist views are limited and often misguided. Clinical reality is not to be seen as a construct derived from unbiased reading of objective *signs* of distress. Rather clinical reality is to be seen as an interpretive construct derived from the interpretation of presented *symbols*. As the interpretive perspective changes, so changes the interpretive construct; i.e., clinical reality.

The symbols that must be clinically interpreted include evident and presented symptoms of patients but just as importantly encompass such meaningful symbols as physiognomy (apparent "race" or ethnicity), the significance of patients' domains of discourse, styles of self presentation, patients' insight into their problems, speech styles and linguistic competence, gender, and a host of other characteristics. I have argued that the psychiatric encounter, like all other social encounters, is an essentially hermeneutic interaction. Through the examination of five cases it has been shown that clinical reality is a product of psychiatric interpretations that may be inadequate or based upon unexamined folk ideas and assumptions. Because of the essentially interpretive basis of clinical reality, it has been possible to show that alternative constructions of clinical reality may be achieved through the application of social-cultural anthropological theory, method, and knowledge in clinical psychiatric practice.

This paper on the whole argues for a particular role of anthropology in clinical psychiatric settings. Although one role of the anthropologist in these settings might be as 'culture broker", or patient advocate as Weidman has argued (Weidman 1980), another role suggests itself as well. It may be appropriate and possible for anthropologists to work as members of health care teams. As a member of a team, the expertise of the anthropologist would be well placed to augment the skills of the biomedical specialist in psychiatry in the construction of clinical realities and in the assessment of the alteration of those realities over time. The appropriate interaction of anthropological and medical sciences would augur well for the promotion of increased understanding of patients and their illnesses and diseases and thereby improve patient outcomes. As Kleinman has noted (Kleinman 1980: 387), the cooperation of anthropology and psychiatry to produce an anthropological psychiatry is essential for the achievement of the "full potentialities of a culturally appropriate, human, integrated practice of clinical care".

ACKNOWLEDGEMENTS

This chapter has greatly benefited from the helpful comments and criticisms of Drs. Mark Nichter, Noel Chrisman and Thomas Maretzki. Any problems which remain are of course my own.

NOTES

1. Anthropology may be divided into five main branches, each branch of which contains numerous subfields. The five main branches are biological anthropology (formerly and

sometimes still referred to as physical anthropology), linguistic anthropology (now often referred to as sociolinguistics), archeology, social and cultural anthropology and applied anthropology. While there may be lessons for clinical psychiatric practice from biological anthropology and from linguistic anthropology (Labov and Fanshel 1977), this paper is concerned only with the application of components of social and cultural anthropology (hereafter shortened to social-cultural anthropology). The reader should note that some anthropologists suggest that applied anthropology is not to be considered a separate field of anthropology but rather designates those instances where aspects of the primary four branches are applied in the pursuit of some practical aim such as those described in this chapter.

2. The names of all persons and those of most places have been changed to preserve anonymity.
3. The data on which this paper is based were collected during the period of September 1978 to October 1979, inclusive, during which time the author was a post-doctoral fellow in the department of psychiatry of a local university.
4. As the reader will note in excerpts of conversations with Bob, he was preeminently preoccupied with pop culture, specifically Rock music. Once it was recognized that his concern for Rock music included his becoming a recording star himself, it was obvious that 1-a-x, the second half of his name (Edlax), referred to the designation of Los Angeles International Airport. Hollywood, and Los Angeles in general, is the site of much of Rock recording, live performances (clubs and concerts) and is the place of residence of a great many artists (both American and British). When I asked Bob if his name did indeed refer to Los Angeles, he was amused and replied that it did. He then told me the meaning of the remaining two letters; these were the initials of two friends with whom he played music. So, his name meant, "Bob, Ed and Don go to Los Angeles." That is, his 'group' (he hoped) would go to Los Angeles and record.
5. The author recognizes that there may be problems of self-disclosure in a closed society such as Hawaii. It would seem that the more anonymous a setting, the less problematic self-disclosure, as advocated here, would be.
6. Low riders are usually, but not always, Latino. The emphasis is upon the appearance of the cars (and drivers), not on performance of the cars as is the case with Anglo high riders or Hotrodders (cf. Sacks 1979). As with the designation Hotrodder, the term is one used by insiders who thereby control the symbols distinctive to it and thereby bestow group acceptance on others (Sacks 1979). The form of the presentation of self of members of the group seems based upon their drugs of choice taken in combination (alcohol and barbiturates) and the notion of maintaining one's cool, being unflappable, as in Black culture.
7. Some weeks after this encounter with Roger and Dr. Seldon, I was informed by several residents that nothing remarkable had appeared in the protocols of psychological tests administered to the Roger by staff psychologists. I believe a recognition of the ethnographic materials might have led clinicians to consider certain neurotic conditions or even personality disorders (histrionic) as appropriate to the case.

BIBLIOGRAPHY

Abram, Harry and Clifton Meador
  1976 Introduction: The Patient, the Physician and the Psychiatrist. *In* H. Abrams (ed.), Basic Psychiatry for the Primary Care Physician. Boston: Little, Brown and Company.
Barth, Frederik
  1969 Introduction. *In* Ethnic Groups and Boundaries: The Social Organization of Culture Difference. Bergen: Universitetsforlaget.
Berreman, Gerald
  1972 Prologue: Behind Many Masks, Ethnography and Impression Management. *In* G. Berreman, Hindus of the Himalayas. Berkeley: University of California Press.

Blu, Karen
1980 The Lumbee Problem: The Making of an American Indian People. Cambridge: Cambridge University Press.
Brill, N. and H. Storrow
1960 Social Class and Psychiatric Treatment. Archives of General Psychiatry 3: 340–345.
Derogatis, L., L. Covi, and R. Lipman, et al.
1971 Neurotic Symptom Dimensions as Perceived by Psychiatrists and Patients of Various Social Classes. Archives of General Psychiatry 42: 454–464.
Dorfman, D. and R. Kliner
1962 Race of Examiner and Patient in Psychiatric Diagnosis and Recommendations. Journal of Consulting Psychiatry 26: 393.
Duehn, W. and N. Mayadas
1967 The Effect of Practice Orientation on Clinical Assessment. American Journal of Orthopsychiatry 46: 629–638.
Edgerton, Robert
1971 The Cloak of Competence: Stigma in the Lives of the Mentally Retarded. Berkeley: University of California Press.
Freidson, Eliot
1970 The Profession of Medicine. New York: Dodd and Mead.
Gaines, Atwood
1979 Definitions and Diagnoses: Cultural Implications of Psychiatric Help-Seeking and Psychiatrists' Definitions of the Situation in Psychiatric Emergencies. Culture, Medicine and Psychiatry 3: 4: 381–418.
1980 Alcohol in Black Culture: Comments on Cultural Considerations. Paper presented at the SUNY Downstate Medical Center's Career Teacher Conference Symposium, "Cross-Cultural Studies of Alcoholism." Joseph Westermeyer, organizer. San Francisco, California. May 1980.
1982 Cultural Definitions, Behavior and the Person in American Psychiatry. In A. Marsella and G. White, (eds.), Cultural Conceptions of Mental Health and Therapy. Dordrecht, Holland: D. Reidel Publ. Co.
n.d. Ethnicity as a Cultural System: Race and Culture in Strasbourg, France. Ms.
Geertz, Clifford
1973 Religion as a Cultural System. In C. Geertz, The Interpretation of Cultures. New York: Basic Books.
Good, Byron
1977 The Heart of What's the Matter: The Semantics of Illness in Iran. Culture, Medicine and Psychiatry 1: 1: 25–58.
Good, Byron amd Mary Jo DelVecchio Good
1981 The Meaning of Symptoms: A Cultural Hermeneutic Model of Clinical Practice. In L. Eisenberg and A. Kleinman (ed.), The Relevance of Social Science for Medicine. Dordrecht, Holland: D. Reidel Publ. Co.
Handlin, Oscar
1957 Race and Nationality in American Life. New York: Doubleday Anchor.
Hiernaux, Jean
1970 The Concept of Race and the Taxonomy of Mankind. In A. Montagu (ed.), The Concept of Race. New York: Macmillan.
Katz, Martin, Jonathon Cole, and H. Alice Low
1969 Studies of the Diagnostic Process: The Influence of Symptom Perception, Past Experience, and Ethnic Background on Diagnostic Decisions. American Journal of Psychiatry 125: 937–947.
Katz, Martin, Kenneth Sanborn and Howard Gudeman
1969 Characterizing Differences in Psychopathology Among Ethnic Groups in Hawaii. In F. Redlich (ed.), Social Psychiatry. Baltimore: Williams and Wilkins.

Kiev, Ari
  1968 Curanderismo. New York: Free Press.
Kleinman, Arthur
  1975 The Use of "Explanatory Models ... "; Appendix to Chapter 36. *In* A. Kleinman, et al. (eds.), Medicine in Chinese Cultures. Washington, D.C.: U.S. Department of Health, Education and Welfare.
  1977 Rethinking the Social and Cultural Context of Psychopathology and Psychiatric Care. *In* T. Manschreck and A. Kleinman (eds.), Renewal in Psychiatry. Washington, D.C.: Hemisphere.
  1980 Patients and Healers in the Context of Culture. Berkeley: University of California Press.
Labov, William and David Fanshel
  1977 Therapeutic Discourse. New York: Academic Press.
Lee, Dorothy
  1959 View of the Self in Greek Culture. *In* D. Lee, Freedom and Culture. Englewood Cliffs, New Jersey: Prentice Hall.
Light, Donald
  1976 Work Styles Among American Psychiatric Residents. *In* J. Westermeyer, (ed.), Anthropology and Mental Health. The Hague: Mouton.
Maretzki, Thomas
  1976 What Difference Does Anthropological Knowledge Make to Mental Health? Australian and New Zealand Journal of Psychiatry 10: 83–88.
Marsella, Anthony
  1980 Depressive Experience and Disorder Across Cultures. *In* J. Draguns and H. Triandis (eds.), Handbook of Cross-Cultural Psychology, Volume 6: Psychopathology. New Jersey: Allyn and Bacon.
Mauss, Marcel
  1970 The Gift. I. Cunnison, trans. London: Routledge and Kegan Paul.
Montagu, Ashley (ed.)
  1970 The Concept of Race. New York: Macmillan.
Morrison, James and Thomas Flanagan
  1978 Diagnostic Errors in Psychiatry. Comprehensive Psychiatry 19: 109–117.
Myers, J. and L. Schaffer
  1958 Social Stratification and Psychiatric Practice. *In* E. Jaco, (ed.), Patients, Physicians and Illness. Glencoe, Ill.: Free Press.
Reynolds, David
  1978 Morita Psychotherapy. Berkeley: University of California Press.
Sacks, Harvey
  1979 Hotrodder: A Revolutionary Category. *In* G. Psathas (ed.), Everyday Language: Studies in Ethnomethodology. New York: Irvington Publishers.
Sanborn, Kenneth
  1977 Perception of Symptom Behavior Across Ethnic Groups. *In* Y. H. Poortinga, (ed.), Basic Problems in Cross-Cultural Psychiatry. Amsterdam and Lisse: Swets and Zeitlinger B. V.
Stocking, George
  1968 Race, Culture and Evolution: Essays in the History of Anthropology. New York: Free Press.
Twaddle, A.
  1974 The Concept of Health Status. Social Science and Medicine 8: 29.
U.N.E.S.C.O.
  1969 Race and Science. New York: Columbia University Press.
Washburn, S. L.
  1972 The Study of Race. *In* J. Jenning and E. A. Hoebel (eds.), Readings in Anthropology. New York: McGraw-Hill.

Weidman, Hazel H.
  1980 Comments on Clinical Anthropology. Medical Anthropology Newsletter 12: 16–17.
Zborowski, Mark
  1978 Cultural Components in Response to Pain. *In* M. Logan and E. Hunt (eds.), Health
        and the Human Condition. North Scituate, Mass.: Duxbury Press.

MARY-JO DELVECCHIO GOOD AND BYRON J. GOOD

PATIENT REQUESTS IN PRIMARY CARE CLINICS[1]

INTRODUCTION

Much of medical education is devoted to introducing students to the vast theoretical and data base of contemporary medical science. Students become physicians rather than basic scientists, however, when they develop a particular way of looking at the world — "the clinical perspective" — and learn to apply their knowledge to the treatment of individual patients.[2] Medical students and residents develop "clinical judgment" as they learn to gather clinical data, make medical decisions and take responsibility for a patient's care, working in the context of uncertainty and severe time constraints. Learning to see the world as a physician requires students to narrow their vision from the natural gaze to the "clinical gaze" (Foucault 1973). They must reorganize their perception and learn new "structures of relevance" (Schutz 1970): they must learn what to consider data, what differences make a difference, how to screen out the irrelevant and focus on data that may reveal pathology. Carlton describes the socialization of clinical perception in this way:

... the use of the clinical perspective ... entails learning a particular mode of seeing — removing some blinders and acquiring others. The student physician learns to read meaning from a patient's shuffling gait, even when the patient is not aware of how he looks when walking. Yet the student physician can also learn to become unaware of the visible signs of social discrimination which surround him or her within the hospital organization. ... one learns to "see" a limited realm of things as problems, as well as a limited range of solutions to those problems. (Carlton 1978: 82–83)

The physician in training is thus taught both what to regard and what to treat as context or background.

Anthropologists who teach in clinical settings, along with liaison psychiatrists, medical psychologists and other social scientists, face a dilemma. On the one hand, it is incumbent upon us to recognize the primacy of the clinical perspective. On the other hand, the student physician is often explicitly taught to disregard many of the issues central to our disciplines. On the one hand, we participate in the socialization of the clinical gaze. At a philosophical and theoretical level, we may challenge the reductionism of biomedicine; we may decry the alienating ideological structure of medicine that robs it of the holism and caring essential to humanistic medical practice. However, a fundamental challenge to the legitimacy of the clinical perspective and to training for clinical judgment would represent a failure to understand the nature of medical practice and healing. On the other hand, phenomena central to the expertise of anthropologists and consultation psychiatrists — the meaningful dimension of subjective experience, the social and psychological aspects of illness — are often viewed as irrelevant to clinical decisions and as disruptive of

275

N. J. Chrisman and T. W. Maretzki (eds.), Clinically Applied Anthropology, 275–295.
Copyright © 1982 by D. Reidel Publishing Company.

the clinical routine for the harried intern or clerk. An anthropologist teaching in clinical medicine ultimately faces this dilemma.

It is our belief that rather than simply attacking the biomedical model or grandiosely arguing for an anthropological medical practice, anthropologists and behavioral scientists *in their role as clinical teachers* should develop clinical models and techniques that may be added to the physician's repertoire. However structural change may occur in medicine, change in clinical practice can occur only as new knowledge is embedded *within* the clinical perspective.[3] During the past five years we have carried out research and teaching – with medical students, clerks, residents, and staff – with this as our goal. We have worked primarily in two clinical settings – a family practice clinic and a psychiatric consultation-liaison service. This paper describes our research around one particular clinical model: the negotiation of patient requests. This chapter briefly outlines the general framework we have developed for our teaching; it describes the negotiation of patient requests in a family practice setting; and it describes the development of an instrument to study patient requests in primary care.

SOCIAL SCIENCES AND CLINICAL TEACHING

The general framework upon which our teaching is based begins with the simple recognition that clinicians use multiple perspectives and clinical models in their work. Carlton (1978) argues that in addition to the "clinical perspective", physicians may assume a "legal perspective" or a "moral perspective", depending on the patient management problems or the clinical decisions they are called upon to make.[4] For example, the physician may assume the legal perspective when electing to order certain laboratory tests to document sound medical practice and avoid a malpractice potential rather than for real diagnostic purposes. The legal perspective may also be assumed in seeking informed consent for routine or experimental procedures or in decisions concerning efforts to sustain life. In the latter two settings, ethical as well as legal issues are raised, and the physician may assume a moral perspective. These three perspectives require collection and analysis of different data and construct quite different perceptions of clinical reality. They dictate quite different modes of negotiation with a patient, and may suggest conflicting clinical decisions (Carlton 1978). Further research will probably reveal the use of still other perspectives, particularly in specialized medical settings – for example, a public health perspective or a socio-political perspective may be assumed by clinicians in alternative clinics (such as those in which food has been "prescribed" for the malnourished) or in industrial safety medicine. In training, however, physicians are socialized into the primacy of the "clinical perspective", while familiarity with alternative perspectives is gained in a haphazard and partial manner.

In addition to these broad "perspectives", physicians develop a repertoire of more specific "clinical models". In their various clinical rotations, clerks and residents learn to use models appropriate to specific clinical syndromes and clinical services. The same patient problem may be perceived quite differently depending on the clinical model selected by the clinician. In psychiatry, a depressed patient may be perceived and treated as suffering from a biochemical imbalance, a stress reaction, an enmeshed family disorder, a developmental disorder, or a lapse into helplessness and hopelessness, depending on the clinical model selected by the therapist. Selection of one or another model will result in quite different therapeutic strategies. A similar diversity of models is available to internists, surgeons, and other clinicians. Any physician thus has available a repertoire of clinical perspectives and models that may be used, depending on the disease or management problem presented and on the training of the physician.

It is our general belief that in our role as *clinical* social scientists, anthropologists should develop specific, limited clinical models and techniques, grounded in the anthropological enterprise, that may be added to the physician's repertoire. Teaching such models has three foci. First, residents or students need to be taught the theoretical framework and data base in which the clinical models are grounded. Second, they need to become aware of their subjective or experiential involvement in the use of particular clinical models (issues of "cultural transference and countertransference"). Most importantly, they need to be taught to use the models in clinical practice, integrate them into their own forms of practice, and learn for what kind of patients or management problems a particular clinical model is most useful. A single experience of success at solving a difficult clinical problem using a new clinical technique is the most important learning experience that can be provided in clinical teaching.

When we began teaching clerks and family practice residents, we began teaching them to distinguish "disease" and "illness" as a clinical tool (Kleinman, Eisenberg and Good 1978). This approach was helpful. It provided a clear, usable clinical tool that focused attention on a variety of social and cultural variables and their relationship to patient problems. It focused attention on the subjective experience of the patient and therefore on the patient's culturally constituted realities. On the other hand, this approach led to diagnosis and enumeration of a variety of psychosocial problems for which social workers, psychologists, and psychiatrists have more specialized treatment skills than do anthropologists. When the family practice program developed a psychological medicine course that ran parallel to ours, we developed a more clearly "cultural" approach to our teaching.

We currently carry out our clinical teaching from the perspective of a "cultural hermeneutic model" (B. Good and M. Good 1981a).[5] We teach clinicians to think of their practice as transactions or negotiations across "medical subcultures," in particular between professional medicine and the popular medical subcultures of patients. In our family practice seminar, we provide residents with experiences with various medical subcultures − the lifestyle and medical subculture specific to American homosexuals; the world of Vietnamese immigrants; spiritualism and spiritualist healing; adolescents (conceived as an American minority group); and other subcultures. We provide readings to demonstrate that an individual's "medical subculture" is grounded in that of a larger social group. Second, we teach the residents to use various clinical techniques that make the patient's meaning structure relevant to their diagnostic and therapeutic work. We teach them to distinguish disease and illness, and elicit illness problems from the perspective of the patients. Residents learn to elicit explanatory models in order to understand the explicit content of patients' understandings of their current illness. We teach them to analyze semantic networks (B. Good 1977; B. Good and M. Good 1981b), to investigate the symbolic and affective associations that provide the implicit context for the patient's experience. They learn to investigate care-seeking patterns (Chrisman 1977), to explore the relationship between the care they as physicians provide and that provided by other support systems. And we teach them to elicit patient requests in order to focus on specific concerns of patients (including hidden agendas) and negotiate issues for attention in each clinical transaction. Our goal is to make residents skilled and comfortable with these clinical techniques, to teach them to integrate parts of the approach into routine history-taking, and to make the cultural hermeneutic model available as part of their repertoire of clinical models.

Elicitation of patient requests is one useful clinical technique that we have integrated into our teaching. In the remainder of this paper we will limit our discussion to the patient request and to our research effort to provide a validated clinical tool for primary care.

PATIENT REQUESTS IN PRIMARY CARE

Aaron Lazare and his colleagues introduced the "customer approach to patient-hood" in reports of research at an outpatient psychiatric clinic at the Massachusetts General Hospital (Lazare, Eisenthal and Wasserman 1975; Lazare et al. 1975; Lazare and Eisenthal 1977). This approach to clinical transactions conceptualizes an initial interview with a psychiatric patient as "a process of negotiation between the clinician and the patient, taking the patient's request as the starting point" (Lazare, Eisenthal and Wasserman 1975: 553). This view is contrasted with the "diagnostic approach", in which clinicians determine the client's disease status and develop a treatment plan based on diagnosis, and with the "suitability approach", in which the clinic screens patients on initial visits for "good therapy cases." In the customer approach to initial interviews, the starting point for the contract between therapist and client is neither the patients' chief complaints nor their ultimate goal (what they would like to accomplish or how they would like to feel). The starting point is rather the patients' "requests": the specific services patients would like the clinic to provide them.

The patient request approach is particularly appropriate for primary care. Unlike clients in long-term psychotherapy, primary care patients commonly bring to a visit a set of requests not previously negotiated or discussed with the clinician. These requests often are not made explicit. Patients may present physical symptoms, which they believe meet the physician's diagnostic model. They often do not readily reveal important factors that triggered their visits (McWhinney 1972) and their "request" or the service they most desire. The patient request may become evident only at the end of a visit in a comment beginning, "By the way, Doc, I was just wondering if . . . " Explicit elicitation of the patient's request allows the physician to deal directly with the problem for which the "customer" is seeking help in a limited amount of time.

Elicitation of patient requests and negotiation of the problems to be addressed in a visit are important clinical techniques associated with a cultural hermeneutic clinical model. The patient request format is patient-centered: it requires the clinician to elicit the client's subjective perspective. Patient requests are grounded in patients' explanatory models and semantic networks. Careful decoding of a patient request will often reveal a network of powerful meanings, affective experiences, and life situations that are troubling the patient and are linked semantically to the illness. Elicitation and negotiation of patient requests thus require a conscious elicitation of the structure of the patient's subjective experience and a negotiation across systems of meaning. Real negotiation requires a sharing of power; it does not require the physician to accept the patient's definition of either the problem to be addressed or the service to be provided, but it requires that the patient's request for a service be seen as legitimate (Katon and Kleinman 1981). This is often experienced by physicians as threatening. At the same time, it may be liberating to the clinician to discover, after eliciting a long list of physical and psychosocial problems, that the patient wants a relatively limited service. Feeling responsibility for all ills of a multi-problem family is overwhelming. Eliciting and negotiating a limited set of requests allows the patient and physician to jointly establish priorities and a realistic problem set.

Family practice residents in our seminar are encouraged to integrate elicitation and negotiation of patient requests into their clinical routine. It is suggested that after the clinician elicits the chief complaints, the history of present illness, and a brief explanatory model, the patient should be asked: "How do you hope (or wish) I (or this clinic) can help you today? . . . Is there anything else? . . . Is there anything else you would like to discuss with me today?" (cf. Lazare, Eisenthal and Wasserman 1975: 554). It is important that these questions not be asked at the very beginning of the interview and that the patient be given genuine support and encouragement to voice what he hopes (not necessarily expects) will happen during the visit. Residents are especially encouraged to explore the patient's questions and the context for these concerns before attempting to provide explanation and reassurance. Too often reassurance is directed at the questions raised for the physician by a set of symptoms, rather than at the question brought by the patient. For example, reassurance that he does not have cancer may be more troubling than helpful to a man fearful of a heart condition like that which recently struck a friend.

A STUDY OF PATIENT REQUESTS IN PRIMARY CARE

Our study of patient requests in primary care had two purposes. First, we wanted to provide a data base for our clinical teaching — to demonstrate the range and clustering of requests, to determine how patient requests in primary care differ from those in a walk-in psychiatric clinic, and eventually to demonstrate the effectiveness of eliciting and negotiating patient requests. Second, we wanted to develop an instrument to document actual demands or desires of consumers of health care.

During the past decade, a wide variety of groups, both consumers and academic critics, have sharply criticized health care for not meeting the needs of consumers. Many have criticized medicine for its increasingly biotechnical focus and its inattention to psychosocial treatment or caring. These views are reflected in the statements of various leaders of health care advocacy groups, who have called for more holistic approaches, for preventive services, for physicians to focus on stress reduction. Others have criticized health care for not adequately responding to the needs of women or for not providing culturally appropriate services for ethnic groups. On the other hand, some have replied that consumers want quality medical care, not psychosocial support. Others argue that patients often come to primary care with inappropriate requests. Physicians, in particular, often believe that many patients primarily seek medication. Debates about these issues are seldom based on much data. It is therefore difficult to determine whether criticisms of health care represent concerns of large groups of consumers or primarily articulate concerns of ideological spokespersons.

A central goal of our research has been to direct attention to persons who are actually seeking medical services. Our approach was to elicit a range of patient requests through direct interviewing, then use these requests to develop an instrument for studying patient requests in various primary care clinic settings. The following pages report the development of the Primary Care Patient Request Form and initial findings from research with the instrument in four quite varied clinics.

PATIENT REQUEST QUESTIONNAIRE FOR PRIMARY CARE CLINICS

A questionnaire to study patient requests in primary care needed to meet several criteria. We wanted to tap a wide range of "requests" of patients rather than their "expectations" of primary care providers. We wanted to elicit requests for both instrumental and affective, both biomedical and psychosocial treatment. Above all, we wanted to create an instrument that would assist us in answering the question *what indeed do ordinary patients in primary care settings hope to gain from their visit to the doctor?*

The development of the questionnaire proceeded through several phases. In the first phase of the research, 100 structured in-depth interviews were conducted and clinical interactions observed with the aim of eliciting patients' requests, their explanatory models, and the extent to which physicians elicited these during the clinical encounters. The requests were extracted from these in-depth interviews and grouped into conceptual categories by four researchers (see Table I). Examples of patient requests include the following: "I want someone to explain the cause of my illness". "I want the results from my tests". "I want the doctor to sit down and talk with me about my problem". These items were augmented by requests derived from observations of doctor-patient interactions in primary care clinics and from items from several categories in the studies by Lazare and his colleagues of psychiatric outpatient requests which appeared appropriate for primary care settings.[6] We designed the initial instrument to include a number of items which tapped the same or part of the same request domain for each of 22 request categories. We also included a general item which subsumed the specific items in each category. The redundancy and use of general items were purposeful and aided us in testing the validity of the instrument. The initial questionnaire included 129 items, which were reduced to 89 items after pretesting. After the analysis of the data from the current study of 460 patients, which included correlation coefficient alphas and factor analysis, the request questionnaire was further reduced to 53 items.[7] For the sake of brevity, redundant items and several conceptual categories were eliminated from the final format. A five-point scale proved to be more useful to the data analysis (and necessary for factor analysis) than a three-point scale, which was first used to designate to what extent a particular request item represented what the patient wanted from the clinic or physician (1 = Not at all; 5 = Exactly).

TABLE I
Patient request categories

Biomedical categories

Check-up	The patient seeks information about his/her "state of health" and wants the physician to do a physical or check a health problem.
Diagnosis	The patient seeks information about the meaning of symptoms and wants the physician to use his/her expertise to label the illness or to conduct appropriate tests.
Explanation	The patient seeks professional medical information on his/her condition, on the etiology, degree of seriousness, and/or course of the illness.
Maternal/child health	The patient seeks information/and or reassurance that the pregnancy is proceeding normally or that her child is developing normally.
Medical advice	The patient seeks guidance as well as information regarding how to treat his/her medical problem.
Referral	The patient seeks instrumental action by the physician required for referral to a specialist.
Rule out feared condition	The patient seeks reassurance from the physician that nothing is physically wrong, and wants instrumental action by the physician, such as a physical exam.
Test results	The patient seeks information from previous instrumental actions of the physician.

Table I (continued)

Treatment explanation	The patient seeks information regarding the physician's treatment plan, including medications and non-drug treatments.
Treatment requests general	The patient seeks instrumental action by the physician for unspecific medical treatment of symptoms or disease.
Medications	The patient seeks instrumental action by the physician in the form of medications or innoculations.

Psychosocial categories

Administrative	The patient seeks legal or quasi-legal assistance from the clinic including medical permission to apply for disability or medical approval for employment or leave.
Community triage	The patient seeks guidance and assistance from the clinic in obtaining help from community social service agencies.
Habit control	The patient seeks instrumental actions by the physician/clinic to assist in controlling unwanted habits such as smoking, drinking, or to lose weight or relax.
Medical treatment for "Nervous" condition	The patient wants instrumental actions, i.e., medical treatment, by the physician to treat nervousness, anxiety, tiredness, weakness or depression.
Psychiatric treatment	The patient seeks counseling from the physician, instrumental action, for self-labeled emotional or interpersonal problems.
Social advice	The patient seeks guidance or advice on social situations self-labeled as problematic, such as interpersonal and family relations, work and financial difficulties.
Social intervention	The patient seeks instrumental action by the physician to use the physician's influence to alter an interpersonal problem.
Succorance	The patient seeks a sense of being cared for and a responsive and comforting physician to whom he/she can talk.

Patient-practitioner interaction categories

Dissatisfaction	The patient seeks to convey a sense of frustration over course of illness or treatment to the physician.
Continuity of care	The patient seeks a family physician who will provide continuity of care to self and/or family.
Legitimation	The patient seeks legitimation from the physician.
Share perspective	The patient seeks to convey beliefs about his/her own problem to the physician and receive positive or confirming response.

The 22 request categories are described in Table I and are grouped into clusters of biomedical, psychosocial, or patient-practitioner interaction requests. Each category can also be characterized as requesting instrumental action, reassurance or affective support, and/or information. Requests for explanation and for information are central to clinical interaction in primary care and not easily classifiable into instrumental or affective requests. Explanation of test results, the likely course of an illness, symptoms, or medication requires a physician to draw on technical or instrumental skills as well as communicative and affective skills.[8]

The internal consistency of each of the request categories was evaluated for the 89-item questionnaire by the computation of coefficient alphas. Interitem correlation matrices were prepared using Pearson's R correlation coefficient, and the coefficient alpha was computed for 18 categories utilizing the Medical Center adult patient sample. Two single item categories — administrative requests and habit control — and two highly specific categories — maternal/child health and continuity of care — were excluded from this analysis. Reliability as estimated by coefficient alpha provided a measure of each category's internal consistency. Overall the internal consistency of the hypothesized request categories was exceptionally high. As noted in Table II, 15 of the 18 categories emerged as cohesive categories with

TABLE II

Coefficient alphas for selected request categories

	Number of Items	Coefficient Alpha
Request categories above 0.70		
Medical		
Diagnosis	4	0.84
Explanation	11	0.93
Medical advice	7	0.83
Referral	2	0.72
Test results	2	0.79
Treatment explanation	5	0.75
Treatment requests (general and medication)	13	0.72
Psychosocial		
Community triage	3	0.70
Medical treatment for "Nervous" condition	7	0.84
Psychiatric treatment	7	0.95
Social advice	3	0.81
Social intervention	2	0.74
Succorance	5	0.75
Patient-practitioner interactions		
Dissatisfaction	5	0.76
Share perspective	3	0.77
Request categories below 0.70		
Check-up	3	0.30
Rule out feared condition	2	0.55
Legitimation	2	0.33

coefficient alphas of 0.70 or above. The three categories with coefficient alphas below 0.70 included *check up, rule out feared condition*, and *legitimation*. In each of these categories, it appeared that the individual items measured separate areas of requests.

THE SAMPLE: CLINICS AND PATIENTS

We hypothesized that the pattern of patient requests in primary care would be influenced in part by the health culture and social location of patients, and in part by the type of clinic and kind of practitioner(s) from whom patients had chosen to seek services. Thus patients were sampled from four contrasting clinics situated in four contrasting community settings. Our findings, which we discuss below, suggest remarkable similarities as well as several differences in request patterns among our four patient samples.

The Four Clinics

The four primary care clinics chosen for the study included a University Medical Center Family Practice outpatient clinic, staffed by residents, attending physicians, and family nurse practitioners, and located in a major urban center; a private practice clinic located in a small rural farm town and staffed by three physicians, two of whom had lived and practiced in the community for over 20 years; a 10 year old Free Clinic for women located in a university town, staffed by volunteer medical students and physicians; and a private practice Holistic Health Clinic located in a wealthy suburb of a major metropolitan area, which was run by two primary care physicians and also staffed by an acupuncturist, a nutritionist, and a Feldenkreis body worker.

Payment plans varied for each of the four clinics. The Holistic Health Clinic served only private pay patients, excluding MediCal patients because they require "too much paper work". In contrast, 80% of the University Medical Center Family Practice clinic population was covered by MediCal, Medicare or clinical teaching funds. The rural private physicians estimated 30 to 40% of their patients to be on MediCal or Medicare, and one doctor noted: "We treat everybody here, no one is turned down". The Free Clinic for women requests a small donation of $6.00 per visit if the person can afford it. The clinic's other funding comes from a variety of community sources and from Title XX federal funding for family planning. Each of the providers in these four clinics have specific and somewhat unique philosophies regarding health, illness and health care delivery. Most, however, hold the view to some extent that ". . . all people have emotional problems associated with illness; you can't separate them" (rural physician). The younger physicians at the Holistic Health Clinic and the Free Clinic, many of the practitioners at the Medical Center, and the new doctor in the rural practice explicitly stated that one of their central purposes was to educate their patients. The content of that "education" varied according to their medical philosophy.

The Patient Sample

A total of 460 patients were interviewed using the 89-item patient request form from August 1979 to October 1980. Table III indicates various demographic characteristics of patients by clinic. In the University Medical Center and rural private practice populations, a percentage of respondents were parents of children who were patients (under 15 years of age).[9]

The Medical Center sample approximated very closely the overall patient population of the clinic. In a previous study conducted by the authors,[10] it was found that adult males accounted for 16% of all visits, adult females for 57% of all visits and children age 15 and under for 26% of all patient visits in a 12-month period. Our Medical Center sample included 19% adult males, 57% adult females and 25% parents of children. Two-thirds of patients who were asked to participate did so. Refusals came primarily from patients who were elderly, illiterate or exceptionally ill or harried. The sample is therefore somewhat biased toward younger and less seriously ill patients.

The patient sample from the Rural Private Practice Clinic included 48% adult women, 32% adult men, and 20% parents of children. Sixty-seven percent of all patients asked to participate did so, although refusals came primarily from the elderly (50% of all refusals were from people over 50 years old) and from a proportionately greater number of men than women (41% of refusals were from males in contrast with 32% of completed questionnaires).

Patients sampled from the Free Clinic for women appeared representative of the general patient population in age and education. Seventy-eight percent agreed to participate and completed the questionnaire. There appeared to be no particular bias due to refusals. Patients sampled at the Holistic Health Clinic also appeared to be representative by age, sex, and education of the general clinic population with no particular bias pattern noted in the refusals.[11]

As indicated in Table III, patients in our four clinics had notable differences in their demographic characteristics. The rural patients were least well educated, but had the lowest percentage unemployed and the highest percentage married. The urban university clinic had a large number of patients who were unemployed and divorced or separated. The Free Clinic's patient population reflected the university community in which it is located in level of education, percentage of students, and overall youthfulness of the patient population. A greater proportion of patients at the Holistic Health Clinic were professionals and college graduates than were patients at the other clinics, although fewer of these patients were married or in a permanent relationship. Ethnic diversity was greatest for the Free Clinic and the University Medical Center.

Table IV illustrates several medical characteristics of the patient sample for each clinic, including the mean number of chief complaints elicited by the interviewer, an assessment of whether the visit was for health maintenance or for treatment of an acute or chronic illness, last visit made to the clinic, and an estimated mean number of visits to any health provider for the past 30 days. As indicated in Table

TABLE III

Demographic characteristics of patient sample by clinic

	Rural private practice clinic	University medical center family practice clinic	Free clinic for women	Holistic health clinic
	$n = 119$	$n = 203$	$n = 110$	$n = 28$
	(%)	(%)	(%)	(%)
Sex of Respondent				
Male	36.1	20.7	– 0 –	46.4
Female	63.9	79.3	100	53.6
Sex/Age of Patient				
Adult Male	32.2 (38)	19 (38)	– – –	46.4 (13)
Adult Female	47.5 (56)	57 (115)	100 (110)	53.5 (15)
Child (parent as respondent = 92% females)	20.0 (25)	25 (50)	– – –	– – –
Marital Status (adults)				
Single	25.6	22.7	51.9	35.7
Married or S.O.	59.0	49.8	37.1 (20.4% have S.O.)	35.7
Divorced, Separated, Widowed	15.3	27.6	11.1	28.6
Education				
< High School	31.9	10.8	12.7	3.6
High School	38.7	31.0	19.1	3.6
Some College	20.2	42.9	21.8	17.9
College Graduate	9.2	15.3	46.3	75.0
Occupation				
Housewife (only)	23.7	33.7	6.5	14.8
Professional	7.6	12.9	28.9	48.1
White Collar	5.1	11.0	11.2	11.1
Blue Collar	50.8	22.3	15.8	14.8
Student	6.8	8.4	31.8	3.7
Other	5.9	10.9	6.5	7.4
Employment				
Employed full time	45.7	19.3	31.8	63.0
Employed part time	14.7	8.9	35.5	7.4
Retired	5.2	5.9	– 0 –	3.7
Other (housewives)	23.7	33.7	6.5	14.8
Unemployed (not housewives)	10.8	32.1	26.2	11.9

Table III (continued)

	Rural private practice clinic	University medical center family practice clinic	Free clinic for women	Holistic health clinic
Ethnicity				
European	75.2	74.6	73.5	84.6
Hispanic/Latin	16.3	8.5	10.8	– 0 –
Asian	– 0 –	1.0	5.0	11.4
Black/African	– 0 –	12.5	6.9	– 0 –
Native American	3.4	1.5	1.0	– 0 –
Mixed	5.1	2.0	2.9	3.8
Religion				
Protestant or				
Christian Scientist	32.8	45.1	20.9	14.3
Catholic	31.9	19.2	18.2	3.6
Jewish	0.9	2.5	6.4	17.9
Other	10.1	3.4	10.9	32.1
No Preference	24.4	29.6	43.6	32.1

IV, patients attending the Holistic Health Clinic had the highest mean number of complaints, the highest percentage of chronic illnesses, and saw the greatest number of health care providers in a 30-day period. The health maintenance patients in the other three clinics included visits for pregnancy, birth control, innoculations, physical check-ups and well baby checks, whereas in the Holistic Health Clinic these patients were seeking nutritional advice to prevent illness. In comparing the disorders elicited by the interviewer on chief complaints, the patients from the holistic health group had the highest percentage who mentioned psychosocial problems (36%), musculo-skeletal problems (43%) and vague symptoms and signs (not otherwise specified) (54%).

Our four sampled patient groups represent a wide cross section of American society. Given these demographic and health status differences, how and to what extent do these patients differ from each other in terms of what they request from their primary care providers?

FINDINGS

Information seeking is a foremost goal of patients in primary care settings, although the type of information sought varies depending on the concerns of particular patients and on the goals of the provider or clinic. A very high proportion of respondents in our study expressed a desire for explanation and medical advice from their physicians, regardless of their sex, the clinic they attended or whether they were patients or parents of patients. For example, patients who wanted their

TABLE IV

Medical characteristics of patients by clinic, sex and identified patient

	Rural private practice clinic	University medical center family practice clinic	Free clinic for women	Holistic health clinic
	n = 119	n = 203	n = 110	n = 28
Mean number of complaints per patient	1.2	1.43	1.33	1.82
Degree of seriousness				
Health Maintenance	11%	36%	60%	18%
Acute	46%	32%	26%	- 0 -
Chronic	42%	19%	9%	82%
Both	1%	6%	1%	- - -
Uncertain	- 0 -	8%	4%	- - -
Last Visit				
New patient	14%	7%	24%	4%
< 1 month	45%	61%	22%	89%
2–6 months	20%	24%	25%	4%
> 6 months	20%	8%	29%	4%
Mean number of estimated visits to any health care provider in past 30 days	0.91	n.a.	1.21	2.54

physicians to explain some things about their illness they currently did not understand (partly or exactly) included 61% of the Rural Clinic, 68% of the University Clinic, 62% of the Free Clinic, and 96% of the Holistic Health Clinic populations. Requests for instrumental action, such as tests and prescriptions, varied by clinic population. Thirty-three percent of respondents in the Rural Clinic and in the University Clinic wanted tests done "to find out what is wrong", whereas only 23% of the Holistic Health Clinic respondents asked for tests. The women attending the Free Clinic were more likely to ask for tests (46%), because one of the chief activities of the clinic is conducting pregnancy tests and pap tests. Requests for medication also varied, with 41% of the Rural Clinic, 43% of the University Clinic, 49% of the Free Women's Clinic, and 7% of the Holistic Health Clinic populations responding partly or exactly to a desire for prescriptions for medication. The vast majority of women at the Free Clinic requesting medication wanted birth control pills.

The variation of the responses to instrumental requests is indicative of the differences in both patient and clinic characteristics. For example, patients who choose to seek care from the Holistic Health Clinic do so because their experience with traditional biomedicine has been unsatisfactory (39%). Many have rejected the instrumental activities of biomedicine and are searching for alternatives, which this clinic offers. In contrast, 63% of the women attending the Free Clinic came for gynecological health maintenance (for contraceptives, pregnancy checks, pap tests), a specialty of the Free Clinic. The other two clinics are more representative of general medicine and general primary care, and their patient request patterns reflect this clinical reality.

Mean Scores Categories

A comparison of the rankings and the mean scores on request categories by clinic population is presented in Table V.[12] Once again the differences by clinic population are noteworthy. The patient respondents from the Holistic Health Clinic have higher mean scores on all six psychosocial categories and on requests for medical explanation, advice, diagnosis, and treatment for symptom relief than any other clinic group, and the lowest scores on requests for medications and test results. Clearly this population of patients is unique in its psychological-mindedness and in

TABLE V
Comparative mean scores on request categories

Request Categories	Rural private practice clinic n = 119		University medical center family practice clinic n = 203		Free clinic for women n = 110		Holistic health clinic n = 28	
	Rank	Mean	Rank	Mean	Rank	Mean	Rank	Mean
Explanation	2	2.67	2	2.74	2	2.57	4	3.57
Diagnosis	5	2.36	5	2.40	4	2.31	8	2.71
Test results	4	2.43	1	3.01	1	2.96	11	1.60
General disease or symptomatic treatment requests	1	3.01	3	2.62	5	2.23	3	3.66
Medications	8	1.93	9	1.76	8	1.95	13	1.06
Treatment explanation	6	2.14	8	2.06	7	2.08	10	2.07
Medical advice	3	2.49	4	2.58	3	2.38	5	3.53
Share perspective	7	1.95	7	2.15	10	1.83	1	3.94
Succorance	9	1.69	6	2.22	6	2.21	2	3.81
Medical treatment of psychiatric disorder	11	1.40	10	1.57	11	1.41	9	2.61
Psychiatric treatment	12	1.34	11	1.48	12	1.39	7	2.87
Social advice	10	1.61	12	1.36	9	1.87	6	2.90
Social intervention	13	1.17	13	1.23	13	1.06	12	1.40

its request pattern. The other three patient samples are more similar in their response patterns. As indicated by the ranking of request categories for these three
samples, requests for information, explanation, advice, and biomedical skills are
most frequent; yet a large proportion of these patients also hope for succorance
from their physicians (58% reported, "I want the doctor to sit down and talk with
me about my problem"), and want to share their perspective regarding their illness
with their physicians (40%). Their responses to the psychosocial request items
were higher on somatic or medical items than on overtly psychological items. For
example, 25% of both the Rural Clinic and the Free Clinic and 33% of the University Clinic (and 79% of the Holistic Health Clinic) respondents noted they were
"feeling tired and weak today and would like medical treatment". In contrast,
only 11% of the Rural Clinic, 17% of the University Clinic, and 7% of the Free
Clinic respondents claimed to want help in dealing with psychological problems.
Eighty-two percent of the Holistic Health Clinic respondents desired such help.
However, when the term "counseling" appeared in the request item, 25% of the
patient respondents from the three clinics noted they partly or exactly desired such
help. The percentage responding partly or exactly to items for psychiatric treatment
and for medical treatment for "nervous conditions" ranged between 10 and 30% of
the adult patient respondents in the three clinics. Again, the Holistic Health Clinic
respondents were both more psychologically minded and also more likely to
request medical treatment of physical symptoms related to "nervous conditions"
than the other respondents. Between 50% and 70% of the respondents checked
partly or exactly on these items.

The differences that appear between the clinic populations, in particular between
the holistic health respondents and others, fit hypothesized expectations that
clinical realities can shape requests. We were struck that the Free Clinic population
was not exceptional in its request pattern, but note that although the financial
and patient education arrangements differ from the other clinics, the medicine
offered is mainstream biomedicine and gynecological practice. The ideology underlying funding of the Free Clinic rather than its medical practice is out of the
ordinary; in contrast, the ideology of health and illness in the Holistic Health Clinic,
rather than alternative payment and funding, is what creates alternative medical
therapeutics.

Analysis of Variance Within Clinic Samples

We hypothesized that patient characteristics, including demographic and illness
related characteristics, would in part account for variations in patient request
responses. Two-way analysis of variance utilizing six independent variables (sex,
age, education, marital status, degree of seriousness of illness — acute, chronic,
health maintenance — and last visit) were computed for six medical and six psychosocial request categories for each clinic subsample.

Several trends that raise questions to be explored in future research emerged
from the analysis. It was expected that patients who are most diffusely "troubled"
— by an undiagnosed or unlabeled illness, by emotional or psychosocial problems,

by chronic illness — would have more requests than would patients with narrowly defined illness problems. Although this appears to be the case, other factors seem to influence request patterns. It appears that the need for assistance from primary care physicians is more diffuse for patients who have fewer resources or are socially isolated.

Mean scores on request categories and the total number of requests appear to vary inversely with education for each of the subsamples, with the exception of the Holistic Health Clinic respondents. The analysis of variance disclosed that level of education was significantly and negatively associated with requests for general treatment of symptoms, medical treatment for nervous conditions, and share perspective for the University Clinic adult respondents, and for explanation, diagnosis, and share perspective for parents of children who were patients. The trend holds for all the categories, although for only six categories was significance greater than 0.05.[13] This consistent pattern was initially surprising, since many physicians assume that requests for explanations and desire to share one's perspective with one's physician is greater among the more highly educated. A similar inverse relationship between education and mean scores on 11 of the 12 request categories emerged for the Free Clinic respondents.[14]

No pattern emerged in the analysis of variance for the Holistic Health Clinic respondents, in part because so few of the respondents had less than a college education. The pattern for the Rural Clinic respondents suggested that the least educated (less than high school) were likely to make more requests of their physicians than other respondents, although the few college educated respondents frequently had higher mean scores on certain request categories than those with some college. Education was not significantly associated (at 0.05 or better) with any of the request categories.

Marital status was associated with differences in request category scores for all of the four samples. Single women and married men and women have consistently lower request scores than do single men or divorced or separated men and women. This pattern holds for all four clinic subsamples, including adult patients and parent respondents.[15]

Education and marital status were thus most useful in analyzing patient characteristics associated with requests. This initial analysis suggests that not only are the less well educated, the unmarried males, and divorced males and females susceptible to a higher incidence of disease, but that they are also in greater need of help from their primary care physicians in a rather global and diffuse way.

Age and sex are less clearly related to number or type of patient requests. In the University Clinic sample, which had the largest age range, the middle-age groups (between 31 and 60) were more likely to have higher scores than patients under 30 and over 60. Significant differences were found for five request categories. In the rural sample, the 40 to 60 age group tended to have the highest scores, whereas for the Holistic Health Clinic sample scores varied inversely with age. However, there were no significant relationships to 0.05. Interestingly, differences between male and female respondents for the three mixed clinic samples were not significant.

Again, this lack of significant difference suggests that female patients are no more demanding of the health care system than are male patients.

Analysis of variance was computed for two additional health related variables — degree of seriousness and last visit. Health maintenance patients score lowest in all clinical settings on all request categories as is expected. No clear distinction emerged between chronic and acute patients, however, although we had hypothesized that the chronically ill would desire more help from their primary care clinics than acutely ill patients. Significant differences (0.05 or better) emerged for nine of 12 request categories for the University Clinic sample but not for any of the other samples. The final analysis, examining last visit, indicated that patients who were new and those who had visited the clinic during the previous month tended to have the most requests. Clearly, however, the demographic as opposed to the health related variables are more powerfully associated with differences in mean scores on request categories for our sampled population.

Psychosocial Requests and Chief Complaints

Most patients in primary care settings do not present to their physicians with a psychosocial chief complaint (8% of the Rural Clinic, 6% of the University Clinic, and 1% of the Free Clinic respondents did so). Even a majority of the most psychologically minded patients in our study, those from the Holistic Health Clinic (64%), did not present with a psychosocial chief complaint. However, when allowed to make a variety of requests, many patients check psychosocial requests. This suggests that patients feel the need to mask requests for psychosocial treatment. Although they may desire that such treatment be provided by their primary care practitioners, they hesitate to be explicit by presenting a psychosocial problem as a chief complaint on admission to a clinic. Rather they choose what is deemed an appropriate problem. Clearly, clinical realities shape what is considered an appropriate problem as is illustrated by the differences in the responses between the Holistic Health Clinic patients and the patients in the other three clinics. Patients still consider the most appropriate ticket of admission to most primary care physician offices to be physical symptoms or complaints.

CONCLUSION

This paper has argued that social scientists teaching in clinical settings need to develop techniques through which new forms of knowledge and perception can be embedded in the clinical enterprise. Following the work of Lazare and his colleagues, we have suggested that the elicitation and negotiation of patient requests is one clinical technique that can lead to changes in perspective and is particularly appropriate for primary care. This approach requires that the patient's reality be taken seriously and treated as legitimate, and that not only knowledge but power relations be negotiated. Our research with the Primary Care Patient Request Form suggests further reasons why this is so. It suggests most clearly that when offered the opportunity, patients in primary care request explanation twice as frequently as medical tests and half again as frequently as medication. Providing help in answering troubling questions and making sense of threatening life conditions is a very fundamental characteristic of medical care. Negotiation of patient requests in primary care sometimes reduces the set of issues to which the physician need respond. However, the physician who openly elicits patient requests must also be prepared to be asked to share and help with some of life's most complex dilemmas. Issues other than biomedical must be faced, and the horizons of the clinical gaze must be broadened. It is for such a reorientation that social scientists in clinical teaching strive.

NOTES

1. This research was funded by a California Policy Seminar Award from the Department of Governmental Studies, University of California, Berkeley. Our thanks to members of the clinics in which we carried out the research, and to Diane Stumbo, Sandra Gifford and James Cooper for their participation in data collection and analysis.

2. See Carlton 1978: 65–83 for a discussion of the "clinical perspective", and Feinstein 1973 for his seminal discussion of "clinical judgment". A more detailed symbolic analysis of clinical practice than we can provide here may be found in B. Good and M. Good 1980a.

3. For a discussion of how "knowledge" is tacitly embedded in the practice of medicine and in medical discourse, see Young 1980.

4. It would be useful to follow Geertz's approach to the analysis of "perspectives" (Geertz 1973), contrasting the clinical perspective with the scientific, the asthetic, and the religious perspectives. Using this language, Carlton's three perspectives would all be considered subtypes of the clinical perspective.

5. We have contrasted the cultural hermeneutic model with the biomedical model, discussed their epistemological assumptions, outlined teaching approaches, and provided case analyses in other publications (B. Good and M. Good 1981a; cf. B. Good and M. Good 1981b; B. Good 1977; and Kleinman, Eisenberg and Good 1978).

6. See Lazare, Eisenthal and Wasserman 1975, Lazare et al. 1975, and Lazare and Eisenthal 1977. Items 4, 55, 60, 63, 70, and 73 from Lazare's Patient Request Form were included in our 83-item Primary Care Patient Request Form.

7. We wish to thank Alberta Nassi, Ph.D., for computing the coefficient alphas and for the factor analysis on the Rural Clinic patient sample. The 53-item questionnaire which resulted from the factor analysis will be used for an NIMH funded study of 1000 primary care patients in rural Northern California. Major factors which emerged included an explanation factor, a psychosocial factor, and a rule-out feared condition/test factor among others which paralleled our earlier request categories.

8. See, for example, Ben-Sira 1976 and Parsons 1951.

9. A parent version of the Primary Care Patient Request Form was devised, using the same requests but referring to patient's request for services to their children. Thus, "I want someone to explain the cause of my illness" became "I want someone to explain the cause of my child's illness".

10. An analysis of 10% of active patient charts in a university primary care clinic (n = 410) was conducted in 1978 and provided base-line clinical epidemiological data for the University Clinic study.

11. The 89-item patient request questionnaire was combined with demographic and health questions. Interviewers asked consecutive patients to participate and interviewing took place in the four primary care clinics between August 1979 and October 1980. The first clinic sampled was the University Medical Center Family Practice Clinic, followed by the Rural Private Practice Clinic, the Free Clinic for women and the Holistic Health Clinic.

Interviewers verbally administered the initial set of questions on demographic background and health status; however, the Primary Care Patient Request Form was usually (97%) completed by the respondent without interviewer assistance.

12. Mean scores for the University Clinic and the Free Clinic studies were adjusted to a five-point from a three-point scale (1 = 1, 2 = 3, 3 = 5) to offer ease of comparability in Table V.

13. Level of education was significantly and negatively associated with requests for general treatment of symptoms ($p = 0.01$), medical treatment for nervous conditions ($p = 0.006$), and share perspective ($p = 0.04$) for the University Clinic adult respondents, and with explanation ($p = 0.02$), diagnosis ($p = 0.04$), and share perspective ($p = 0.02$) for parents of children who were patients.

14. For Free Clinic respondents, education and mean scores were related at the 0.05 level for diagnosis ($p = 0.03$), medications ($p = 0.03$), treatment explanation ($p = 0.006$), medical advice ($p = 0.004$), share perspective ($p = 0.006$), medical treatment for nervous condition ($p = 0.03$), and psychiatric treatment ($p = 0.003$).

15. Significant associations between marital status and request category scores for the University Clinic adult patients occurred for explanation ($p = 0.002$), diagnosis ($p = 0.004$), medical advice ($p = 0.07$), test results ($p = 0.04$), treatment requests ($p = 0.003$), and medical treatment for nervous condition ($p = 0.02$). Two-way interaction effects between sex and marital status were also significant for diagnosis ($p = 0.025$), test results ($p = 0.04$), and share perspective ($p = 0.02$). Significant differences in request category scores emerged for the Free Clinic sample for medications ($p = 0.04$), diagnosis ($p = 0.03$), test results ($p = 0.04$), share perspective ($p = 0.05$) and medical treatment of nervous condition ($p = 0.02$). For the Rural Clinic sample, significant differences in request category scores associated with marital status occurred for test results ($p = 0.001$), general treatment ($p = 0.001$), and for the holistic health sample, treatment requests ($p = 0.001$).

BIBLIOGRAPHY

Ben Sira, Zev
  1976 The Function of the Professional's Affective Behavior in Client Satisfaction: A Revised Approach to Social Interaction Theory. Journal of Health and Social Behavior 17: 3–11.
Carlton, Wendy
  1978 In Our Professional Opinion: The Primacy of Clinical Judgement Over Moral Choice. Notre Dame, Indiana: University of Notre Dame Press.
Chrisman, Noel
  1977 The Health Seeking Process: An Approach to the Natural History of Illness. Culture, Medicine and Psychiatry 1: 351–377.
Feinstein, Alvan R.
  1973 An Analysis of Diagnostic Reasoning, Parts I and II. Yale Journal of Biology and Medicine 46: 212–232, 264–283.
Foucault, Michel
  1973 The Birth of the Clinic. New York: Vintage Books.
Geertz, Clifford
  1973 Religion as a Cultural System. Chapter 4 in The Interpretation of Cultures. New York: Basic Books.
Good, Byron
  1977 The Heart of What's the Matter: The Semantics of Illness in Iran. Culture, Medicine and Psychiatry 1: 25–58.
Good, Byron and Mary-Jo DelVecchio Good
  1981a The Meaning of Symptoms: A Cultural Hermeneutic Model for Clinical Practice,

In Arthur Kleinman and Leon Eisenberg (eds.), The Relevance of Social Science for Medicine. Dordrecht, Holland: D. Reidel Publ. Co., pp. 165–196.

1981b The Semantics of Medical Discourse, *In* Everett Mendelsohn and Yehnda Elkana (eds.), Sociology of the Sciences, Volume 5. Dordrecht, Holland: D. Reidel Publ. Co., pp. 711–712.

Katon, Wayne and Arthur Kleinman
   1981 Doctor-Patient Negotiation and Other Social Science Strategies in Patient Care, *In* Arthur Kleinman and Leon Eisenberg (eds.), The Relevance of Social Science for Medicine. Dordrecht, Holland: D. Reidel Publ. Co., pp. 253–279.

Kleinman, Arthur, Leon Eisenberg, and Byron Good
   1978 Culture, Illness and Care: Clinical Lessons for Anthropologic and Cross-Cultural Research. Annals of Internal Medicine 88: 251–258.

Lazare, Aaron, Sherman Eisenthal and Linda Wasserman
   1975 The Customer Approach to Patienthood. Archives of General Psychiatry 32: 553–558.

Lazare, Aaron et al.
   1975 Patient Requests in a Walk-in Clinic. Comprehensive Psychiatry 16: 467–477.

Lazare, Aaron and Sherman Eisenthal
   1977 Patient Requests in a Walk-in Clinic. Journal of Nervous and Mental Disease 165: 330–340.

McWhinney, Ian R.
   1972 Beyond Diagnosis: An Approach to the Integration of Behavioral Science and Clinical Medicine. New England Journal of Medicine 287: 384–388.

Parsons, Talcott
   1951 The Social System. New York: The Free Press.

Schutz, Alfred
   1970 Reflections on the Problems of Relevance. Richard M. Zaner (ed.), New Haven: Yale University Press.

DAN BLUMHAGEN

THE MEANING OF HYPER-TENSION

Sick people seek out physicians to tell them of their ailments and learn what they
need to do to regain their health. Physicians ask questions about their patient's
illness, and then advise – prescribe – actions which will lead to the sick regaining
their health. In the midst of this recounting, questioning, and advising, it seems
strange that problems of communication would arise, but apparently they do.
Issues surrounding the transmission of information about health and illness are
being discussed more frequently in the biomedical literature, and the debate is even
spilling over into the lay press. Poor communication is blamed for a variety of the
ills besetting health care: at the least it is seen as a major factor in lack of compliance with medical regimens (Hulka 1979; Svarstad 1976), lack of satisfaction
with medical care (Roter 1977; Wooley et al. 1978) and the increase in malpractice
suits. If it is true that problems in communication do lie at the bottom of these
and similar issues, social science disciplines which scrutinize the process, content
and significance of verbal interaction should be able to provide at least tentative
solutions.

Before looking at the content and the significance of the information passed
between patient and practitioner,[1] it may be useful to look at the forum that a
classical biomedical encounter has. From the practitioner's point of view there
are three phases in such an encounter. In the first, the patient, under the guidance
of questions by the practitioner, describes his experiences with health and illness.
This is known as the *medical history*, and is regarded as the single most important
element in achieving a diagnosis (Beeson 1979: 3). Indeed, Feinstein describes
history taking as the most complex and sophisticated task that a practitioner must
perform in the medical encounter. Paradoxically he finds that skills for accomplish-
ing this feat are rarely taught (Feinstein 1967: 299). In this phase, practitioners
often assume that their patients present with a jumble of experiences which must
be reordered into a structure suitable for biomedical interpretation. As has been
amply demonstrated in the social science literature (Chrisman 1977; Freidson
1970; Helman 1978) what the patient brings a healer is not simply a random
jumble, but the result of a more or less extended period of sorting, interpreting,
and negotiating the significance within their own health beliefs and those of their
lay health networks. Thus, as they enter the doctor's office, they have already
determined definitions of what is normal, what is abnormal, which events are
significant and therefore to be reported, and frequently have even come to a
diagnosis which the provider is expected to confirm and treat; a diagnosis decided
by the illness beliefs of a patient and his social network.

We can see the potential for conflict. The patient often implicitly assumes that
the physician's beliefs are the same (albeit more extensive) as his own, and only

297

N. J. Chrisman and T. W. Maretzki (eds.), Clinically Applied Anthropology, 297–323.
Copyright © 1982 by D. Reidel Publishing Company.

wishes to tell of those events which his own beliefs indicate are significant. The physician assumes that the patient has biomedical beliefs at best (and none or incorrect ones at worst) and only wishes to hear those things that he can fit into a biomedical framework.

The second phase of this protypical biomedical encounter deals with gathering physical data, such as performing a physical examination or doing a variety of laboratory of radiological procedures. Ostensibly, there is no interpersonal communication (other than grunts and grimaces when the patient's abdomen is palpated) but there is a significant danger that both patient and physician may use the examination as a substitute for communication. A patient often feels that all the doctor needs to do is order the right test and that will show why he is sick. The physician is often seduced by the scientific aura and pseudoprecision of laboratory tests, and will order them in a "shotgun" fashion, hoping to find something wrong without the necessity of an often tedious dialogue. In fact, very little information is gained during this phase that should not have been indicated by the medical history.

The final phase involves transmitting the practitioner's findings and conclusions to the patient, and often involves an explanation of the illness events and the significance of particular abnormal findings. This is usually coupled with recommendations and negotiations about treatment options.

There is clearly a wide variability in the extent to which each of these three parts is present in any particular patient-practitioner encounter. Some of this is due to the type or duration of problems being addressed: a person with a broken leg will have a very different encounter with a practitioner than someone with a chronic anxiety neurosis. Even more variance may be introduced by the personalities of either the patient or provider. Nonetheless, this summary encapsulating the features involved in much of biomedical diagnosis and treatment focuses on the fact that information must flow in both directions: first from the patient to the provider and then from the provider to patient. Too often communications research has neglected looking at the initial flow of information (which may set the tone for the entire encounter) and has concentrated on what the provider tells the patient (Hulka 1979). Such an approach will necessarily give skewed, incomplete answers to the difficult questions being addressed in this type of research.

The medical encounter usually takes place in the doctor's office or a hospital, which may be considered the temple of faith in biomedicine. Regardless of how much a patient may voice agreement with a doctor, after the patient returns home, the personal and lay network health beliefs as they have been modified by an encounter with a practitioner are the final arbiter of which interpretation of the illness is accepted and which treatment options are used. As Freidson has speculated (1970), if there is close association between the interpretation offered by the physician and that of a cohesive social network, the physician's prescriptions may be followed. On the other hand, if such a social network rejects a particular biomedical interpretation, the treatments will likewise often be rejected. All of this affects the outcome of any medical encounter, but is rarely explored. Because of this importance of popular health belief systems and lay health networks, it is imperative that health professionals be aware of them and be taught to elicit information about them and negotiate diagnostic and treatment options in the light of this information.

While the goal of bettering communication between patient and practitioner may well be an end in itself, most clinicians will not be interested in incorporating such skills into their practices unless tangible results can be demonstrated. This point is extremely important for social scientists working in a clinical setting. It is futile — or worse, academic — to construct elaborate hierarchies of "native beliefs" and social and kinship networks unless these constructs and the communications based on them can be shown to affect illness behavior. Yet, as anthropologists have learned, a researcher cannot rely only on an individual's report of his behavior — that behavior must in some way be observed. Illness behavior in American cultures is very difficult to observe because of high value placed on individual privacy. To replace direct experimental observation of illness behavior, two main proxy measures have developed: "satisfaction", any one of a variety of scales and instruments which report how satisfied a patient is with a particular health encounter; and "compliance", various measures of the extent to which a patient adheres to the practitioner's advice [2]. Unfortunately, even these proxy measures of illness behavior have proven to be extraordinarily refractory to the quantification and standardization necessary to assure the level of reliability and replicability needed for a scientific instrument [3]. Despite these shortcomings, some measure of compliance and satisfaction is useful for comparing different studies.

There have basically been two types of study which have examined communication in medical settings. The first of these has ignored the content, and instead focused on the interactive *process*, using Bales Interaction Process Analysis (Davis 1968, 1971; Korsch et al. 1968; Freeman et al. 1971). These have led to mutually contradictory results, Davis concluding that passive patients were more compliant while Korsch concluded that active patients were more compliant.

The second research approach has examined cognitive models and has attempted to link belief with behavior. The most widely used of these has been the Health Belief Model (Becker 1974). The main elements of this model are diagrammed in Figure 1. It grew from psychological theories of decision making that "hypothesize that behavior depends mainly upon two variables: (1) the value placed by an individual on a particular outcome and (2) the individual's estimate of the likelihood that a given action will result in that outcome" (Maimon and Becker 1974: 336). It was primarily developed to explain why people undertook or neglected certain preventive health behaviors. The theory argues that whether or not an individual will undertake a recommended health action is dependant upon that individual's perception of: (1) level of personal *susceptibility* to the particular illness or condition; (2) degree of *severity* of the consequences (organic and/or social) which might result from contracting the condition; (3) the health action's potential *benefits* or efficacy in preventing or reducing susceptibility and/or severity; and (4) physical, psychological, financial and other *barriers* or costs related to

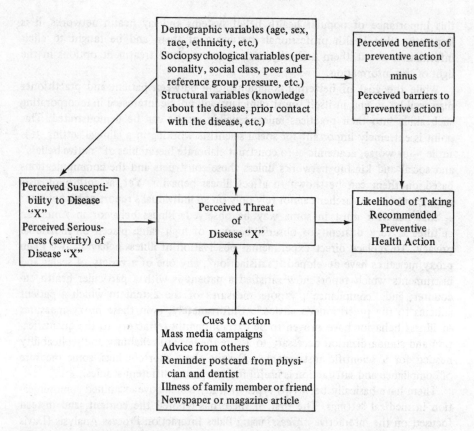

Fig. 1. The "Health Belief Model" as predictor of preventive health behavior (Becker 1974).

initiating or continuing the advocated behavior. The Health Belief Model also stipulates that a *cue to action* or stimulus must occur to trigger the appropriate behavior by making the individual consciously aware of his feelings about the Health threat (Becker et al. 1979: 78–81).

To this point, the Health Belief Model is the best and most widely accepted of the cognitively based theories of health and illness behavior. It has been used extensively as a theoretical underpinning for health services research, and has generally fared well with predicting preventive health behaviors. But how well has it done when predicting such things as compliance in chronic disease? An excellent example is Taylor's work on hypertension (1979). In this he found that the health beliefs predicted by the Health Belief Model before the onset of treatment were unrelated to compliance with a medical regimen six and twelve months later. This indicated that beliefs developed along the course of the illness. The same set of beliefs studied at six and twelve months were statistically correlated to compliance, but together only explained 15% of the variance in levels of medication taking. This degree of association is *not* clinically useful.

Hershey et al. (1980) found similar results when using the Health Belief Model to predict compliance, with control over health matters, perceived barriers, and duration of therapy significantly related to compliance. While these factors correlated well with those patients who reported taking *all* their medications as directed, it is unclear how well they correlate with lesser degrees of compliance. On the other hand, Nelson et al. (1978) found in a very similar study that perceived severity of hypertension, other medications prescribed for other chronic conditions, and older age were predictive of compliance.

If the results generated by social science theories have not been proven clinically sound, where do we turn? In my mind this problem illustrates the fallacy of depending too much on what theories will predict as being important, and too little on what the people involved *themselves* think is important. Despite this caveat, in the search for what important determinants of behavior *are*, rather than what they ought to be, it is necessary to use the existing social science descriptive literature if we are to build our knowledge. Over the past decade, Kleinman has performed extensive reviews of the medical ethnographic literature and has found that there are five core issues that all health care systems seek to address, regardless of the culture in which they are found. For any illness, people seem to seek an explanation for its (1) etiology; (2) time and mode of onset; (3) pathophysiology; (4) course, including both the degree of sickness and the type of sick role − acute, chronic, impaired, etc.; and (5) treatment (1980:105). Beliefs which incorporate some or all of these features and which are formulated and used in coping with a *particular* episode of sickness are termed "Explanatory Models".

An individual's explanatory model should not be viewed as something that is necessarily unchanging. Instead, it is a concise statement of the individual's illness beliefs that are deemed relevant to a particular aspect of that person's experiences at a particular time. As the aspect of interest is changed, as the experiences change, the explanatory model will change, sometimes with amazing rapidity. Thus, for example, if one inquires about the physical causes of an illness, an explanatory model may be given which will be radically different from the explanatory model given by the same individual if one then asks about spiritual or social causes of the same illness. Since explanatory models usually contain treatment options, the presence of different explanatory models for different aspects of the same illness means that an individual may be involved in a variety of treatment options, which appear to be mutually contradictory to the outside observer, without feeling a cognitive strain (Kunstadter 1975). This is repeatedly observed in settings where there are competing healing systems: in Taiwan an individual may use the remedies of a Western physician, a traditional Chinese doctor and a religious shaman at the same time (Kleinman 1980). Questions about the compatibility of these treatments are usually only raised by the ethnographer.

Although it is important to avoid reifying explanatory models, it is also important to recognize that these seem to provide the justification for therapeutic action. Thus, even though they are ephemeral, they are a substantive link between the individual's belief systems and the actions that are undertaken as a result of those belief systems.

When we speak of individual belief systems, particularly as these are applied to lay people, there is a danger that we will be seduced by the term "system". Systematic coherence and interdependence are aspects of professional belief systems. It is an unusual individual (lay person or practitioner) who has worked out all the interconnections of his belief system so that it has become an integrated whole (Berger and Luckmann 1967). It is more likely that a person will have a set of beliefs about illness that are only loosely interconnected, if at all. The connections between the isolated beliefs may be supplied to meet the need to explain a particular situation. In addition, in a situation, both the interconnections and the items of individual beliefs appear to be continuously reworked (in part through the construction of a series of explanatory models) to provide a framework for dealing with a particular illness (Amarasingham 1980). It is only in this sense that we can speak of an individual illness belief system: it appears in fact to be a set of beliefs, a potential system that can be operationalized to cope with a particular experience. Because time and experience are required to work the isolated beliefs into a functioning system, it may not be useful to question people about their explanatory models for hypothetical situations. Unless there has been some reason to work through their beliefs, what will be elicited is only the first, most tentative, most generalized shaping of the belief data.

One of the more important aspects of lay or popular health belief systems is that they are linked to everyday reality or common sense knowledge. Good (1977) demonstrates this when he shows that in Iran the lay health system has its own view of clinical reality which is grounded in the exigencies and experiences of everyday life despite partial acceptance of the three high traditions of medicine – Galenic-Islamic, Sacred Quranic and biomedicine. Because of this the meanings ascribed to illness terms in popular health belief systems are drawn from the meanings of everyday language rather than professional jargon (Berger and Luckmann 1967). Too often we tend to look at the expert definition – since it is most readily available – and then assume that lay people (if they use the term at all) use the same definition. Since the same term may be grounded in expert theories of the causation of disease on the one hand, and in common sense perceptions on the other, we must be cautious to avoid this danger.

Illness terms, or labels, function in a variety of ways. In the first place, the label itself implies a narrowed range of potential explanatory models. Good's (1977) description of heart distress, previously referred to, is an excellent example of the type of explanatory models that an illness term can imply, and how these are interconnected. The label thus serves to link a set of beliefs about the causes and significance of particular types of illness problems with a set of health care seeking choices of available treatment options for these types of illness problems (Kleinman 1980: 108).

However, because the primary effect of an illness is on the person and on that individual's social role, many popular illness terms tend to be linked with psychological and social implications that are associated with the illness. Thus the illness term will link what are seen as typical symptoms and psychological processes with the typical social problems associated with any particular type of illness problem (Kleinman 1980). Through this process of definition, both the behavior and the social role of an ill person will be culturally directed.

These are two problems that arise from this formulation of the social construction of illness. The first of these concerns how people actually use the popular and expert systems of knowledge in conjunction with their own idiosyncratic interpretations and their personal experiences to generate explanatory models. In Good's work, for example, we learn that "heart disease" is associated with "sadness, worry, anxiety". Is this simply a subconcious free association on a societal scale, or are specific mechanisms postulated that would indicate potential interventions? Further exploration is needed to clarify this issue.

The second problem refers back to the issues of communication. If patient beliefs are drawn within a socio-psychological framework, how can they even begin to talk with physicians who use materialistic, mechanistic, stochastic explanations for the occurrence of disease? Yet we know that although communication here may be strained, it has not broken off completely. To understand this we must look at the *content* of words used by patients and practitioners.

STUDY DESIGN

To address some of these issues, particularly as they arise in a complex urban setting, I designed a study exploring some of the illness beliefs of mainstream Americans. In part, my research interests derived from the practical question that faces me as a physician: what is — and should be — the role of a healer in our rapidly changing society? An aspect of this concerns what it means to be "sick" or to be "healed" in America. My approach to unraveling these knotty issues is strongly influenced by my interdisciplinary educational career in medicine, public health, and anthropology, with each field contributing to the design and analysis of my investigation of hypertension.

This research, which forms the basis for my doctoral dissertation in anthropology, was carried out among outpatients in a hypertension clinic. One hundred and seventeen people were interviewed using a semi-structured interview schedule that followed the 'explanatory model' format (Kleinman 1980: 106). The research was conducted over a twelve month period beginning in September, 1977. Other aspects of the findings have been published elsewhere (Blumhagen 1980, 1982) and augment what is reported here.

There are a number of methodological issues which affect the generalizability of the results and must be discussed. Since I was primarily interested in illness beliefs in an urban setting, traditional anthropological techniques to identify a study population (the isolated village) could not be used. Population sampling was beyond my financial and time constraints. As a result, I elected to study a population that was defined biomedically and administratively. These were individuals who were attending a clinic at the Seattle Veteran's Administration Medical Center. The only other formal criterion was that they have been attending the clinic for at least six

months. This time restriction was set to allow the patient's illness beliefs to come
into equiliorium with a new clinic environment as well as to permit retrospective
study of medication compliance.

These restrictions would be expected to affect the data. Probably the most
important effect concerns the distribution of illness knowledge in the study group
as opposed to the population at large. People who have elected to seek and remain
in medical care probably have explanatory models that are less likely to conflict
with the professional's model. Popular health beliefs that conflict with biomedical
models of illness are likely to be less important to this group of people and are
less prevalent among them. Therefore, if popular health beliefs are found, it may
indicate that they are even more prevalent among the population at large than
among the group studied here.

Administratively, only those individuals who have served in the United States
Armed Forces are eligible for health care through the Veterans Administration. This
results in a preponderance of males: thus, only 2 of the 103 individuals finally
included in the study were women. I cannot estimate the effect of this skewed sex
ratio on the data. In addition, minority groups were underrepresented. Of the
103, 90 were white (including both women), nine were black, there were two
American Indians and two Filipinos. The effects of minority group models of illness
will be discussed later in the paper. Since the primary interest is in the health beliefs
of mainstream Americans, this sample serves our purposes.

Other sociodemographic characteristics of this group are as follows: mean age
was 55.4 years with a range of 22 to 79. Mean educational achievement was 11.9
years, with a range from 3 years to a Ph.D. candidate. Mean occupational status
measured by the seven point Hollingshead scale was 4.55 with a range of 1 (highest)
to 7 (Bonjean et al. 1967). To summarize these data, the population consisted of
predominantly white middle aged men with a high school education who were
employed in a middle class occupation.

The reason for selecting a particular clinic was to ensure that all individuals had a
similar physiological experience and that they were all given the same professional
explanatory model. Hypertension was selected as the index medical condition partly
for administrative reasons: i.e., there was a clinic in operation whose staff was
amenable to the research. However, a second important reason is that uncompli-
cated hypertension can exist as a chronic condition without significant numbers of
other coexisting medical problems. This is not as true for heart disease, diabetes, or
chronic lung disease, for example. Individual health beliefs are not neatly segregated
into disease specific packages, and I felt that the task would be much simpler if the
discussion were limited to the experience of a single illness.

A 19 item semi-structured interview schedule based on Kleinman's Explanatory
Model questions (Kleinman 1980: 106) was developed and pretested on six individuals who were not part of the study. The resulting revised interview schedule was
then given to 117 patients in the clinic. I was introduced as a graduate student in
anthropology and therefore someone who was administratively unrelated to the
clinic. The interviews lasted ten to thirty minutes. All interviews were tape recorded

and transcribed. Fourteen of the recordings were technically inadequate for tran-
scription (usually due to electrical interference) and were eliminated, leaving 103
people in the study.

Compliance was calculated from the pharmacy records of refills for each
individual over the 200 days preceding the interview. Since each refill has enough
medication for 30 days, the interval between the end of a 30 day refill and the next
refill were summed for each drug over the study period and divided by 200. This
can be easily transformed into a percentage which represents the "percent of days
which drugs could not be taken" or a "minimum of non-compliance." When this
figure is subtracted from 100 it yields a percentage of maximum compliance.[4]

Similarly, to measure satisfaction, a twenty item questionnaire developed, standardized and validated for this clinic population by Inui et al. (1979) was given to
each participant at the close of the interview. The interview structure and the
satisfaction questionnaire are reproduced in the appendix.

RESULTS: INTERVIEW DATA

Each interview was analyzed to determine the individual's explanatory model of
hypertension. Using the person's own words as much as possible, these models were
diagrammed as a set of 'nodes' and 'arrows' where nodes are important factors in
explanations of etiology, pathophysiology and outcome, and the 'arrows' represent
the causal relationships that were said to exist. Individual models contained a mean
of thirteen nodes with a range of four to twenty-six. Thus we are dealing with fairly
complex, sophisticated models. As would be expected, the models were not necessarily internally consistent. On occasion individuals gave two or more parallel, non-
integrated models at different periods in the interview. When inconsistencies were
pointed out, a typical response was: "I never thought of it that way", suggesting
that the inconsistencies were not problematic to the person interviewed. The models
also had points of merger, where several strands jointed in a single outcome; and
branchings, where a single factor could result in a variety of outcomes.

A manual sorting and grouping technique was devised whereby nodes which
were in structurally similar locations in the various individuals' models and which
had similar semantic content were grouped for the entire sample of 103 individual
explanatory models. This technique allowed the 103 individual nodes to be
collapsed into a set of 59 categories. The categories which occurred in more than
20% of the individual models were selected as being indicative of a portion of a
more general cultural model. These were combined with their first order arrows to
give a summary diagram which I call the Cognitive Domain of Hypertension (Figure
2). In this figure the width of the arrows and the size of each node are proportional
to the number of people who gave that item in their individual models. The nodes
in the cognitive domain model can be further classified as causes, intermediate
mechanisms and outcomes of hypertension. The number of people who included a
particular node in their individual models is shown in Tables I–III. The nodes of
the summary diagram account for 90% of all the nodes given in the individual

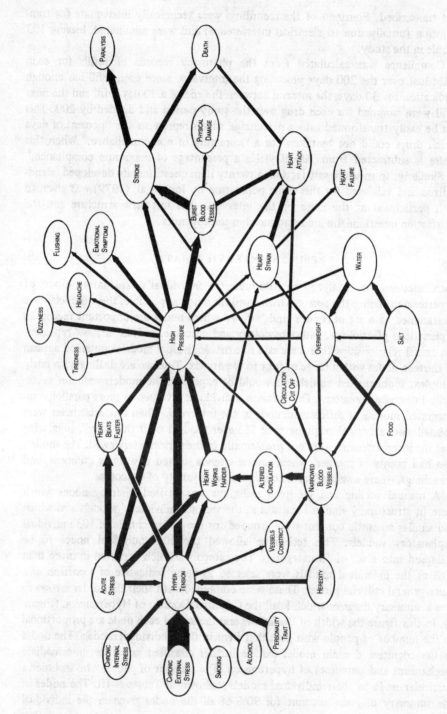

Fig. 2. The cognitive Domain of Hypertension

TABLE I
Causes

	N	%
Acute Stress	57	56
Chronic External Stress	50	49
Chronic Internal Stress	14	14
Smoking	15	15
Alcohol	16	16
Personality Trait	17	17
Heredity	25	25
Food	33	32
Salt	56	55
Water	43	42

TABLE II
Intermediate mechanism

	N	%
Hypertension	63	62
Vessels Constrict	12	12
Heart Beats Faster	23	23
Heart Works Harder	34	33
Altered Circulation	31	30
Narrowed Blood Vessels	43	42
Circulation Cut Off	16	16
Overweight	48	47
High Pressure	48	47
Heart Strain	33	32
Burst Blood Vessel	29	28

TABLE III
Outcome

	N	%
Tiredness	18	18
Dizziness	28	27
Headache	21	21
Flushing	31	30
Emotional Symptoms	29	28
Stroke	68	67
Physical Damage	29	28
Heart Attack	46	45
Heart Failure	33	32
Paralysis	17	17
Death	26	25

Totals are greater than 100% because some respondents listed multiple items.

nodes. However, 56% of the people interviewed had at least one concept which is not presented here, so that only 44% of the individual models can be entirely mapped onto the nodes of the cognitive domain.

The arrows linking the nodes are more difficult to interpret. To be included they had to be given by at least 5% of the sample, and the largest was only included by 39%. During the interviews I gained the impression that whereas the concepts expressed here as nodes are fairly stable elements of the individual's belief system, the links drawn between them are not, and were amenable to being shifted around in response to a different line of questioning. Theoretically, this is what we would expect. Nonetheless, the wide range of individual variation coupled with the inherent ambiguities of these links make it impossible to estimate the "completeness" of this aspect of the cognitive domain.

Given this method of generating a model of the cognitive domain of hypertension, it is important to examine the content of some of the nodes. The ones that are not discussed are either self explanatory and have little internal variation, or are relatively unimportant to the overall schema.

There are two major sets of causes of this illness. These are roughly divided into psycho-social causes on the left of the diagram, which result in a state called Hyper-Tension; and a set of physical-hereditary factors shown at the bottom which affect the pressure in the body. Many of the people interviewed gave elements of both systems. These results correlate well with those found by Johnson (1979).

PSYCHO-SOCIAL CAUSES AND MECHANISMS

The most important of the psycho-social causes of the illness 'Hyper-Tension' fall into a category called 'Chronic External Stress'. Nearly half of the people interviewed said that this was a significant factor in the production of their illness. As can be seen from Table IV this category was used to group three types of social and environmental stresses: first was a single episode of extreme stress, such as being at Pearl Harbor during the Japanese raid in 1941, or in the 1964 Alaskan earthquake. Secondly, there were a set of stressors related to employment: a particularly demanding occupation, such as being a submariner. Disagreeable colleagues or just too much hard work, such as manual labor, were also considered to be significant causes. Finally, an accumulation of stress of normal living is also often given as a reason for developing hypertension. The important difference between this category and the next, which I call 'Chronic Internal Stress', is that here the stressors seem to originate outside the individual and his immediate family network. For a variety of reasons, the two categories seemed to segregate differently and therefore are kept apart in the diagram.

Chronic internal stress (Table V) relates to either psychiatric problems — such as chronic schizophrenia — or long-standing intrafamilial problems. A nasty mother-in-law or an unfortunate marriage with a messy divorce are examples of this. Interestingly this differed from the category labeled 'Personality Trait' which is an expression of the idea "I've always been a high tension person". Despite the fact

TABLE IV
Chronic External Stress
$N = 50$, 49% of Total

	N	Category %
I. *Single episode of extreme stress*	5	10
II. *Job stresses*		
Work too hard	7	14
Specific occupation	5	10
Job stress	13	26
Unemployment	2	4
III. *Buildup of normal stresses*		
Life's stress and strain	9	18
Tension	11	22
Worry/anxiety/nervousness	9	18
Pressure	4	8
Insufficient rest	4	8

Totals are greater than 100% because some respondents listed multiple items.

TABLE V
Chronic Internal Stress

	N	Category %
Psychological problems	7	50
Family or interpersonal problems	9	64

Totals are greater than 100% because some respondents listed multiple items.

TABLE VI
Acute Stress
$N = 57$, 56% of total

	N	Category %
I. *Physical overexertion*	8	14
II. *Internal stress*		
Worry/anxiety	12	21
Nervous	7	12
Emotions	5	9
Anger	5	9
III. *Social stress*		
Stressful situation	27	47
Excitement	11	19
Social demands	6	11

Totals are greater than 100% because some respondents listed multiple items.

that this is an innate characteristic of the individual, it is not seen as inherited; i.e., derived from a parental trait. People actually said "I've always been a tense person and my mother was too, but I don't think it was inherited".

Acute Stress (Table VI) is any situation which is seen as temporarily affecting the individual. Examples of this were becoming angry with someone, being stopped by a policeman, or having sex. People viewed themselves as having been made more vulnerable to becoming "hyper-tense" in such situations. A long series of such circumstances could result in an altered physical state, but would then be classified under 'Chronic External Stress'.

THE MEANING OF HYPER-TENSION

All of these causal factors resulted in a state I call 'Hyper-Tension'. This must be distinguished from the biomedical definition of hypertension, which refers to a sustained elevation of the hemodynamic pressure in the systemic circulation of the body. Since lay terminology is related to everyday English instead of professional jargon the natural translation of this term would be "excessive tenseness". This is what was found when people were asked to describe what they meant by 'Hyper-Tension.' Table VII gives the descriptive terms that were used. Although many of these occurred too rarely to be statistically significant, when they are put together they paint a graphic picture of this illness. There are, however, two components

TABLE VII
Hyper-tension: Descriptive terms

	N
Nervousness	15
Irritated nerves	2
Tenseness	4
Fear/anxiety/worry	6
Overactive	4
Anger/upset	5
Exhaustion	3
Frustrated	1
Mind working	1
Emotional	1
Deterioration	1
Grinding teeth	1
Impatience	1
High stress	1
Excited	2
Being up tight	1
High strung	1
Shook up	1

to 'Hyper-Tension'. In the first place it is a state characterized by the experience
of nervousness, fear, anxiety, worry, anger, upset, tenseness, overactivity, exhaus-
tion and/or excitement. Secondly it is a condition brought on by the psychosocial
factors already discussed which makes the individual more susceptible to becoming
'hyper-tense'.

Despite the psychological sound of the experiences associated with 'Hyper-
Tension', it is considered to be a physical and specifically not a psychological
disorder. It is not an illness which is "all in a person's head", but appears to involve
a physical change in the person, although the nature of this change is not specified.
Thus, for example, despite the fact that tenseness is a central part of the illness,
tranquilizers are not considered to be appropriate therapy.

The state of 'Hyper-Tension' manifests its existence in various ways. The primary
action is on the heart, which may pump faster or harder resulting in an increase in
pressure both on the blood (high blood pressure) and on the body as a whole. Many
informants explicitly made this distinction between 'Hyper-Tension' and high blood
pressure. As one person said:

My interpretation is that the Hyper-Tension moves into high blood pressure and causes high
blood pressure. I think that's where it really gets its momentum from, to cause the blood pressure to to up.

[Hyper-Tension] is nervousness, a condition, a pressure . . . I have a fast moving pressure
thing. Like on a treadmill, moving all the time, fast, I think . . . and then there's some nervousness about it, some nervousness, some worry and concentration that the load is too heavy for
the mind to carry it, . . . it overloads someplace, causes a short circuit.

I didn't know it was high blood pressure. [Note the shift in terms.] I got shortness of breath.
I'd walk up a short ramp and I was out of breath. Went to the doctor for something else . . . and
he discovered that my blood pressure was way up . . . [The doctor said] 'stabilize your body,
you had it stabilized and it should stay there.' It's just like a spring if you had it down now if
you release it [by not taking medication] it'll go back up and damage your heart.

HEREDITARY-PHYSICAL CAUSES OF HIGH BLOOD PRESSURE

In addition to the people who believed that stress caused their Hyper-Tension there
were a substantial number in this study who felt that their illness was caused by
physical or hereditary factors, and not psychosocial ones. Here the primary model
was that a narrowing of the blood vessels could be caused by a variety of factors
such as heredity, salt which would cause deposits in the blood vessels, or excessive
weight squeezing the blood vessels. Whatever the cause, this alteration in blood flow
was seen as making the heart work harder and thereby increased the blood pressure.

Similarly, too much food was seen as causing a person to become overweight,
which would then stress the whole body system. This would occur either by narrowing the blood vessels as has been described, by putting an additional workload
on the heart, or simply by increasing the body's 'pressure'. Fatty food and salt were
felt to be particularly dangerous in this regard. Salt reportedly holds on to water,
which either makes one overweight, or simply increases the fluid pressure in the

'system'. The concept of 'water' contributing to overweight appears to be wide-spread, and probably is due to the well-known phenomenon of premenstrual weight gain and to the similarly well-known effect of water retention during weight loss. Since hypertension is universally treated with diuretics ('water pills') which are also popularly used for premenstrual edema and weight loss, this professional practice supports a popular cognitive system not directly related to the professional cognitive system.

THE EFFECTS OF HIGH PRESSURE

As Figure 2 indicates, most of the effects of this illness work through the interme-diate mechanism of high pressure. Just as there are psychosocial as well as physical causes of high pressure, there are psychosocial and physical results. The psychosocial effects are shown at the top of the diagram and consist of the categories tiredness, dizziness, headache, flushing and emotional symptoms. Most of these categories are self-explanatory. It must be noted that despite intensive clinical research, no con-sistent correlation can be established between the blood pressure as measured by a physician using a sphygmomanometer (blood pressure cuff) and these symptoms (Kaplan 1978). This includes headaches. These symptoms must therefore be considered to be symptoms of a popular or folk illness and not part of the patho-physiology of (professionally defined) high blood pressure.

The only one of these symptoms that requires further discussion here is the category of 'emotional symptoms', listed in Table VIII. These include altered psychological states as well as the changed social status. If this table is compared with the tables describing Acute Stress and Hyper-tension (Tables VI and VII) it is immediately obvious that many of the factors which are said to cause Hyper-Tension are also seen as the result of Hyper-Tension. Some of the individuals recognized this and explicitly called attention to a vicious cycle or positive feedback loop which tends to exacerbate their situation. Thus, for example, the inability to meet social demands which is viewed as a result of their high blood pressure is believed to feed back as an acute stress further exacerbating the person's illness.

Similarly, people recognized a set of permanent, physical results from their ill-ness. These primarily consist of stroke, heart attack, and a wide variety of other results which are grouped under the classification of 'physical damage'. Problems with blood vessels were prominent in this category: varicose veins, 'poor circulation' resulting in leg pain, and aneurysms were frequently mentioned.

Given the high proportion of social causation, it is interesting that of the two conditions that result from these permanent changes, paralysis and death, the former was more widely feared. Death was considered preferable to a state of permanent invalidism, where people were perceived as being totally dependent on others, with no opportunity to exercise any meaningful social role. Physical death is preferable to social death.

A third group of effects existed that could not be easily fit into one of these two

TABLE VIII
Emotional symptoms

		N
I.	*Psychological symptoms*	
	Nervous	8
	Temper	3
	Irritable	8
	Anxiety/worry	3
	Upset	1
	Feel stress	1
	Gets up tight	1
	Changed behavior	1
	Tension	2
	Hyperactivity	1
	Loss of sleep	1
	Easily distracted	1
II.	*Changed social function*	
	Unable to meet social demands	3
	Unable to work as well	3
	Unable to show restraint	1
	Ill at ease	1
	Altered behavior	1
	Relationships deteriorate	2

classifications because the interviews yielded data which were too divergent or too fragmentary. Included in this was a single individual whose ethnic background and illness belief system were typical of humoral or hot/cold beliefs of illness causation which are frequently found in Spanish speaking countries (Fabrega, 1974: 228) He believed that eating many kinds of food, especially different kinds of meat would fill his stomach up and never allow it to go down. This in turn would cause his body to "flood up and get hot", resulting in dizzyness or sleepiness but being unable to sleep. To treat it he would take as bath in cold water, but this was dangerous because it occasionally caused him to catch cold.[5] The nurse practitioner was aware of this belief but was unable to negotiate with it. According to pharmacy records he rarely took his medication. Interestingly, the other individual from his country accepted the Hyper-Tension model.

COMPLIANCE AND SATISFACTION DATA

If we take the types of models of illness which emerge in this study and compare them to compliance and satisfaction, we find that those who believed that hypertension is Hyper-Tension (n = 73) had a higher compliance (78%) than those who believed it to be caused by heredity or physical factors. (n = 23, compliance = 64%, $p < 0.01$) The third group (n = 7) who could not be classified either because I could not elicit a model, the model was too fragmentary, or, as above, was too divergent to be included, had yet lower compliance (54%, p not significant because the numbers were too small).

To further define the relationship between the various elements of the model and compliance, a stepwise multiple regression analysis was performed where "compliance" was the dependent variable and the model nodes were the independent variables. Race, sex, age, occupation and education were entered into the regression equation first, to control for sociodemographic factors that are said to influence compliance. These accounted for only 8% of the variance. Factors in the cognitive model, ten nodes and an arrow (Table IX), accounted for an additional 40% of the variance yielding a total $R^2 = 0.48$.

TABLE IX
Compliance regression analysis

		Direction of correlation[+]	Cumulative percent of variance
(1)	Demographic variables*	N.A.	8
(2)	Stroke	+	25
(3)	Vessels contrict	−	36
(4)	Heart Attack	−	43
(5)	Satisfaction Score[‡]		48

*　Race, sex, age, education, occupation.
+　Positive correlation indicates that the presence of that item in an individual's model correlated with a higher compliance score.
‡　Higher satisfaction score indicates more dissatisfaction.

The satisfaction score was derived from a Likert scale questionnaire with twenty items that were scored from 1 "most satisfied" to 5 "most dissatisfied". The possible range was thus from 20 to 100, where the lower score indicates greater satisfaction. The actual range obtained was 20 to 47. In all, 93 satisfaction questionnaires were completed, and had a mean score of 29.46. The two groups with the models of "Hyper-Tension" and "hereditary or physical factors" had means that were identical with the overall mean: 29.81 and 28.37. However, the group whose illness beliefs could not be classified were much less satisfied with a score of 36.2. Interestingly, although compliance is not significantly correlated with satisfaction directly, when the intervening variables are controlled, compliance becomes significantly correlated with satisfaction ($p = 0.026$).

The satisfaction score was also subjected to a similar stepwise multiple regression analysis. The results are given in Table X. The total R^2 was 62.4.

These results should be compared with the results that were discussed earlier under the Health Belief Model. Using those items as predictors of compliance, only 15% of the variance could be statistically explained. The level of correlation in

TABLE X
Satisfaction regression analysis

		Direction of correlation+	Cumulative percent of variance
(1)	Demographic variables*		7
(2)	Narrowed blood vessels	+	16
(3)	Chronic External Stress	+	25
(4)	Physical Damage		34

* Race, sex, age, education, occupation.
+ Positive correlation indicates that the presence of that item in an individual's model correlated with a *lower* satisfaction score (i.e., more satisfied).

my results has not been found with any previous examination of the determinants of compliance or satisfaction. Unfortunately, however, I cannot explain *why* the results come out this way. Why, for example, does the fear of a stroke lead to greater medication compliance, while fear of a heart attack does not? Why is the perception of vessels constrictory as a cause of hypertension associated with greater satisfaction? These answers must come from much more carefully controlled experiments that delve further into this fascinating field.

APPLICATIONS TO CLINICAL TEACHING

A major goal of clinically applied anthropology is to bridge the gap between social science theory and research on the one hand and medical practice and clinical teaching on the other. Clearly, the use of this model to elucidate significant determinants of compliance and satisfaction is a demonstration of its practical utility, but I wish to turn from this to the nitty-gritty problems that occur when this is used either in practice or education.

To begin with, the Explanatory Model questions (Table XI) or their functional equivalent must be part of every patient encounter until they become second nature. I make no claims about their theoretical validity, but as (a) a clinical tool, (b) an educational technique, and (c) a research methodology, they have no parallel. Obviously social science instructors should not attempt to teach them to clinicians until the teachers themselves are thoroughly familiar with their use in patient interviews. While experience is the best teacher, some practical comments can be made. Many patients will initially counter with responses such as "I don't know — you're the doctor!" This seems to be a reflection of the expectation many people have when entering the medical complex that they *will be told* about their illness, not required *to tell* what is wrong with them. If they are pushed — particularly people who have been sick a long time — they will frequently give suprisingly complex personal illness belief models. A second problem in clinical application

TABLE XI

Explanatory Model questions*

(1) What do you call your problem? What name does it have?
(2) What do you think has caused your problem?
(3) Why do you think it started when it did?
(4) What does your sickness do to you? How does it work?
(5) How severe is it? Will it have a short of a long course?
(6) What do you fear most about your sickness?
(7) What are the chief problems your sickness has caused for you?
(8) What kinds of treatments do you think you should receive? What are the most important results you hope to receive from the treatment?

* From Kleinman 1980: 106.

reflects a point made ealier — patients often assume that the models and the words they use are identical to those used by their practitioners and are quite surprised when questioned on this. Word definitions and linkages in semantic networks of illness beliefs are usually tacit, and some effort is required to make them explicit. One of the most helpful things I have found to do is to attempt to reconstruct the patient's model in my mind, look for discrepencies and discontinuities, and then attempt to get the person I am interviewing to clarify these. One should also be prepared to meet contradictions and use them as a lead to a deeper under-standing while at the same time not expecting the individual to be able to resolve all inconsistencies.

As experience with using explanatory models is gained, illness descriptions such as the one used here can be exceptionally useful both in patient interviewing and in teaching. A knowledge of what the popular beliefs are around a common illness condition can lead to more intelligent questioning. Thus, for example, a person with hypertension could be asked "Some people think that nervousness is associated with this illness. How do you see that applying to yourself?" A person who was delivering (almost by rote) a biomedical model can sometimes be shifted to a deeper, more significant layer of illness belief explication by this type of question.

Similarly, understanding what the patient *means* when he refers to some illness problem leads to a host of ways to enlarge upon the understanding of the illness and negotiate a wider range of treatment options. Implicit understandings are more easily made explicit. For example, among patients who feel their hyperten-sion is an expression of nervousness there is the danger that medication will only be taken when the person feels nervous. One of the approaches I use in these cases is to say: "It's true that your blood pressure goes up when you feel nervous. That's normal and won't hurt you. But what sometimes happens is that blood pressure doesn't always come back down when you're relaxed, and you *can't* feel that. So you need to keep taking your medicine even when you don't feel tense".

This approach can sometimes be used with spectacular effects in teaching rounds. In such situations, the biomedically inclined physicians and students may present a patient who is proving to be a problem in medical management, and turn to the social scientist and skeptically say: "What can you offer to the care of this patient". In one such situation the patient being presented was a Chinese woman who was found to have one of the rare treatable causes of hypertension. She had angrily refused surgery, was not compliant with her drug management, and even went so far as to take two trips to Taiwan where she underwent traditional Chinese therapy. With skillful and patient handling by a Family Medicine resident eventually she was convinced to undergo an invasive, but non-surgical, procedure to correct her problem. She was then selected by the anthropologists to be presented at a large conference to illustrate how successfully social science could contribute to patient care. During the interview which was part of the conference, she was asked to respond to the Explanatory Model questions, apparently for the first time. Her response was that she believed that her hypertension was caused by sibling arguments and family stress in her youth. This led to the question "How can surgery help problems caused by family tension?" The obvious answer, that it could not, drove the interview to the conclusion that she believed that she still had her underlying condition, her *Hyper-Tension*, despite the fact that surgery had cured her *hypertension*! Suddenly the "cure" we had been congratulating ourselves on vanished, to be replaced by a deeper, more accurate understanding of this woman's problems. This episode demonstrated to us not merely the efficacy of the technique in promoting patient-practitioner understanding (some of those in attendance even claimed that the question had been a "plant") but also that social scientists could be shortsighted and fall into the traps of the biomedical paradigm! Other ways that patients use this model of Hyper-Tension, which suggests other approaches to treatment negotiation are described elsewhere (Blumhagen 1982).

CONCLUSION

At the outset I described the clinical encounter as a set of communications which perhaps should be viewed as a series of transformations: an individual translates unusual *sensations* into *symptoms* of illness; the physician translates the symptoms into *signs* of *disease*. The disease is then translated into a set of indications for therapy, and so on. Unfortunately, the participants are rarely aware that a translation is occurring, or even that multiple languages are being used. This is particularly true when laymen and practitioners refer to the same *term* in their discourse, not recognizing that the expert use and the lay use of the same word may be far apart. And thus it has proven to be with the terms hypertension and Hyper-Tension. Even if no other conclusions could be formulated, the explanatory model approach has clarified this muddy water. What has been presented here can be used as the first approximation of both a dictionary and a grammar of the language of illness.

As such, the use of the explanatory model interview may well be useful in facilitating communication between practitioners and patients. If so, there may be good fruits of the endeavor, including improved compliance and greater patient satisfaction. But a caveat should be introduced: to date, medicine has discovered no therapy which does not have side effects. We know nothing of the *dangers* of increasing our knowledge of what people believe about their illness. One such danger may be predicted from Balint's work: "What [practitioners] resented most was that their work and their responsibility had not been made easier by their new experience and their newly won skill . . . As they learnt to see more, more exactly and more deeply, their work becomes more complicated, their responsibility heavier" (Balint 1964: 293). In addition we do not yet know when it is *inappropriate* to use the technique. This knowledge will come with greater clinical experience.

Despite this, we now have a powerful tool to use in exploring the problematic areas linking professional consultations with popular and individual illness beliefs and illness behavior. The skillful use of this technique has only begun to explore the riches of the function of illness in society. The results in clinical consultation as well as the striking ability it provides to understanding compliance and satisfaction with health care services has already been demonstrated to overcome the skepticism of many "hard research" clinicians.

ACKNOWLEDGEMENTS

The research was supported by the Robert Wood Johnson clinical scholars program at the University of Washington and the Health Services Research and Development Affiliation Program of the Seattle Veterans' Administration Medical Center. Opinions expressed in this paper are those of the author and not necessarily those of the Robert Wood Johnson Clinical Scholars Foundation. An earlier version of this paper was presented to the American anthropological Association in Cincinatti, Ohio, December 1, 1979.

APPENDIX A: STUDY INSTRUMENTS

INTERVIEW SCHEDULE

(1) Why did you come to the clinic today?

(2) What is the name that you usually use for this problem? Have you ever heard it called something else? What is the difference between these names?

(3) When did you first know that you had this problem?

(4) What do you think caused it?

(5) Why do you think it started when it did?

(6) What do you think your problem does to you? What is going on inside you?

(7) How severe is your problem? How long do you think it will last? Do you think it will develop into something more serious? What are the main difficulties your problem has caused you? What do you most fear about it?

(8) What is your most important health problem? Why is this more important than the problem you are being seen for now?

(9) Can you tell when your problem is doing better or worse? How do you know? What do you do when you know your problem is worse?

(10) How are you treating your problem? How do these treatments work? What are the most important results you hope to receive from these treatments?

(11)   Do you ever get medications anywhere other than the V.A. pharmacy?
(12)   Do you think that there is anything that would help your problem that your doctor or nurse hasn't told you about? How do these work?
(13)   Are there people other than doctors or nurses who might be able to help this kind of problem? What do they do? Do you know anyone who has been to see one of them?
(14)   What part of the country do you come from?
(15)   How much schooling have you had?
(16)   What is/was your occupation?
(17)   What is your religious affiliation?
(18)   When was the first time you were treated in a V.A. facility?
(19)   Have you or anyone else in your family worked in a health care institution?

APPENDIX B: SATISFACTION QUESTIONNAIRE

Here are some things people sometimes say about Nurse Practitioners and medical care. Please read each statement carefully and give us your reaction to it. Circle one of the numbers on each line to indicate whether you *Strongly Agree* with the statement, *Agree* with it, are *Uncertain, Disagree*, or *Strongly Disagree* with it. There are no right or wrong answers. We just want your opinion.

When completing this questionnaire, think ONLY about the medical care you have received at the hypertension clinic *over the past six months*.

	Strongly agree	Agree	Uncertain	Disagree	Strongly disagree
(1) My Nurse Practitioner is very careful to check everything when examining me.	1	2	3	4	5
(2) My Nurse Practitioner seems to be very competent and well trained.	1	2	3	4	5
(3) My Nurse Practitioner *misses* important information which I give her.	1	2	3	4	5
(4) My Nurse Practitioner is *not* as thorough as she should have been.	1	2	3	4	5
(5) The medical problems I have had in the past have been *ignored* during my visits.	1	2	3	4	5
(6) There are things about the medical care I have received that *could be better*.	1	2	3	4	5
(7) I think my Nurse Practitioners have a good understanding of my past health history.	1	2	3	4	5

(*continued*)

	Strongly agree	Agree	Uncertain	Disagree	Strongly disagree
(8) I have a great deal of confidence in the Nurse Practitioners who have treated me.	1	2	3	4	5
(9) I am very satisfied with the medical care I have received.	1	2	3	4	5
(10) My Nurse Practitioner has really seemed to care about me and my health problems.	1	2	3	4	5
(11) My Nurse Practitioner has explained things in words I could understand.	1	2	3	4	5
(12) My Nurse Practitioner let me tell her everything I thought was important.	1	2	3	4	5
(13) I would *not* feel comfortable asking my Nurse Practitioner questions.	1	2	3	4	4
(14) My Nurse Practitioner has *not* explained my medical problems to me.	1	2	3	4	5
(15) My Nurse Practitioner has had a complete understanding of the things that are wrong with me.	1	2	3	4	5
(16) My Nurse Practitioner has known what I thought were my most important health problems.	1	2	3	4	5
(17) My Nurse Practitioner has known what health problem I have wanted to talk about.	1	2	3	4	5
(18) I think all the health problems we have discussed are important.	1	2	3	4	5
(19) My Nurse Practitioner has not had a complete understanding of the things that are wrong with me.	1	2	3	4	5
(20) I have health problems which should have been discussed at the hypertension clinic but were not.	1	2	3	4	5

NOTES

1. Throughout this paper I often use the term "practitioner" rather than "physician". It is my observation that the behavior described herein, while often attributed to physicians, is the *modus operendi* for the entire spectrum of biomedical practitioners — nurses, osteopaths, technicians, etc. Indeed, I suspect (without data) that this is a characteristic of "expert-client" behavior for all consultations in Western culture.
2. It should be pointed out that the practitioner's satisfaction with a particular encounter is rarely studied, nor the extent to which practitioners do what their patients want them to (but see Helman 1978)!
3. The research literature, particularly that on compliance, is vast and contradictory. Haynes, Taylor and Sackett (1979) have written an encyclopedic review which is invaluable for serious research, but Stone (1979) and Roter (1977) are easier introductions.
4. For example, if a patient's prescription had been refilled on day 1 of the 200 day study period, and then again on day 35, 65, 90, 125, and 170, there would have been insufficient medication for five days between days 1 and 35; and 15 days between days 125 and 170. The apparent gaps between days 90 and 125 is made up by a shorter period between days 65 and 90. This leads to a total of 20 days missed out of 200, or a maximum possible compliance rate of 0.90. In all cases, prescription dates preceding the 200 day interval were gathered to ensure that the estimate of pills available at the beginning of the study interval was as accurate as possible.
5. This individual's explanatory model partially validates the use of this instrument and the results of the interviews. One of the frequent (and appropriate) criticisms of survey techniques is that by forcing responses to specific questions, they create their own results, which may be far removed from what the respondant really believes. Finding an Explanatory model so radically different from the rest of the individuals in the study, but which is congruent with the extensive literature on humoral medicine, indicates that, to some extent, this technique taps the individual's true illness beliefs.

REFERENCES

Amarasingham, L. R.
    1980 Movement Among Healers in Sri Lanka: A Case Study of a Sinhalese Patient. Culture, Medicine, and Psychiatry 4: 71–92.
Balint, M.
    1964 The Doctor, His Patient, and the Illness. New York: International Universities Press.
Becker, M. H. (ed.)
    1974 The Health Belief Model and Personal Health Behavior. Health Education Monographs 2: 323–508.
Becker, M. H., L. A. Maiman, J. P. Kirscht, D. P. Haefner, R. H. Drachman, and D. W. Taylor
    1979 Patient Perceptions and Compliance: Recent Studies of the Health Belief Model. In R. B. Haynes, D. W. Taylor and D. L. Sackett (eds.), Compliance in Health Care. Baltimore: The Johns Hopkins Press.
Beeson, P. B.
    1979 On Becoming a Clinician. In P. B. Beeson, W. McDermott and J. B. Wyngaardens: Cecil Textbook of Medicine. Philadelphia: W. B. Saunders.
Berger, P. L. and T. Luckmann
    1967 The Social Construction of Reality. Garden City, New York: Doubleday and Co.
Blumhagen, D.
    1980 Hyper-Tension: A Folk Illness with a Medical Name. Culture, Medicine, and Psychiatry 4: 197–227.

1982 Speaking of Illness: Popular Conceptions of Hypertension in American Culture.
      Unpublished Ph.D. Dissertation. Seattle, University of Washington.
Bonjean, C., R. J. Hill, and S. D. McLemore
  1967 Sociological Measurement: An Inventory of Scales and Indices. San Francisco:
        Chandler Publishing Co.
Chrisman, N. J.
  1977 The Health Seeking Process: An Approach to the Natural History of Illness. Culture,
        Medicine, and Psychiatry 1: 351–378.
Davis, M. S.
  1968 Variation in Patients' Compliance with Doctor's Advice: An Empirical Analysis of
        Pattern of Communication. American Journal of Public Health 58: 274–288.
  1971 Variation in Patient's Compliance with Doctors' Orders: Medical Practice and Doctor-
        Patient Interaction. Psychiatry in Medicine 2: 31–54.
Fabrega, H.
  1974 Disease and Social Behavior: An Interdisciplinary Perspective. Cambridge, Mass.:
        The M.I.T. Press.
Feinstein, A. R.
  1967 Clinical Judgement. Huntington, New York: Robert E. Krieger Press.
Freeman, B., V. Negrete, M. Davis, and B. Korsch
  1971 Gaps in Doctor-Patient Communication: Doctor-Patient Interaction and Patient
        Satisfaction.
Freidson, E.
  1970 Profession of Medicine. New York: Harper and Row.
Good, B.
  1977 The Heart of What's the Matter: The Semantics of Illness in Iran. Culture, Medicine,
        and Psychiatry 1: 25–58.
Good, B. J. and M. D. Good
  1981 The Meaning of Symptoms: A Cultural Hermeneutic Model for Clinical Practice. In
        A. Kleinman and L. Eisenberg (eds.), The Relevance of Social Science for Medicine,
        Dordrecht, Holland: D. Reidel Publ. Co.
Haynes, R. B., D. W. Taylor and D. L. Sackett
  1979 Compliance in Health Care. Baltimore: The Johns Hopkins Press.
Helman, C. G.
  1978 'Feed a Cold, Starve a Fever' – Folk Models of Infection in an English Suburban
        Community and their Relation to Medical Treatment. Culture, Medicine, and Psy-
        chiatry 2: 107–138.
Hershey, J. C., B. G. Morton, J. B. Davis, and M. J. Reichgott
  1980 Patient Compliance with Antihypertensive Medication. American Journal of Public
        Health 70: 1081–1089.
Hulka, B.
  1979 Patient-Clinician Interactions and Compliance. In R. B. Haynes, D. W. Taylor, and
        D. L. Sackett (eds.), Compliance in Health Care. Baltimore: The Johns Hopkins Press.
Inui, T. S., R. A. Jared, W. B. Carter, D. S. Plorde, R. E. Pecoraro, M. S. Chen, and J. J. Dohan
  1979 Effects of a Self-Administered Health History on New-Patient Visits in a General
        Medical Clinic. Medical Care 17: 1221–1228.
Johnson, S. S.
  1979 Health Beliefs of Hypertensive Patients in a Family Residency Program. Journal of
        Family Practice 9: 5: 877–883.
Kaplan, N.
  1978 Clinical Hypertension. Baltimore: Williams & Wilkins.
Kleinman, A.
  1980 Patients and Healers in the Context of Culture. Berkeley: University of California
        Press.

Korsch, B. M., E. K. Gozzi, and V. Francis
  1968 Gaps in Doctor-Patient Communication: Doctor-Patient Interaction and Patient Satisfaction. Pediatrics 42: 855–871.
Kunstadter, P.
  1975 Do Cultural Differences Make Any Difference? Choice Points in Medical Systems Available in Northwest Thailand. *In* A. Kleinman et al. (eds), Medicine in Chinese Cultures: Comparative Studies of Health Care In Chinese and Other Societies. Washington, D.C.: U.S. Government Printing Office for Fogarty International Center, DHEW Publication (NIH) #75-653.
Maiman, L. A. and M. H. Becker
  1974 The Health Belief Model: Origins and Correlates in Psychosocial Theory. Health Education Monographs 2: 336–353.
Mechanic, D.
  1976 The Growth of Bureaucratic Medicine. New York: John Wiley and Sons.
Nelson, E. C., W. B. Stason, R. R. Nenton, H. S. Solomon, and P. J. McArdle
  1978 Impact of Patient Perceptions on Compliance with Treatment for Hypertension. Medical Care 16: 893–906.
Roter, D. L.
  1977 Patient Participation in the Patient-Provider Interaction: The Effects of Patient Question Asking on the Quality of Interaction, Satisfaction and Compliance. Health Education Monographs 5: 281–315.
Stone, G.
  1979 Patient Compliance and the Role of the Expert. Journal of Social Issues 35: 34–59.
Svarstad, B.
  1976 Physician-Patient Communication and Patient Conformity with Medical Advice. *In* D. Mechanic (ed.), The Growth of Bureaucratic Medicine. New York: John Wiley and Sons.
Taylor, D. W.
  1979 A Test of the Health Belief Model in Hypertension. *In* R. B. Haynes, D. W. Taylor, and D. L. Sackett (ed.), Compliance in Health Care, pp. 103–109. Baltimore: The Johns Hopkins Press.
Waitzkin, H. and J. D. Stoeckle
  1972 The Communication of Information about Illness. Advances in Psychosomatic Medicine 8: 180–215.
Wooley, F. R., R. I. Kane, C. C. Hughes, and D. D. Wright
  1978 The Effects of Doctor-Patient Communication on Satisfaction and Outcome of Care. Social Science and Medicine 12: 123–128.

BARBARA GALLATIN ANDERSON, J. RAFAEL TOLEDO, AND
NANCY HAZAM

AN APPROACH TO THE RESOLUTION OF MEXICAN-AMERICAN RESISTANCE TO DIAGNOSTIC AND REMEDIAL PEDIATRIC HEART CARE

INTRODUCTION

When physicians and other medical personnel first began to think in cultural terms it was with the conviction that where barriers to acceptance of Western (cosmopolitan, international) medicine existed, they were rooted in the ways of reticent populations. Anthropologists, particularly those working in early international public health programs, shared this view. We believed that the answers to most problems of acceptance lay in penetrating health-related beliefs embedded in the social and cultural forms of recipient peoples. We assumed that once we obtained this knowledge we would be in a position to translate the relevant dimensions of Western medicine in such a way that decimating diseases could be treated and adverse health conditions eradicated. "By understanding (and in appropriate situations perhaps even utilizing) the hot/cold belief system of Hispanic patients (Harwood 1971) or the yin/yang system of Chinese patients (Kleinman 1975) it has been reasoned, Western health professionals would be better able to enforce compliance with treatment" (Kleinman 1978: 86).

At the same time, anthropologists saw themselves as champions of the people-at-risk, mediating the confrontations of dissimilar health systems. We measured the success of our intervention by our ability to affect minimal cultural change with maximum health advantage. In all of this the dynamic unit was the "target group". It was the locus of change. The target group and its practices were manipulated into medical adaptation. To the extent concessions were made within Western medicine it was with a kind of conspiratorial charity and the sense that the exigency of the situation overrode obvious common-sense procedures. Conventional clinical posture was never significantly altered and it was a rare participant who argued that it should be.

Physicians and other medical personnel generally have been attentive, if not always receptive, to what anthropologists have told them about the customs and beliefs of the people with whom they work. Why shouldn't they be? After all, the problem has been identified as being "out there" with the patients. And like most of us, physicians prefer to believe that frustrations in performance are due to factors over which they have no control. Many have genuinely agonized over the unwillingless or inability of patients to help themselves when the proper course of action had been made clear to them and they had only to follow it. In hospitals physicians, as the most prestigious of personnel, have set the tone, creating an environment faithful to professional standards and values. It is an environment not marked by easy patient communication, and one in which procedures that threaten the standards and values of the patient-world arise unrecognized in their impact, or

N. J. Chrisman and T. W. Maretzki (eds.), Clinically Applied Anthropology, 325–350.

if detected are seldom reviewed from the perspective of effecting change in clinical procedures.

Yet, with time anthropologists have grown more receptive to the disquieting thought that "at least as many of the resistances of scientific medicine are rooted in the medical profession and in health bureaucracies as in the target peoples" (Foster and Anderson 1978: 233). Recent literature abounds in evidence that medicine's clinical assumptions, the statuses of its practitioners, its bureaucratic organization, its view of patients – all these, and additional factors *of its own creation*, inhibit the successful practice of scientific medicine (Foster 1976; Taylor 1970; Kleinman 1980; Foster and Anderson 1978: 223–262).

In the last ten years we have moved from criticisms of the ethnocentric and reductionist views that characterize the biomedical model (in which biological processes alone shape the "real" world of clinical medicine) to the articulation of alternative models for the interpretation of clinical phenomena and for clinical treatment (Fabrega 1974; Kleinman 1980). These models emphasize a systems approach to illness and healing. From a holistic posture, radical to much of medicine but always implicit in medical anthropology, they direct attention to the need to appreciate, explore, and document the cultural meanings and social relationships that shape health care systems. Within these models physicians *like* patients are recognized as embedded in culturally derived experiences, activities, and expectations, in mutually affecting, if sometimes differing contexts.

Within the medical community, appreciation of this systems approach remains limited, particularly since medical anthropologists have been slow to document its clinical utility or to devise methods by which clinicians can use ethnomedical concepts, such as the prognostic value of familiarity with divergent constructions of clinical "reality". We need outcome studies to demonstrate what impact, if any, is realized by making clinical care more culturally appropriate. "Thus far there is little systematic research that demonstrates improved outcomes in patient compliance and satisfaction, for example, following ethnomedical interventions" (Kleinman 1978: 88).

THE CLINICAL PROBLEM

This paper describes the course of physician-initiated research into patient resistance to clinical procedures. It documents the interaction of medical anthropologists and physicians in restructuring the focus of research so that the inherent adversary model was abandoned for one of allied patient/physician effort. Anthropologists were involved as a consequence of a telephone call from the chief-of-staff of a large hospital in the American Southwest who said that, like Marcel Proust who confided to the French Academy that he "knew poetry was important; he just didn't know what it was important for", *he* knew medical anthropology was important and invited us to help him determine *what for* in the context of a vexing clinical problem. We were asked to join an extant multidisciplinary team investigating Mexican-American resistance to diagnostic and remedial pediatric heart care.

In association with the staffs of the hospital (private) and a state sponsored heart program, a team of two pediatric cardiologists, two psychologists, one sociologist, and two medical anthropologists collaborated for a two year period in the study of 398 Mexican-American families with children diagnosed as having heart disease. The sponsoring organizations have been bringing specialized health services to a 27,000 square mile area for the last twenty years. They maintain a hospital-based urban clinic and have established 12 "satellite clinics" in rural areas close to the Mexican border. The families served are among the poorest in the Southwest.

The initial goal of the project was "to evaluate the effectiveness of an education program directed to provide parents of children with heart disease with information they could easily interpret and utilize when making decisions related to their child's illness" (Toledo 1979: 1). Previous observations by hospital and heart-program staffs had suggested that "explaining the heart's anatomy, physiology, and pathology" would "significantly improve parental comprehension, retention, and retrieval of relevant information" (Toledo 1979: 1). The first year of the project was in progress and had as its goal to evaluate the effectiveness of existing approaches to parental education. The second year would be directed to the development of a new heart-education program that would redress noncompliance and make possible Mexican-American utilization of the appropriate diagnostic and remedial hospital procedures.

The clinical challenge, then, as initially defined was to find ways to convert recalcitrant parents through better explication of the intricacies of heart disease and heart surgery. An underlying premise was that the education of parents would put an end to noncompliance; once parents of cardiac children could be made to understand the goals of the physician or surgical team (on behalf of their diseased children) compliant behavior would follow.

These assumptions proved to be erroneous. Two years later the research team knew why and could demonstrate what *was* necessary for the modification of *staff and patient* behavior so that both parents and staff might make optimal use of clinic and hospital facilities. Today logistical problems remain. However, we have developed and tested a new and effective clinical approach to the treatment of heart disease among Mexican-American cardiac children. In the following pages we trace the shifting interpretations of the clinical challenge and the insights that channeled our research efforts and shaped our conclusions and recommendations. Studies of this nature, involving both theoretical and applied efforts directed to the resolution of a (here) clinical problem and the implementation of a procedure that redresses the problem, are research-and-demonstration projects. Ours was supported by a federal grant from the Office of Child Development of the Department of Health, Education, and Welfare.

A first step in the development of a workable clinical procedure was the redefinition of the clinical issue. Embedded in the initial hospital-based, physician formulated research design was an unarticulated, but manifest syllogism:

In the life-and-death world of pediatric cardiology the doctor knows best.
The complying patient understands that the doctor knows best.
Therefore, the non-complying patient must be made to understand this too.

Education was seen as the obvious vehicle for removing this deficiency in insight on the part of the patient's family. This posture, it needs to be understood, reflected the deep concern of the medical community for untreated children with heart disease, as well as the realization that a serious barrier existed between them and the children's parents. The medical community wanted the problem resolved and were acting as innovatively as they knew how to resolve it.

The medical ideal, Stimson tells us "is that the patient should obey or comply with what the doctor says. It is an ideal of the patient as a passive and obedient recipient of medical instructions" (Stimson 1974: 99). Where noncompliance occurs, the patient is seen as in conflict with the physician and impeding the scientific resolution of a problem which falls within the domain of the physician as legitimate arbitor of medical decision-making. That the patient's perspective is different from the physician's may be readily recognized by the physician, and *was* in the case of these Mexican-American families who had been referred to the clinics by general practitioners or, as was more often the case, by school nurses who in routine examinations had detected some basis for suspected heart disease. The children who appeared for the clinic visit usually were asymptomatic. Their parents arrived already fearful and confused by the guarded explanations of referring physicians and nurses. Although hectic, the clinic atmosphere exuded a sense of ordained but rarely voiced medical authority. Parents usually faced long, unexplained delays, moved from desk to desk, room to room, while in the words of Constancia Morales "everybody gets information from us and we get information from nobody".

Already the "realities" of heart disease and its treatment are different for patient families from those "realities" shaping a progression of physician-initiated clinical events. And from the beginning in silent, unwitting signals as well as explicit directives, the medical community makes evident their priorities. It makes evident, too, the medical consensus that a logical first step in remedying discrepancies between parent expectations for their children and clinic-based expectations must be the recognition of the physician as expert. "Sickness-parenting", as one M.D. termed it, is the physician's domain. And this "fact" legitimately moves care of the child from conventional family supervision to that of the physician-supervised clinical staff.

Full understanding of the medical problem is not considered achievable; however parents are expected to strive for sufficient insight to act "responsibly". Education — some form of simplified and authoritative instruction — follows as the obvious vehicle for removing whatever deficiencies in understanding may contribute to parental resistance to recommended clinical procedures. The intractable noncomplier is seen as irrational or deviant. Further, the complier/noncomplier dichotomy is often translated as an ethical dichotomy in which, in the case of heart disease (by definition *serious*), the responsible parent chooses life for the child; the irresponsible parent, the risk of death or permanent disability.

MAGNITUDE OF THE PROBLEM AND REVIEW OF RELATED
CLINICAL LITERATURE

The problem of noncompliance is a major medical issue. Despite a proliferating medical technology enhancing the physician's ability to prevent, diagnose, or treat a multitude of health disorders, a large segment of the population fails to utilize available resources. With minority groups the situation is often grave (Toledo, Sims, and Hughes 1979). The magnitude of the problem was documented by Davis who in a comprehensive review of contributions to the Journal of Public Health concludes that "at least a third of the patients in most studies failed to comply with doctor's orders", and further that in one in three studies noncompliance rates reached 50 per cent (Davis 1968: 274). In an excellent assessment of more than 300 clinical articles Sackett and Haynes (1976) concluded that compliance with short-term medication could be expected to decline from day to day and that about fifty per cent of patients on long-term medication regimens were noncompliant. The reported rates of noncompliance vary widely across the studies reviewed, influenced not only by factors such as length of therapy, severity of symptoms, and doctor/patient relationships, but also as a consequence of the differences in methodology from study to study. Nevertheless, the percentages reported are consistently elevated.

In spite of the prevalence of the problem, the search for specific factors associated with noncompliance has not been a very productive endeavor. Many factors have been investigated; few have proven significant. Reviewing clinical literature, Marston reports that researchers could demonstrate little or no association between demographic variables and noncompliance (Marston 1979). Age, sex, race, socioeconomic status, education, and religion were not found to be significant. Researchers have investigated the relationship between noncompliance and the severity of illness (Watts 1966). These studies show little evidence that children with serious illnesses such as rheumatic fever (MacDonald, Hagberg and Grossman 1963), or patients with arthritis (Parker and Bender 1957), ulcers (Roth and Berger 1960), or cardiac problems (Johannsen, Hellmuth and Sorauf 1966) were significantly more compliant than others with less serious illnesses. Prolonged treatment has been shown to have an inverse relationship with the rate of compliance (Luntz and Austin 1960; Bergman and Werner 1963; Bonnar, Goldberg and Smith 1969; Ireland 1960; Johnson 1975; Francis, Korsch, and Morris 1969).

The variable most consistently associated with noncompliance was the quality of physician/patient relationship (Waitzkin and Stoeckle 1972; Ley and Spelman 1967; Sackett and Haynes 1976). Noncompliance is most likely to occur when the patient perceives the physician as formal or rejecting, or when the physician requests information or elicits action without offering the patient an *acceptable* rationale for patient response (Davis 1968; emphasis added).

REDEFINING THE CLINICAL ISSUE

Noncompliance, as defined by our study, was the refusal to accept recommended cardiac catherization, or to proceed with recommended cardiac surgery, or failure to keep three or more scheduled appointments. The initial working hypothesis was that if parents could "see" the rationale behind medical recommendations, parental non-compliance with health regimens would vanish or be minimized.

At the time the medical anthropologists (Anderson and Hazam) joined the research team, an exploratory survey on patient comprehension of the clinical problem had been completed by two psychologists. Work had begun on techniques for reducing the scientific complexity of pediatric cardiology to a level and form appropriate for patient consumption. The heart, well and damaged, was explained in simplified printed matter, on tape, and in oral exchanges with the patient and parent. Physicians, nurses, social workers consecutively and jointly participated. Parents were instructed, urged, cajoled, and variously enticed to participate. The results were disappointing. One of us (Toledo) tested the effect of these efforts on 200 parents, and was able to demonstrate that even with the acquisition of knowledge (accurate or inaccurate) compliance was in no way better assured. His findings support those of Greene (1970), and we could agree with Leventhal that the arousal of fear about an illness may cause an increase in the probability the patient will become noncompliant (Leventhal 1965: 1144). Further, although we could not document it to our satisfaction, consensus was that a surprising number of parents did not *want* to be educated into the complexities of heart disease which, as one informant put it, "must be tough enough for doctors to understand."

THE ROLE OF THE ANTHROPOLOGISTS

The difficulties in working with the premises, or even the terminology of "noncompliance" suggested experimentation with a different approach. Throughout the project, the research team, including the anthropologists, was given full access to all medical facilities. This was an enormous advantage. Without a sense of the full theatre in which hospital and clinic personnel function and within which medical decisions are made, the anthropologists certainly would have found themselves as bereft of data as they would be if they could not venture beyond the housefronts of a village they wished to study. We now ventured beyond the progammed study of Mexican-American comprehension of heart disease to the analysis of beliefs, experiences, and values that might affect convictions related to health care in general, and heart disease and heart care in particular. This research brought us into the lobbies and treatment rooms of the hospital and rural clinics, into consulting rooms, the intensive care unit, the cafeteria and kitchen. We followed children and parents throughout their routines. And we left the hospital for the barrios and homes of concerned families.

Our attention turned to the ways in which parents (the word parent as used hereafter means the caretakers of children and includes the affected child) receive and process input in decision-making *separate* from, but *coexistent* with, that of the medical community and on the basis of which decisions are made regarding health and illness, action or inaction. In this health-care-systems context, compliance and noncompliance become complex multifaceted interactions between (in this case) Mexican-Americans and their culture on the one hand, and the medical community and its culture on the other. Further, with heart disease a joint focus, each group or "community" was facing intrusion upon its cultural sphere by the other, "alien", group or community on a more than casual level – one which the medical community had labeled as life/death related. The issue of compliance at this level of interaction evokes in each group value-laden decisions. We found that in those cases where individuals are not complying with prescribed medical treatment, they are in compliance with other social, emotional, or economic factors more central to well-being in a crisis situation than are medical priorities.

We instituted a shift in terminology from that of compliance/noncompliance to adoptive/nonadoptive. It was a semantic change of some importance in that it respects the legitimacy of parental decision-making in a medical context. We hoped to influence physicians to: (1) reevaluate their interpretation of the basis for nonadoptive (noncompliant) behavior, and (2) to assist in the development of a more parent-effective approach to heart care procedures. The combination, we hypothesized, would accomplish the goals of the research: reversal of nonadoptive (noncompliant) behavior.

RESEARCH AND FINDINGS

We were not alone in our reassessments. Information collected by the team sociologists, psychologists, and above all by the physician/principal investigator (Toledo) influenced the restructuring of the research design. The study was divided into five phases: (1) an exploratory phase to identify the major antecedent variables influencing parental decision-making; (2) assessment of the relative frequency of identified variables among a group of nonadopters and a control group; (3) interviews of parents of cardiac children who *had* undergone catherization or surgery to document motives behind the decision to adopt cardiac procedures; (4) exploration of parent/physician/health personnel relationships and parent assessment of the hospital and clinics – we also documented parent views of the heart and its function; and (5) the development and testing of a structured approach for the management of nonadoption.

The theoretical framework behind our approach to the resolution of Mexican-American resistance to diagnostic and remedial pediatric heart care follows closely the Health Belief Model theory described by Rosenstock (1975). This model bases the predictability of health behavior on the following elements: (1) the individual's perceived susceptibility to the disease and its severity; (2) his/her perception of potential benefits versus barriers if action is taken; (3) internal and external "cues" to action; and (4) psychosocial variables which interact in the decision-making process. The elements are not independent of one another but do provide a framework for examination of contributing influences on health behavior.

The medical anthropologists participated most actively in the first and fourth phases of the project and assisted in the design (and observed the administration) of the approach tested in phase five. We developed special interviews, questionnaires, and a sentence completion test, working in depth with 40 families. We joined the "flying doctor" teams in monthly visits to four clinics. We followed parents into hospital facilities and documented their reactions to prescribed treatment over an 18-month period. We participated in the regularly scheduled meetings of the cardiology staff and of the research team. We submitted quarterly subdisciplinary reports, and assisted in the preparation of those joint reports that went forward to the supporting agencies as well as in the final 375-page report.

Findings of the research project were copious. It would be impossible here to attempt even cursorily to do justice to the insights of participating colleagues of other disciplines. These have been reported upon elsewhere. As anthropologists we established our own priorities within the research and were fortunate to have staff encouragement to pursue them. We were concerned particularly with ethnic attitudes and with the patterns of physician/parent interaction in the context of heart disease or its threat. Since 90 per cent of the hospital and clinic clientele are Mexican-American, our research was focused on this group. However, for comparative purposes, information was documented on Anglo families as well. In presenting our findings we take a combined topical and chronological approach, reviewing sequentially: (1) variables antecedent to parental decision-making, (2) parental attitudes in the clinical context, and (3) parent and physician interaction.

1. *Variables Antecedent to Parental Decision-Making*

Long before initial contact with the cardiologist, parental attitudes toward health care and medical practices have been established and firmly enmeshed with other cultural beliefs and behaviors. This interdependence has been widely documented in the medical anthropological literature on Medican-Americans (Saunders 1954; Clark 1959, Rubel 1960; Madsen 1961 and 1964; Madsen and Martin 1966; Romano 1965; Kiev 1968; Gonzales 1976; Kay 1978).

Mexican-American parents may sense a differentness in the outlook of the Anglo medical community, but nevertheless often unwittingly assume that in the critical area of life and death, particularly as it relates to helpless children, most of us have the same priorities. The medical community too recognizes that attitudes toward the heart, life and death differ between the more traditionally-oriented Mexican-American and their own scientific community, yet regards itself as the legitimate and final arbitor in the admittedly grave dimensions of pediatric cardiology. From the beginning a perceptual dichotomy influences behavior.

Although we were prepared by the literature and fieldwork for the religiosity of Mexican-Americans, our interviews and particularly the sentence. completion test graphically brought home its influence on the clinical issue. Mexican-Americans come to the physician and hospital with little empathy or preparation for a secular view of heart disease. Rather they are conditioned to the sacred dimensions of illness in general and of the heart in particular. God is the final arbitor of sickness and health. As one informant put it: "The health of my child is most important to me. I told my husband, ask God to help Pablo get better. God first — and then the doctors". God plays an ongoing and essential role throughout the course of heart disease. Prayers are often to the "Sacred Heart" (another name for Jesus) who ultimately manages the child's illness through an M.D., a curandero, a faith healer, or the intercession of the Blessed Mother, or sometimes simply through prayer alone without the need for medical intercession. *He* exercises veto power over *any* medical decision-maker.

Although the same intensity characterized Anglo requests for supernatural assistance, these are coupled with a feeling that one should deal with one's own problems, a conviction that God helps those who help themselves, a need to meet more rigid societal expectations on self-reliance. Coupled with this Anglo hesitation to charge God personally with the responsibility of cure is a more mechanistic view of heart disease as an illness requiring expert scientific attention.

For the Mexican-American parent, "logic" or "common sense" (frequently appealed to by clinicians) derived from a different world view, inferring causality which from a scientific perspective, i.e., that of the physician, was indefensible. We had parents who thought a congenital heart defect "could be filled with love", or that a cardiac lesion was caused by "susto" (fright), or that a defective heart was God's punishment for something *they*, the parents, had done wrong. It was clear to them that they could not share these concerns with the physician.

Even when parents *want* a scientific diagnosis, the climate is often not right for its acceptance. In the case of three families, the child's condition had been variously diagnosed as no more than flu, tonsillitis, or fatigue induced by the common cold. These experiences have negative implications for parent-faith in subsequent clinical pronouncements. In five cases parents and their ill child had gone from hospital to hospital seeking a definitive diagnosis.

Symptomatology plays a critical role, and a symptom is culturally relative in the degree of perceived ambiguity (Apple 1960), severity (Zborowski 1969), and acceptability (Foster and Anderson 1978: 156–157). Symptoms, says Suchman "will be recognized and defined not in medically diagnostic categories, but in terms of their interference with normal social functioning" (Suchman 1965: 115). What is a symptom to the pediatric cardiologist is not necessarily a symptom to the parent — even when the manifestation may seem clinically evident. If a child can not walk or breathe without difficulty medical help of some kind *will* be sought. But, if there are no visible symptoms to serve as clues, the immediacy of the problem fades despite staff insistance to the contrary. Parents of children with heart problems may eventually adjust even to a "blue", or cyanotic child, and cease to recognize the condition as symptomatic. On the other hand, "sad eyes" may necessitate immediate medical consideration.

Surgery is a radical step, and the rationale has to be clearly manifest. The premature or untimely mention of any kind of surgical procedure may induce panic or withdrawal. Parents "turn off listening", as one women put it. Catheterization is subsumed by most under the rubrics of surgery despite explanations to the contrary by staff. While physicians judged the efficacy of a laboratory test by the accuracy and reliability of its results, parents looked at the number of trials required to puncture the vein to obtain blood. Any surgical procedure, even the insertion of a catheterization tube, however expertly, constitutes mutilation.

Our fieldwork indicates that in daily social intercourse the family remains a critical unit among Mexican-Americans. Effective familial ties may extend over three generations. At the same time, the nuclear family stands out in sharp relief from the rest of kin. It is the nuclear rather than the extended family which plays the major role in the decision-making process with regard to health care. Generally decisions relating to medical diagnosis and treatment are joint decisions by husband and wife. Illness suggests that something is wrong within the family unit and arouses collective fear and joint action. Thus, when the physician outlines a course of treatment for a sick child (catheterization, surgery, the parents go home, consider the situation, and invite the counsel of relatives. But commitment to follow or to disregard the physician's advice, to adopt or not to adopt a course of clinical procedures, is parental. The *machismo* syndrome of male dominance and its concomitants, pervasive in Latin-American culture (Madsen 1964: 18–21), would appear to be less operative in the health care sphere than in other arenas of social control. While there are cases where treatment of the child-patient is rejected by the husband over the wife's objections, there are also cases where the wife, lacking the support of her husband, arranges surgery for her child.

In an atypical development, final decisions on heart surgery were in two cases left to the child-patients themselves. Such a situation may in actuality represent a negative decision on the part of one or both parents, a decision reflected in the children's subsequent refusals to permit surgery. However, it is also possible that parental abdication of decision-making is an outright rejection of the life-death responsibility. Unfamiliar or uncomfortable with Western health care, the Mexican-American parent may hesitate to commit himself/herself to a foreign medical system — better to let the child make the decision and be led by God's will.

Although this form of withdrawal from health care responsibility is a phenomenon worthy of further study, in the majority of traditional Mexican-American families it is parents who determine the course of their child's heart care. Their decision, in most cases, receives strong support from kin. In fact, it is in this supportive role that the influence of the extended family is clearly to be seen. Sisters, brothers, aunts, uncles, and grandparents serve as baby-sitters when parents leave for the hospital, take over household chores, and alert distant kin of the need for prayer, financial support, or the emotional reassurance of their presence. A serious operation is likely to call forth the entire extended family. In one instance where a 18-year old was undergoing surgery, his wife, mother, father, two sisters, aunt, uncle, great aunt, grandmother, and two female cousins all came to wish him well and be present during the operation. Such familial aggregations would appear to provide valuable parental as well as patient support.

2. *Parent Attitudes in the Context of the Hospital/Clinic Structure*

Mexican-American families shared with Anglo families a negative impression of the hospital and/or clinic experience. All reported uneasiness and discomfort. This holds as much for parents as for the child-patients themselves. The hospital in particular projected an antiseptic and fear-promoting atmosphere. In the Sentence Completion Test we are told: Hospitals . . . "are places we don't want to go" . . . "are scary to me" . . . "make me cry". In hospitals: . . . "everything goes so slow" . . . "first they take your money and *then* they take care" . . . "there is no one to talk to."

Mexican-Americans, often initially shy and restrained, welcomed the opportunity to discuss with us their reactions to the hospital environment. The fact that we were not members of the hospital staff seemed to cast us often into the role of confidant, so that they shared with us pent-up aggravations. There was praise, too. The data can perhaps be dichotomized into attitudes toward the hospital: (1) as a medical entity, and (2) as a person-to-person, care-dispensing center. There was almost uniform respect and praise for the former, but reserve and an expressed sense of depersonalization for the hospital experience itself. These "very efficient" places are awesome. It is striking how vibrantly parents communicate the sense that they have moved into a different, mysterious, technologically advanced world in which integration is impossible if not unthinkable. Doctors and nurses come and go, sometimes wordlessly, on little-understood missions. Language, garb, furnishings — even neighbors — are strange to them. They feel uncomfortable and parents are reluctant to leave their children's sides.

Parents are easily intimated by what appears to them the overwhelming regimentation of the hospital. This is communicated to them in a number of specific contexts. Hospital food, typically enough, is unpopular. Menus cater to Anglo food preferences rather than those of the Mexican-American patients who are in the majority. Concessions that are made are rarely effective. In response to a nurse's remark that her child must surely like rice, one mother commented: "Julio does like rice, but the rice he eats at home is made with tomato, onion, and spices". To the nurse's consternation, the mother displayed no concern with the hospital goals of dietary regulation. The child would eat none of the unfamiliar food. It might have helped if the mother had been advised about the dietary rationale (and the taste consequences) of her son's salt-free diet. At the same time, the blander food would have been easier to accept if presented as an effort at compromise with more conventional Mexican cuisine. It definitely did not help that the dietician viewed the hospital experience as an opportunity to expose families to the nutritional benefits of "basic food groups". Trays of liver and broccoli, whole grain bread, and apple juice were returned untouched. Distraught parents sneaked home-prepared or "fast-food" tidbits to their children.

In interpersonal contacts not directly related to medical care, parents sense an aloofness. A reserved people trying to negotiate in a foreign situation, Mexican-American parents often shut down communication altogether on receiving a negative response from the staff. When a nurse informed Mrs. Davalos that she could not remain with her son the night before his operation, Mrs. Davalos did not confront her. But the resentment was there and erupted as bitterness after death following surgery.

Mrs. Nuñez's request for a blanket for a night's sleepover in the hospital lobby was only grudgingly granted and when her sister also remained for the night, the two huddled under one blanket rather than make any more requests. As Mrs. Nuñez put it, "I thought I'd gone far enough and was afraid to ask them".

Mr. and Mrs. Jerome, an Anglo couple, had a similarly unhappy experience on their first visit to the hospital. On arriving they were told to be seated on a wooden bench. When finally interviewed three hours later, Mrs. Jerome complained about the hard seats. When it was pointed out to her that the clinic waiting room with cushioned chairs was only two feet away from the bench, she responded that she, her husband, and baby were specifically asked to sit on the bench adjacent to the staff's headquarters. They were not about to risk their place in line by moving.

Still other communication barriers arise because parents are fearful of being embarrassed or penalized for expressing their traditional beliefs. A mother, checking her child for "empacho" (a clogging of the stomach and upper intestional tract) was discovered by a Mexican-American nurse and subjected to a thorough interrogation. The disdain felt by the nurse for her more traditional sister was painfully obvious both to the shamed mother and to a witness of the incident (personal communication).

Many nurses received praise from the parents. Nurses generally are considered hardworking — often overworked, and able to meet only serious parent demands. Nurses are next to doctors in importance. They are as close as parents can hope to come to a guide and interpreter within the hospital universe. "The nurses make you feel better mentally when they come in the room, when they tell you 'everything is going to be all right'." Parents do not want to fall out of favor with nurses.

In sum, for Mexican-Americans who find themselves so uncustomarily alone, the strained hospital context does not provide an atmosphere for the expression of deep-rooted health concerns, for emotional and physical support. Several women reported feeling thoroughly disoriented on finding themselves in a strange place in an unfamiliar city. Many were fearful of leaving the hospital, even for a walk. They did not know where the nearest shopping center might be, and were dependent on the limited cafeteria hours (or food-dispensing machines — often out-of-order) for a chance to leave the child's bedside for nourishment of their own. It was not uncommon for husbands and wives to live for days in the parking lot, out of a borrowed car or truck. These circumstances, however, did not seem to them problems that they might or should verbalize.

The cumulative pressures did not make for receptive, informed, optimistic, or adoptive responses when parents found themselves in decision-making positions about medical procedures advocated by the physician.

3. Parent Relations with Physicians in the Hospital

Physicians who worked 12-hour days in rural clinics were often puzzled by the apparently erratic decisions made by Mexican-American parents in the face of the threat of serious heart disease. It was frustrating to delay — to the child's disadvantage — "obvious" hospital procedures. It was time-expensive for the physician. With those parents impervious to explanations and directions, harassed physicians could slip easily into an adversary stance. This was sometimes communicated to the parent in emphatic exchanges and thinly veiled denigration of parental judgment. More graphic to the Mexican-American were the non-verbalized cues that restrained parents from voicing the nature of their reservations, even if they could do so in a context comprehensible to the physician. The situation was exacerbated by the minimal to non-existent command of Spanish on the part of the medical staff, and the comparable English limitations on the part of some parents.

In no time at all both "sides" are confirmed in their negative anticipations. Misunderstanding abounds and channels of communication may wholly break down. One "noncomplier" commented that he became disenchanted when his child's doctor announced, with little elaboration, that he wished to do an additional catheterization. In the parent's assessment of the situation the doctor's treatment was bringing no visible relief or change in the child's condition. Further, the physician seemed ready to risk catheterization again without having explained to the parent's satisfaction the rationale behind his treatment. In another instance, the father brought the child to the hospital unprepared and emotionally unready for an unmistakeable assumption on the part of the examining physician that the boy was to overnight at the hospital. The father withdrew the boy without a word at the first opportunity.

Unfortunately, in most cases such as the above, the Mexican-American parent's dissatisfaction is never verbally communicated to the physician. Adequate and accurate communication between patient and physician remains a stumbling block. The problem is in large part a basic one relating to language fluency or the causal use of complex (in the parent's view) medical terms. Utilization of interpreters alleviates but does not entirely allay this problem. Few parents recall with any clarity the scientific explanation of their child's ailment, even with the use of charts or diagrams. Simple hand drawings, made on the spot, by the attending physician were best received, and months later some patients produced them from purse or wallet to show to us. The use of medical vocabulary by physicians and hospital personnel created a significant communication barrier for Anglo patients. However, it is a barrier compounded for many Mexican-Americans who have only a limited familiarity with English, and none with technical medical terms.

It is not easy to gauge optimum timing of vital communication between parent and physician or to determine just how much information should be provided in any one exchange. Parent anxiety is very high at the initial realization of the medical problem. A mother or father who has just been informed that a child suffers from severe cardiac malfunction may not be able to handle additional more precise medical input at that time. Possibly not for days. As Mrs. Tomasina, mother of a young heart patient explained:

"When the doctor told me the baby had a murmur, I just about fell through the floor; I didn't hear another thing he said. All I could think was, how serious was it? Could it be corrected? How was my husband going to take it? Oh God! Oh God!"

In such situations the timing of information becomes critical. Continuing elaboration may merely raise the parent's anxiety level, and the information imparted will probably have to be repeated in any case. One woman pleaded not to be told anything more until some other family member was with her.

Unlike traditional Mexican-American curers, the physician comes from outside the social and economic class of his patient. He is rarely from the same home community. This vast social gulf creates a certain uneasiness that further widens the communication gap and reduces doctor/parent rapport. A doctor's maintenance of religious neutrality under life-death situations may also serve to weaken his influence with some parents. On the other hand, gestures of empathetic concern, the personal touch — these are appreciated and remembered and have a powerful effect on doctor/parent relationships. "When the doctor told me about it, I couldn't say anything", one father recalled, reconstructing how he received the news of his three-year old son's grave condition. "He put his hand on my shoulder and just kept it there a full minute. That guy really cares."

Mexican-American and Anglo patients alike have enormous faith in Dr. X. He is considerate, empathetic, skilled, and concerned. Though his Spanish is minimal he takes the time to counsel with distraught parents and makes the extra visit to the bedside of ailing children. His long hours and dedication to his work are obvious to both clients and staff. In the opinion of all he rates the respect and authority he commands.

Dr. X is providing what many of his Mexican-American patients seek most in a doctor. Someone to guide and protect them, someone to ameliorate and share their pain and suffering. Where the individual touch and small gesture are important health care values, Dr. X proves his worthiness. For instance, the morning Alma left her room for surgery, her mother placed a crucifix on her chest. When, as the cart moved into the hospital corridor, the crucifix fell to the floor, Dr. X picked it up and taped it to her leg. It is not difficult to imagine the trust and gratitude felt by Alma's parents when Alma and crucifix both returned intact following the operation.

The burden upon Dr. X is obviously great and can create bottlenecks in the larger medical system within which he functions, despite the accessibility of other gifted and dedicated staff physicians. If it were possible to spread his charismatic mantle to include other medical and support staff — and it should be — greater protection would be provided for him and for his patients, who do not easily cope with his absence.

PROPOSAL FOR THE RESOLUTION OF THE CLINICAL PROBLEM

On the basis of our research and with the information gleaned by all members of the research team, a structured approach was designed to induce Mexican-American nonadopters to reconsider their decisions to reject proposed medical treatment for their cardiac children. Also a set of specific procedures was recommended for the improvement of general staff relations with Mexican-American patients and was submitted to the administrative staff of the hospital.[1]

These developments marked a significant juncture: the transition from the research to the demonstration phase of our project. For the anthropologists, excitement that the clinical applicability of their cultural interpretations would now be put to the test was tempered with the realization that the product of that testing, if successful, would suggest a reappraisal of existing hospital and clinic regimens. These were eventualities, the reader will remember, not envisioned in the initial research design which was geared to achievement of the desired goal — reversal of Mexican-American noncompliance — almost solely through parent-group adaptations.

What we were espousing would require considerably more time "up front", in initial clinic encounters with nonadopters. We believed this investment by hospital staff would pay for itself by avoiding the greater expenditure of time and effort necessary once some parents got locked into hard-core nonadoption. In the long-term picture we saw a procedure that would intercept the seeds of nonadoptive behavior and establish a continuing climate of optimal physician/parent interaction as well as smoother clinic and hospital routines.

At this juncture of the project we wanted to make the best case we could for the program we were advocating. We asked for and got 12 of the most recalcitrant, unreachable, long-alienated pediatric cardiology cases. Also, though we believe the proposed approach adapts to use by a range of health providers (physician-assistants, staff psychologists, nurses, medical anthropologists) we made use of the physician (Toledo) as hospital protagonist in the test of the clinical procedure. And it cannot be denied that, with the Mexican-American sample at least, the presence, authority, and impact of the physician as a concerned actor in the confrontation strengthened the hospital's case.

We discuss now the 4-step management program which we developed for the conversion of nonadopters, presenting sequentially: a bare-bones outline of the program, a procedural guide to its administration, and illustrative case histories of its use.

OUTLINE OF MANAGEMENT PROGRAM FOR MEXICAN-AMERICAN NON-ADOPTERS

(1) Establish informed rapport with parent(s). In hard-core cases this involved the physician going to the home of the patient.

(2) Explain the purpose of what the physician is there to do. The physician wants to:

(a) understand the parents' feelings,
(b) help them with their concerns and fears,
(c) make sure he has an accurate perception of their view of the child's physical condition, and that they have an accurate perception of the hospital's view, after which they will be disturbed by no further visits unless they want them.
(d) Make sure they understand that the hospital is not "after their business". They will be assisted in having catheterization or surgery done in another hospital if they wish.

(3) Estimate the family's actual perception of the cardiac problem. (At this point we found them receptive to both informal and formal questions and tests.)

(4) Provide the clinical explanation and proposed plan of cardiac treatment with one member of the hospital staff (named) charged with following through on the psychosocial as well as medical programming needs of the family.

PROCEDURAL GUIDE TO ADMINISTRATION OF THE MANAGEMENT PROGRAM

The general procedures utilized in dealing with the nonadoptive families builds in some of its dimensions on the Health Belief Model described by Rosenstock (1966).

(1) *Establishing informed rapport.* Prior to the meeting the physician (or alternate) with the necessary staff assistance examines all available health records (including those provided by the referral source), talks to other health professionals with whom the patient has already had contact, confirms that the necessary medical regimen will be available if and when the family is willing to comply, confirms that the appropriate physician is available to participate in the management as necessary, and is assisted in the evaluation of all sociocultural influences (here predominantly Mexican-American) on parental/child behavior.

The physician's meeting with the parents must establish a climate of unconditional positive regard on the part of the physician. Positive regard for the parents' belief system is not synonymous with positive sanction or approval. It means communicating to the parent a genuine caring that is not conditional on the parent producing feelings or thoughts that are acceptable to the health provider. Accurate empathy is dependent on the ability and willingness of the "interviewer" (here, physician) to receive all of the messages the parent gives, both verbal and nonverbal, explicit and implicit.

The physician (or health provider) must be what he is, without front or facade, openly accommodating the feelings and attitudes that are flowing in him at the moment. He must establish a genuine relationship with the parent. This earnestness must be communicated to the parent through such behavior as refusing to play the traditional role of medical counselor, being spontaneous, being oneself, being nondefensive.

Specific approaches of demonstrated effectiveness in working with Mexican-American parents include: self-disclosure which helps the patient identify with the physician, the verbal restatement in different words of the meaning or attitude or emotional tone which the parent seems attempting to convey, unpatronizing use of the patient's level of language, humor and knowledgeability in nonverbal skills such as good eye contact, sitting close to the parent, nodding. Particularly effective was the ability to create a context in which the parent could comfortably interview "the interviewer". Such a context will be dependent on the medical community's awareness of and interest in the cultural values and priorities of the patient families.

(2) *The purpose of the interview* must be made clear, emphasizing that a decision will not be forced. The physician communicates his understanding that the parents are worried, that this worry about their child's condition is inevitable and shared by all parents of cardiac children. The physician wants to discuss their situation. He makes clear that part of the reason for his being there is *to listen* to the family and to learn from them how he can better understand their position, and he asks that he then be allowed to explain the medical (clinical) view of the situation. Once this goal is accomplished, the parents will be left alone unless they wish further assistance. The staff does have many resources to help them, for example, in coping with their natural fears, in providing tours of the hospital and its cardiac facilities. Parents of other cardiac children have used these resources and have expressed their willingness to meet with them and share their experiences, both good and bad.

Assure the family that a particular physician or institution is not going to be imposed, and if they choose another hospital, they will be assisted in the transition in any feasible way.

(3) *Determine where the family is now as far as perception of the problem* is concerned. Persons ultimately responsible for decision-making affecting the cardiac child should be included in the discussion. When the interview is conducted in the home, this sometimes involves asking that a grandmother (in the kitchen) or a god-parent (down the street) be sent for. When the meeting is scheduled for a hospital or clinic office, the invitation to include family members must be earnestly extended beforehand by phone or visit when possible and in any case by a carefully worded letter reflecting medical interest in broad familial input.

Establish the family's perceived view of the health status of the child. Do they think the child has a health problem? The medical assumption that noncompliant Mexican-American parents *must* realize a problem exists but cannot or will not follow medical guidance in its resolution, we had learned, was a false assumption in a great many cases. And without a sense of problem, parents understandably were repulsed by medical pressure to resolve it.

Parents and relatives need time, unharassed by interruption or correction or thinly veiled ridicule, to voice their thoughts. Many have had little practice in communicating with physicians, particularly with specialists whose domains and privileges are unclear to them. Our experience was that the presence of several relatives led to exchange between them on the history of their travails in unraveling the basis of medical interest in the patient — in the course of which their own perceptions of the child's condition were clarified.

If and when a problem is acknowledged, the interviewer proceeds to explore the family's perceptions of the benefits of and barriers to some form of action. Some families long have recognized that a child is ill. Some have sought alternate forms of treatment. Do they believe the condition is going to improve without complying with hospital recommendations? Are they afraid of procedures? Do they think the child will undergo great pain, be hurt, crippled, die? Does care impose hardships (transportation, cost, other priorities)? Are recommended procedures against their moral, religious, familial, or other cultural convictions?

The interviewer listens uncritically. At this point, if we expressed the need for a better understanding of their view of the situation, none resisted more formal testing (sentence completion, draw-a-heart). Often it provided a good basis for ending the interview and establishing a second get-together. On three occasions subsequent meetings were established, at the parents' suggestion, that included a meal or coffee with the family.

(4) In *providing the clinical explanation and proposed plan of treatment*, a first phase was the demonstration of the existence of the heart problem to introduce a foundation for a clinical interpretation. This meant utilizing appropriate (and available) auditory, visual, and tactile explanatory approaches. Using well siblings (or parents) together with the cardiac child (whose presence we had requested), we offered all possible sensorial evidence of the heart condition to the family; e.g.: (a) auditory: with the aid of a stethoscope let them listen in turn to a well heart and then a heart murmur; (b) visual: as appropriate, describe and denote cyanosis, clubbing, carotid pulsation, dyspnea, edema, thoracic deformity; (c) tactile: let the parents or relatives distinguish the feel of the rhythm of a normal heart versus trills, ventricular heave, diffuse apical impulse, pounding pulses. Explain that resources such as chest X-rays, electrocardiograms, echocardiograms, stress tests (whatever is relevant to the case) are designed to present additional evidence of the same kind of activity.

Explanation of the proposed management technique for the cardiac child was adapted to our assessment of parental receptivity and, of course, to the cardiac condition. For the most part we combined a "rational approach" which stressed a mini-lesson on the particular dysfunction and the required procedure (if such a dysfunction were found to exist), with a "relationship approach" which emphasized the continuing trust relationship. A focus on the positive outlook of the situation, that the patient actually may not need surgery but a cardiac catheterization is needed to determine that for sure, paves the way for easier receptivity to the explanation of *that* diagnostic procedure. Medical explanations should be done in a manner the family can most readily understand, through the use of simple analogies and diagrams. Periodic checking — O.K.? Clear so far? Maybe I could make that clearer — is necessary to make sure the desired clarification is being achieved and that the family's problems are kept track of. (If parents do recognize the need to bring their fear under more manageable control before considering a decision, another health professional, the psychologist, can be introduced into the situation by the physician.)

Finally the parent needs to be advised of the time frame within which action — if action is decided upon — needs to be initiated in the child's best interest. We found that informing the parents that a choice between two appointment dates was available to them often provided an acceptable trigger for decision-making.

Case Study — Juan Montoya

Juan Montoya was a 10-year old Mexican-American boy who underwent a cardiac catheterization at age six. As a result, he was diagnosed as having an atrial septal defect including a significant left to right shunt. He was the youngest of four children. His mother was a 44 year old widowed housewife with little formal education. When Juan was diagnosed at age six, surgical correction was recommended and refused by his mother. At nine years of age, another catheterization was performed and again surgery was recommended and refused. The family later moved to another community within the state and was visited by a nurse who recommended that Juan be seen for a medical check-up. The case was referred via a satellite clinic to one of the authors (Toledo).

After a review of the case, the first interview was scheduled. Once rapport had been established, Mrs. Montoya was asked about her view of the situation. She stated that she was very upset, and was totally opposed to cutting up the heart. She was afraid that Juan would die and she did not want to make the decision by herself. She did have trust in the doctor and she believed that Juan had a heart problem. However, she was terrified that something "would go wrong" if surgery were performed. Even so, she felt guilty and very upset whenever she was approached by the nurses and doctors. The physician empathized with her concerns and told her that he wanted to help her cope with the situation.

Concerning the heart itself, she had some notion of its functioning and the lesion affecting Juan. She stated that "too much blood was being pumped by one side of the heart and it makes it tired". She reiterated her fear of surgical repair. Emotional support through empathy and positive regard was given and Mrs. Montoya appeared comforted. She stated that she was appreciative of the understanding and concern that the physician had shown for her feelings. However, she was by herself and she just could not make such a decision alone. The physician offered to help her seek broader familial input. She accepted and another appointment was set.

The second contact was scheduled to take place at the family residence. This was done to allow other family members and close friends to be present and to share in the responsibility of the decision. Juan, his sister Rachel, Mrs. Montoya, and her best friend were present. The physician chatted briefly with them and established a casual and friendly rapport. When he introduced the problem at hand, he first asked Juan to express his feelings about the situation. Juan stated that he did not have strong feelings either way about the surgical procedure. Rachel asked for more specific information about the heart. The physician explained the heart's functioning by making analogy to a water pumping station. He explained to her how this related to her normal heart and how in Juan's case due to the large blood flow to the lungs, pulmonary hypertension could develop and Juan's chances for successful surgical correction would decrease. With that Rachel stood up and said to her mother, "What are we waiting for? Don't you see that the longer we wait, the greater the risk?" Mrs. Montoya agreed. The surgery was scheduled and performed one moth later.

Case Study – Olga Ramirez

Olga Ramirez was an 8-year old Mexican-American girl who was diagnosed as having a valvular pulmonic stenosis in need of corrective surgery. She had three younger sisters. Her mother was a 27 year old housewife who had six years of school. Her father, a 32 year old mechanic, also had had six years of formal education. Olga underwent a cardiac catherization at age six and a moderate stenosis was revealed, however no surgery was indicated. By age 8 the lesion had increased to the point that surgical repair was recommended. The case was referred to Toledo after Olga's parents refused to consent to surgery over a two-month period.

The first interview was held with Mr. and Mrs. Ramirez and Olga. Olga's father could not believe that his daughter needed heart surgery. "She runs and plays and never gets tired. Besides, they didn't say anything about surgery after the first catheterization." The mother stated that she knew that Olga needed surgery but was afraid "just like my husband" that she would die during or as a result of the operation. They were hoping that time or maybe some new medication or even prayer would solve the problem. The physician reflected their feelings and told them that they were not alone as many other parents felt the same way.

Concerning their knowledge of Olga's problems, Mr. Ramirez said, "They say the vein going to her lungs is plugged but I don't know how that can affect her since she never gets sick." Mrs. Ramirez declined comment. Realizing that their understanding of the problem was poor, the physician explained their daughter's problem, using a water-pump analogy, in terms that they were more readily able to understand. He supplemented his verbal explanation with more tangible evidence. He allowed Mr. and Mrs. Ramirez and Maria to listen to Olga's heart and then to compare it to the sound of the normal hearts of two of Olga's sisters. He empathized with their feelings of emotional stress concerning such a serious decision and offered to be of any possible assistance in making the decision. They stated that they felt a lot better about the situation and the physician's concern and understanding was appreciated. A second appointment was arranged.

At the second session Mrs. Ramirez surprised her husband by stating that she was ready to consent to the surgery. Although Mr. Ramirez was reluctant he finally agreed. The date was set and the surgeon and hospital psychologist were advised that the family needed additional emotional support to get them smoothly through the hospitalization. Maria underwent a successful surgical correction five weeks later.

DISCUSSION

Of the 12 families on whom the approach has been used, 10 have adopted the proposed management of the child's condition. The average time of resistance to surgical intervention had been 35.5 months (or almost 3 years) in spite of efforts to convince them of the benefits of the proposed therapy. The 10 families became "adopters" (i.e., compliers) after an average of two physician encounters and 2.5 months between initial contact and the date of acceptance of prescribed medical procedures.

Our results suggest that a program of direct but informed intervention can be clinically effective in reversing patterns of nonadoption among Mexican-American parents of cardiac children. However, success in it requires a better comprehension of the basis for parental rejection of prescribed diagnostic and remedial heart care than is presently evident in general clinic procedures. Critical also is the establishment of a more equitable balance between expectations of hospital staff and those of parents. Such a balance is achievable. It requires modification of patient-directed behavior on the part of clinicians as well as planned and empathetic assistance to parents toward the optimal appreciation of clinical goals. We suggest that without staff initiative the elevated rate of Mexican-American "noncompliance" is unlikely to lower.

Too often the deeply embedded beliefs, experiences, and activities that perpetuate the health system of Mexican-Americans surface in the pediatric cardiology clinic under circumstances highly charged with tension. Heart disease in children is viewed by parents as a perilous but capricious and sometimes unverifiable condition. Basic cultural values are drawn into an unreceptive medical spotlight. In the judgment of Mexican-American parents, answers — the right answers — to complex issues come too swiftly, too surely to the physician. Procedures seen by physician and staff as clinically evident arouse in parents anxiety, chilling premonitions, and all too often the solace of flight. Stress operates to justify the faith of all participants in the legitimacy of their respective health systems.

We have suggested that effective clinical communication with Mexican-American parents of children with congenital heart disease take into account the following: their distinctive and pervasive religiosity, their reticence and reserve in the face of institutional regimentation, their traditional cultural priorities (particularly those in conflict with hospital or clinic priorities) the critical family support system, communication barriers, and expectations of empathetic concern.

Rapport and trust can be developed by focusing on the family, by acknowledging their feelings, and by adapting pre-catheterization and pre-surgical procedures to specific case situations. The 4-step management procedure advocated for nonadoptive parents, however, would probably not be optimal in emergency situations in that it may take a considerable amount of time to implement. On the other hand, where opposition remains obdurate, the procedure has demonstrated considerable success within a limited test situation.

Although what has been proposed clinically is not a simple, mechanical, clonable process, the methodological approach and case examples could be used as a framework for training health professionals. With some alterations, the approach should be adaptable to other clinical confrontations with nonadoptive behaviors. We hypothesize that, with refinement, the approach would work regardless of the nationality of the physician, provided there was some meeting ground of language proficiency. Its adaptability to use by nurses, physician's assistants, etc., needs to be studied.

Ultimately, the procedure or some version of it could be built into regular health delivery systems for the *prevention* of conflict rather than as a system to negotiate the *consequences* of it. Research is indicated in order to identify and incorporate the necessary and sufficient components of the method. A more complete clinical training manual is also needed.

It may be that, as in this report on Mexican-American parental reaction to the esoteric course of clinical pediatric cardiology, we are reaching the point where: (1) medical technological development does not lend itself to literal translation for many Americans, regardless of ethnicity, (2) fear must be considered as an inevitable side-effect blocking education as more and more medical practice takes on death-related therapies, and (3) the interjection of technologically complex procedures at the asymptomatic stage of disease – or even in the absence of disease – creates long-lasting reservations about medical intervention. And finally, it must be observed that patient "compliance" is all the more qualified when there is no ready evidence that their priorities are at least understood, if not shared, by the medical community which exercises such awesome control over them.

What our research team has developed in effect constitutes *a total management program*. It may be that this *is* needed to counteract the multiple psycho-cultural assaults of what we have referred to elsewhere as "medical overdevelopment" (Anderson, Hazam and Toledo 1979). If this is the case, the approach may have promise in the context of other complex medical interventions, such as cancer therapy, pregnancy termination, and renal dialysis and the clinical procedures that are being advocated for them.

NOTES

1. We suggested consideration of the following approaches to improved health education and health care within the clinic context:

(A) *Inhouse seminars*
Lecture/discussion sessions for all hospital staff with joint input of experience. Guest lectures by specialists on needs of hospitalized children and their parents, ethnic concepts of health and disease, how to cope with the threat of death or disability.

(B) *Projective tests*
The development of health-adapted versions of projective tests would tap many of the barriers to health care that are repressed, or not easily verbalized by our subejcts. We began experimentation with modified Thematic Apperception Test cards.

(C) *Interviews with physicians and nurses*
Our research objectives focused on parents of cardiac children. A valuable research complement would be in-depth interviewing of physicians, nurses, and other health personnel.

(D) *Language training*
Some proficiency in conversational Spanish should be actively encouraged for all hospital personnel.

(E) *Improved facilities for parents and relatives within the hospital*
Needed are more flexible access to the cafeteria, a "coffee cart", a map of the hospital, a map of the area surrounding the hospital marking shopping areas and restaurants, blankets and folding cots.

(F) *Simple literature and drawings of the heart*
Presentations of the well heart/the sick heart. Parents did not seem to benefit greatly from detailed, scientific presentations. They *did* like personalized line-drawings and the opportunity to review them informally at home. Descriptive literature should be available *in Spanish*.

(G) *Parent/Parent contact*
Parents were buoyed by the opportunity to meet with other parents who were undergoing or had undergoine the same experience. They understood one another's anxieties and often relayed simple information about hospital procedures and facilities otherwise unexplained to the parent. Sometimes they found a bilingual translator/confidant.

(H) *Ombudsman*
Abortion clinics have experimented successfully with a kind of "ombudsman" who greets the patient and family on arrival, remains with them until they are comfortably settled, may be contacted to answer questions, is present (if wanted) before and after surgery, and intervenes on the patient's behalf in the resolution of conflicts. He/she is medically knowledgeable, enjoys access to physicians, and has their respect. Some modification of this approach could prove adaptable in the context of the cardiac clinic program.

REFERENCES

Anderson, Barbaro Gallatin and Nancy Hazam
 1978 Cultural Factors Influencing Diagnostic and Remedial Heart Care Among Mexican-Americans. Paper read at the 1978 Annual Meetings of the Society for Applied Anthropology, Merida, Yucatan, Mexico.
Anderson, Barbara Gallatin, N. Hazam, and J. R. Toledo
 1979 Confrontation with Medical Overdevelopment: Crisis and Resolution in South Texas. Paper read at International Congres of Anthropological and Ethnological Sciences, Poona, India.
Apple, Dorrian
 1960 How Laymen Define Illness. Journal of Health and Human Behavior 1: 219–225.
Bergman, A. B. and R. J. Werner
 1963 Failure of Children to Receive Penicillin by Mouth. New England Journal of Medicine 268: 1334.
Bonnar, J. A. Goldberg, and J. A. Smith
 1969 Do Pregnant Women Take Their Iron? Lancet, March: 457.
Chrisman, Noel J.
 1976 American Patterns of Health-Care-Seeking Behavior. *In* W. Arens and Susan P. Montague (eds.), The American Dimension: Culture Myths and Social Realities, New York: Alfred Publishing Co., Inc. pp. 206–217.

Chrisman, Noel and A. Kleinman
    1980 Health Beliefs and Practices. *In* Harvard Encyclopedia of American Ethnic Groups.
          Cambridge, Mass.: Harvard University Press.
Clark, Margaret
    1959 Health in the Mexican-American Culture. Berkeley, Calif.: University of California
          Press.
Davis, M. S.
    1968 Variations in Patients' Compliance with Doctors' Advice: An Empirical Analysis of
          Patterns of Communication. American Journal of Public Health 56: 275.
Fabrega, Horatio
    1974 Disease and Social Behavior: An Interdisciplinary Perspective. Combridge, Mass.:
          M.I.T. Press.
    1978 Ethnomedicine and Medical Science. Medical Antrhopology 2: 2: 11–24.
Foster, George M.
    1976 Medical Anthropology and International Health Planning. Medical Anthropology
          Newsletter 7: 3: 12–18.
Foster, George and Barbara Gallatin Anderson
    1978 Medical Anthropology. New York: John Wiley and Sons.
Francis, V., B. M. Korsch, and M. J. Morris
    1969 Gaps in Doctor-Patient Communications: Patient's Response to Medical Advice. New
          England Journal of Medicine 280: 535.
Gonzales, Elena
    1976 The Role of Chicano Folk Beliefs and Practices in Mental Health. *In* Hernandex,
          Haug, and Wagner (eds.), Chicanos: Social and Psychological Perspective. St. Louis:
          C. V. Mosby.
Good, Byron
    1977 The Heart of What's the Matter: The Semantics of Illness in Iran. Culture, Medicine
          and Psychiatry 1: 25–58.
Greene, L. W.
    1970 Should Health Education Abandon Attitude Change Strategies? Perspectives from
          Research. Health Education Monographs 30: 25.
Harwood, A.
    1971 The Hot-Cold Theory of Disease: Implications for Treatment of Puerto Rican Pa-
          tients. Journal of the American Medical Association, 216: 1153–1158.
Ireland, H. D.
    1960 Outpatient Chemotherapy for Tuberculosis. American Review of Respiratory Disease
          82: 378.
Johannsen, W. J., G. A. Hellmuth, and t. Sorauf
    1966 On Accepting Medical Recommendations: Experiences with Patients in a Cardiac
          Work Classification Unit. Archives of Environmental Health 12: 63.
Johnson, W. J.
    1975 Conformity to Medical Recommendations in Coronary Heart Disease. Paper pre-
          sented at the American Sociological Association Annual Meeting, Chicago, Illinois.
Kay, Margarita A. with Anita Stafford
    1978 Parallel, Alterantive or Collaborative: Curanderismo in Tucson. *In* B. Velimirovic
          (ed.), Modern Medicine and Medical Anthropology in the U.S.–Mexico Border
          Populations. Washington, D. C.: Pan American Health Organization, Scientific
          Publication PAHO No. 359.
Kiev, Ari
    1968 Curanderismo: Mexican American Folk Psychiatry. New York: The Free Press.
Kleinman, Arthur
    1975 Medical and Psychiatric Anthropology and the Study of Traditional Medicine in

Modern Chinese Culture. Journal of the Institute of Ethnology, Academica Sinica 39: 107–123.

1978 International Health Care Planning from an Ethnomedical Perspective: Critique and and Recommendations for Change. Medical Anthropology 2: 2: 71–96.

1980 Patients and Healers in the Context of Culture: An Exploration of the Borderland Between Anthropology, Medicine, and Psychiatry. Berkely: University of California Press.

Kleinman, A., L. Eisenberg, and B. Good
1978 Culture, Illness and Care. Annals of Internal Medicine 88: 251–258.

Leventhal, H.
1965 Fear Communications in the Acceptance of Preventative Health Practices. Bulletin of New York Academic Medicine 41: 1144.

Ley, P. and M. S. Spelman
1967 Communicating with the Patient, London: Staples Press. pp. 45–87.

Luntz, G. R. and R. Austin
1960 New Stick Test for P.A.S. in Urine: A Report on Use of "Phenstix" and Problems of Long-term Chemotherapy for Tuberculosis. British Medical Journal, May: 1679.

MacDonald, M. E., A. M. Hagberg, and B. J. Grossman
1963 Social Factors in Relation to Participation in Follow-Up Care of Rheumatic Fever. Journal of Pediatrics 62: 503.

Madsen, William
1961 Society and Health in the Lower Rio Grande. An analysis of conflicting cultural attitudes toward disease with recommendations for implementing public-health programs in Hidalgo County, Texas. Austin, Texas: The Hogg Foundation for Mental Health.

1964 The Mexican-Americans of South Texas. New York: Holt, Rinehart, and Winston.
Madesen, W. and H. W. Martin
1966 Folk Disease among Mexican-American: Etiology, Symptoms, Treatment. Journal of the American Medical Association 196: 2: 147–150.

Marston, M. V.
1970 Compliance with Medical Regimens: A Review of the Literature. Nursing Research 19: 312.

Parker, L. Burton and Leonard F. Bender
1957 Problem of Home Treatment in Arthritis. Archives of Physical Medicine 38: 6: 392–394.

Romano, Octavio V.
1965 Charismatic Medicine, Folk Healing, and Folk Sainthood. American Anthropologist 67: 1151–1172.

Rosenstock, Irwin M.
1966 Why People Use Health Services. Milbank Memorial Fund Quarterly 44: 94.

1975 Patients' Compliance with Health Regimens. Journal of the American Medical Association 234: 4: 402–403.

Roth, J. P. and D. G. Berger
1960 Studies on Patient Cooperation in Ulcer Treatment: Observations of Actual as Compared to Prescribed Antacid Intake on a Hospital Ward. Gastroenterology 38: 630.

Rubel, Arthur J.
1960 Concepts of Disease in Mexican-American Culture. American Anthropologist 62: 795–815.

Sackett, D. L. and R. B. Haynes (eds.)
1976 Compliance with Therapeutic Regimens. Baltimore: The Johns Hopkins University Press.

Saunders, Lyle
  1954 Cultural Difference and Medical Care. New York: Russell Sage Foundation. pp. 141–
        173.
Stimson, G. V.
  1974 Obeying Doctor's Orders: A View from the Other Side. Social Science and Medicine
        8: 97–104.
Suchman, Edward A.
  1965 Stages of Illness and Medical Care. Journal of Health and Human Behavior 6: 114–
        128.
Taylor, Carol
  1970 In Horizontal Orbit: Hospitals and the Cult of Efficiency. New York: Holt, Rinehart
        and Winston.
Toledo, J. R.
  1979 Cultural Variables Affecting Health Care Outcome. Adjusting Health Provider/
        Recipient Interphase to Encourage Patient Acceptance. Final Report. Grant #90–C–
        907 from the Office of Child Development, Department of Health, Education and
        Welfare.
Toledo, J. Rafael, J. Sims and H. Hughes
  1979 Management of Noncompliance to Medical Regimens in Ethnic Groups. In J. R.
        Toledo: Cultural Variables Affecting Health Care Outcome. Final Report, Grant
        #90–C–907 from the Office of Child Development, Department of Health, Educa-
        tion and Welfare.
Waitzkin, F. and J. D. Stoeckle
  1972 The Communication of Information about Illness. Advanced Psychosomatic Medicine
        8: 180.
Watts, D. C.
  1966 Factors Related to the Acceptance of Modern Medicine. American Journal of Public
        Health 56: 1205.
Zborowski, Mark
  1969 People in Pain. San Francisco: Jossey-Bass, Inc., Publishers.

LINDA ALEXANDER

ILLNESS MAINTENANCE AND
THE NEW AMERICAN SICK ROLE

INTRODUCTION: THE CLINICAL PROBLEM

A superficial understanding of the social science concept of the sick role might suggest that it is considered to vary culturally, but within a specific culture to be relatively fixed. In this chapter the implicit assumption of "a" sick role is challenged on the basis of cultural change in the total pattern of illness experiences and illness construction. The underlying changes are as much a product of medical technology developments as they are of social and cultural conditions for the prevention and control of illness. They raise major questions about the meaning and nature of curing.

Physicians, nurses, and other health practitioners in the United States are trained primarily to cure. A very traditional *curative premise* underlies most of the Euro-American or Western institutional and clinical medical purposes. The curative premise consists of an implicit and explicit mandate to heal, and if not to heal, at least not to hurt. Its explicit expression may be found in many times and many places.

I will use treatment to help the sick according to my ability and judgement, but I will never use it to injure or wrong them. (Hippocratic Oath, circa 460 B.C.)

I will maintain the utmost respect for human life; even under threat, I will not use my medical knowledge contrary to the laws of humanity. (Declaration of Geneva, Physician's Oath, 1948.)

In Western society, where disease is presumed to yield to application of scientific method, the doctor is regarded as an expert, a man professionally trained in matters pertaining to sickness and health and able by his medical competence to cure our ills and keep us well. (Fox 1979: 20)

But its explicit statement, both in medical training contexts and in systems of institutional care, is far less potent than its implicit expression in the organization of these facilities. Hospitals and medical clinics are designed to serve acute and transient disorders. Their patients are anticipated to pass through the system, not to remain within it. Intense and extensive human and technical resources are mobilized to treat the ailing individual in these contexts, at large human and monetary expense. Third party carriers, public and private, the medical entrepreneurs, impose constraints on the time and cost of service that may be provided any patient.

Health care practitioners and students in the healing professions are motivated to seek rewards for their efforts in patient outcomes, rather than in monetary gain or in peer group approval. Thus a demand, as well as a wish, that patients get well and confirm the efficacy of medical interventions is instituted. Yet, for reasons offered below, the curative premise is largely obsolete. Chronic and redundant illness characterize much of the population presenting themselves for help from the health care system.

351

N. J. Chrisman and T. W. Maretzki (eds.), Clinically Applied Anthropology, 351–367.
Copyright © 1982 *by D. Reidel Publishing Company.*

Compared with other program categories, chronic illness is by far the largest area of service — and the least defined . . . combined with aging, chronic illness serves as a 'dumping ground' for a miscellany of unspecified conditions which fail to fit under other program headings. Without legitimacy as a speciality in its own right, chronic illness receives scanty and peripheral attention. (Zuckermann 1977: 52)

The curative premise has been invalidated by numerous changes in recent decades, yet it persists as a major medical motivation. A dissonance on two levels occurs, creating two kinds of clinical problem. For health care professionals, the contradictions inherent in the combination of their intent and their achievement lead to frustration, disillusionment, and cynicism (Fox 1979). For patients, the discrepancy between the curative expectation and their continuing sick role state leads to anger, distrust, and sometimes litigation. For social scientists working in medical contexts with patients, students, and professionals, the dissonance creates a clinical problem at an ancillary level. The "patient" for the social scientist is the health care system itself; its dissonance and internal contradictions are its pathology. This is a "second-order" pathology and our task here is to determine whether or not the social scientist should adopt a curative premise to deal with it. Perhaps dissonance and contradiction are inevitable and necessary chronic states in health care systems.

Various changes in the American sick role and in patient populations have developed in the last fifty years (Kassebaum and Baumann 1965). We will explore several here, keeping in mind that each single explication is simplistic. Ours is a large, complex, heterogeneous society and simple causal patterns are improbable.

We must note a linguistic change in connotations of ailing and healing that may correlate with the increase of urban populations and labor specializations. Generally people have shifted from a discriminating reference about their health states to a mutually exclusive definition of "ill" and "well". It is colloquial and common to elicit, by asking "how are you", a categorical response: "I'm fine", or "I'm sick". The latter state may be expressed as "I feel lousy, I've got a cold", or "my head aches." The reference is to a total state of ill-being and does not distinguish within a spectrum of sensation. Seldom do we elicit a reply, "I'm 10% uncomfortable with a cold and 90% well with other circumstances". Or, "my broken leg aches today but the rest of my soma feels super". In urban contexts, perceptions of wellness and illness have become mutually exclusive: a person is one or the other, not both. In rural society, a continuum of ailing and feeling well is more common because the ailment is tested against overall function and work. A "small ow" is one that does not preclude fulfillment of one's work responsibilities. Amputated fingers, flu, colds, hangovers, headaches, menstrual pain and other discomforts do not, in green collar or rural enterprises, disqualify one from work. In occupations where sick leave is provided, on the other hand, illness is an all-or-none formula for sanctioned work avoidance. A stuffy nose does as well as a hysterectomy for calling in sick.

Not only have references to illness become more global, but the category of what constitutes illness and ailing has enlarged. In the last few decades an elevated public consciousness of health and illness seems evident. The kinds and numbers of signs and symptoms constituting sickness have increased. The mutually exclusive category of sensations and feelings defined as wellness has diminished. Illich has characterized this change as the "medicalization of health". "Life turns from a succession of different stages of health into a series of periods requiring different therapies." "People have become patients without being sick" (Illich 1975).

Without conceding that medical institutions cause this change in perception, we must note a corollary in the increased need for, and use of, medical facilities and an expansion of medical entrepreneurship and third party intervention. In Bateson's terms, an accelerated cycle of increased consciousness → increased demand → increased supply → increased consciousness results and is diagnosed as schismogenesis. Schismogenic relationships are escalations, exponential in their character. "These potentially pathological developments are due to undamped or uncorrected positive feedback in the system" (Bateson 1972: 324). The breakdown in familiarity and communication between patients and practitioners is well-documented in the medical and social science literature and need not be repeated here. What is important is to note that the breakdown consists of diminished negative feedback loops. Increased medical supply should result in diminished illness consciousness: i.e., the need should be met or satisfied. Instead, while increasing their use of medical facilities, "the general public has demonstrated an increasing disenchantment with the present health-care delivery system" (Rushmer 1975: 15).

Another gross change in patient populations relates to the expansion of the category of signs and symptoms to include new criteria for ailing, which now subsume illnesses for which there are no medically justified bases. This phenomenon is called variously "psychosomatic", "hysteria", "hypochondriasis", "malingering". Persons who present themselves for treatment without medically sanctioned symptoms are called variously "hysterics", "hypochondriacs", "malingerers", "somaticizers", "problem patients", "crocks", and "gomers" in the medical vernacular (George and Dundes 1978; Mannon 1976; Luborsky et al. 1973; Carlson and Alexander 1979; Groves 1978).

Circumstances which foster the inclusion of imaginary and/or deceitful complaints in the illness category are extensive and complicated. Several factors can be unequivocally identified and described. One factor is the increased number of social rewards for illness behavior. These include monetary gain — from disability insurance, workman's compensation, private medical insurance, and litigation; interpersonal gain — sympathy, attention, assurance of personal importance, excuse for inept or unsuccessful interpersonal performance; freedom — sanctioned release from onerous responsibility, from work and employment, and from reality by means of mood and mind altering medications. Such rewards are called "secondary gains" in the literature. Illness in instances of manifest or suspected secondary gain is thought to be motivated and socially deviant (Wooley et al. 1978).

Another factor operating to encourage illness behavior in our society is stress. Stress is thought to contribute to an individual's propensity to somaticize. Intrapsychic disorder and an "inability to cope" serve as explanatory constructs for theories of stress leading to psychosomatic illness (Langner 1962). Predisposition and personality are also offered as intervening constructs (Freidman 1969). Additionally, notions about social alienation, job pressures and dissatisfactions, and cultural and/or economic deprivation are offered to explain why stress leads to illness for some and not for others (Kasl and Cobb 1966). Indirectly, smoking, drinking, and obesity are offered as stress indicators or stress responses, and these also lead to illnesses (e.g., Kaplan and Kaplan 1957).

There is another way in which the American sick role has modified and challenges the health care profession's curative premise. Rapid and major advances in medical technology and public health programs during the last few decades have radically changed the character of the general patient population. More than any other influencing factor, medical interventions have become more effective and more contributive to a large chronically-ill or redundantly-ill population. Lethal illnesses are less lethal; terminal diseases are prolonged. Conditions that previously identified patients as acute, or kill them, are now modified by treatment, arrested by therapy, or set in remission or suspension by medical regimens. Some examples are tuberculosis, Hansen's Disease, diabetes, renal failure and schizophrenia. Palliation has become an alternative to cure. In almost all instances of prolonged medical intervention and palliation, symptoms secondary to treatment emerge. These secondary symptoms or "side effects" are sometimes more severe and/or destructive than the disease their treatment was intended to modify.

In sum, changes in medicine and in medical populations have increased the numbers of organic, psychogenic, sociogenic, and iatrogenic complaints which are criterial for admission to the health care system. Many of these complaints are not curable: nor are they lethal. To a growing extent, American medicine has become an illness maintenance system. In spite of these changes, a curative premise continues to motivate or underlie most medical interventions and patient expectations. Failure to cure and failure to get well result in contradiction and dissonance in the context of healing and ailing.

A set of questions emerges. What are the attributes and character of the new American sick role when it becomes a permanent, not a transient, assignment? What axiom can replace the medical caretakers's curative premise? How can the healer fail to cure with sanctity? How can the sick person fail to get well with grace? How can illnesses be maintained creatively and productively?

THE THEORETICAL FRAME

Talcott Parsons' formulation of the sick role remains seminal and has the advantage of familiarity. Because it posits illness as social deviance, it is especially apt here, where our concern is with chronic illness which deviates from curative expectations.

Medical sociologists have defined as the 'sick role' that set of attitudes towards the self which lead a person to claim the privileges afforded to the 'sick' and to initiate corrective actions. (Mechanic and Volkart 1961)

The underlying assumptions of Parsons' theory are:

That there are uniformities in the constitutions of all human groups at the organic level goes without saying, and hence that many of the problems of somatic medicine are independent of social and cultural variability. (Parsons 1958: 168)

Nevertheless, illness is invariably seen by all societies as immoral in its nonsomatic aspects:

The stigmatizing of illness as undesirable, and the mobilization of considerable resources of a community to combat illness is a reaffirmation of the valuation of health and the counter-vailing influence against the temptation for illness, and hence the various components which go into its motivation, to grow and spread. (Parsons 1958: 177)

With Renee Fox, Parsons goes on to add:

As we have already emphasized, illness is very often motivational in origin. Even in those instances where the *etiology* of the disorder is primarily physico-chemical, the nature and severity of symptoms and the rate of recuperation are almost invariably influenced by the attitudes of the patients. (Parsons, Fox 1952: 237)

There are proposed four components of the sick role: two obligations or respon-sibilities, and two rights or privileges. Rights include the sick person's exemption from other role obligations for the duration of the illness, and the claim that he/she is irresponsible for the state of sickness; i.e., illness is involuntary.

Responsibilities require that the sick person actively cooperate in altering his/her sick state, and that he/she be motivated to evacuate the sick role.

A distinction between illness and disease is not expressed in Parsons' formulation, but it is implied. The attitudinal and motivational aspects of illness are clearly cultural and contextual variables, not somatic variables. Kleinman et al. provide a clear statement of the distinction and its significance:

Modern physicians diagnose and treat *diseases* (abnormalities in the structure and function of body organs and systems), whereas patients suffer illnesses (experiences of disvalued changes in states of being and in social function; the human experience of sickness). (Kleinman et al. 1978: 251 their reference omitted.)

Chrisman points out that:

Illness-related shifts in role behavior imply a 'bargaining' process in which modified rights and obligations are established with others in the social environment ... Unambiguous acute symptoms place the individual in the strongest position for attaining the fullest extent of modifications in role behaviors and place upon him the strongest obligations to get well. On the other hand, ambiguous or chronic problems are not nearly so compelling. (Chrisman 1977: 357 his references omitted.)

And Kleinman et al. continue:

Illness and disease, so defined, do not stand in a one-to-one relation ... Illness may occur in the absence of disease (50% of visits to the doctor are for complaints without an ascertainable biologic base); and the course of a disease is distinct from the trajectory of accompanying illness. (Kleinman et al. 1978: 251 their references omitted.)

Paraphrased to express the disease-illness distinction, Parson's model reads as follows:
(1) The sick person is exempt from other role responsibilities for the duration of the *disease*.
(2) The sick person is not responsible for his/her *disease*.
(3) The sick person must seek and cooperate with resources to eliminate his/her *illness*.
(4) The sick person must be motivated to abandon his/her *illness*.

Parsons' model has a terseness and durability that many other characterizations of sickness do not. It has been criticized for its overgenerality and dependence on the concept of regression (Alexander 1981). It has also been challenged on the basis of its major assumption: that illness is motivated and socially deviant. Pflanz and Rhode argue that being ill is an expectable event in every human's lifetime and thus not socially deviant: in fact it is normative. With respect to its motivation, they say:

... since by definition all social behavior is motivated, in Parsons' view illness is motivated, too. Thus, illness can be traced already in the motivational system being deviant motivation. And this point of view fits neatly into psychosomatic theory. Each and every illness would be, then, to some degree 'mental' on the basis of being motivated. (Pflanz and Rhode 1970: 650)

Their argument, like Parsons', suffers by its lack of distinction between disease and illness. Clearly the covert presence of an undetected virus or fever is not social behavior: this, their basic point is incontestable. But *any* report about or response to a physiological condition *is* social and *is* behavior. As such, the behavior is subject to. social manipulation and control. The disease is one of the *referents* of illness behavior and in any language reflects a nonnormal state of the organism. The illness behavior, on the other hand, may or may not be normative: but to the extent that any behavior is motivated, so must be reports about and responses to disease. Any reduction of motivation to "mental" is unfortunate and trite. Motivation is inspired by context, circumstances, fortuitous events, errors, and the expectations of others. It is guided by collective and cultural events and may or may not be subjectively conscious and/or mental.

The essential issues devolve on the concept of deviance. It is an ambiguous term, having two general senses. We may mean by deviance a divergence from a norm: the sense is then statistical and relative. A range of normality is implied and those events or acts that fall outside the range are deviant. Or we may mean by deviance any behavior or events that are exceptional with respect to some absolute. In this sense, "pretending" to be sick in order to obtain monetary compensation is deviant, meaning "bad", no matter how many people do it. Szasz would have it so: "The 'malingerer' is one who cheats in a game which is a segment of 'real' life". (Szasz 1956: 442) But if the curative premise constitutes a rule of the game of healing and ailing, anyone who does not "get well" is then a malingerer.

We will explore the issue of deviance below, by means of the Parsonian model, adjusted as above. The Parsonian assumption that deviance is regressive will be ignored; it is not essential to the model.

THE RESEARCH

For about four years and ending in 1977, I directed a unique nonmedical clinic for diagnosis and treatment of patients with hard core chronic illness patterns of behavior. The clinic operated on the basis of social science approaches and principles and is described in detail elsewhere (Alexander 1979). One hundred and fifty patients were referred by physicians during the clinic's period of operation. Half were men; half were women. The patients ranged in age from sixteen to seventy-five years. They spanned all kinds of occupations and all levels of economic and educational achievement. Ethnically and subculturally, they were white, Japanese, Chinese, Korean, Portuguese, Hawaiian, Puerto Rican, Filipino, Micronesian, and cosmopolitan. The major common trait shared by these persons was their puzzling, persistent claims of pain and/or illness. Multiple tests, treatments, and interventions characterized most of their histories. Some had medically ascertained organic disease to justify some of their presenting behaviors; but none had sufficient organic pathology to explain their chronic, unremitting sick role status. Some had no discernible physical bases for their complaints.

In short, these were the "hysterics", "hypochondriacs", "malingerers", "somaticizers", "problem patients", "crocks", and "gomers" mentioned earlier. Research with the group consisted of a compressed, topical ethnographic collection of data about each patient. Most of the investigation was done in their homes, places of work, and places of recreation. An initial interview in the clinical setting permitted comparisons of their self-presentation in that environment and in other nonclinical contexts. Each patient was followed for eight or more weeks. Family members, friends, co-workers and important others were part of the inquiry and supplied important perspectives on the patient's problems. Medical and nonmedical parameters were thoroughly reviewed and a holistic composition of the person's ailing and wellness behavior was elicited, both by questioning and observation, and by review of records. Additionally each patient kept a log or diary during a portion of the research period, reporting every four hours his/her physical status and sensations, affect, medication intake, sleep patterns, and eating activity. The diaries were surprisingly complete, considering the demand they made on the patient.

I studied a second kind and group of patients from 1969 to 1973. These were patients undergoing hemodialysis as inpatients and outpatients in a general acute care hospital. They numbered seventy, ranged in age from eight to sixty-six, and were half males and half females as a sample. In their cases, the organic bases for their ailments were unequivocal and clear. The necessity of treatment eight hours a day, three days a week involved them in ongoing and interminable sick roles. Research with these patients consisted of participant observation, interview, psychological testing, and record review. A detailed report of the research is provided elsewhere. (Alexander 1977, 1981).

Both groups of patients — those referred for suspected malingering to the clinic, and those treated with hemodialysis for renal failure, were involved in an intense and explicit effort to define and justify their identities in terms of unremitting sickness. They were hardcore chronics who remained sick and who elaborated, rather than evacuated, their sick roles. They accepted the rights but not the responsibilities of the sick role, and they couldn't, or wouldn't, get well. In the cases of both, the medical community tended to react as to exaggeration. These patients were thought to complain *in excess* of their ailment. Their illnesses exceeded those behaviors thought appropriate to their diseases. This was so whether or not they had a discernible organic pathology.

A typical case is presented by Mr. O, a 48 year old man who was referred to the clinic as a probable malingerer.

Mr. O

Mr O was injured at work two years before his referral to the clinic. At the time of the injury to his right leg, when bricks fell off a platform and hit it, he delayed going to a doctor for a week. He explained that he thought he would jeopardize his job if he didn't continue working: however he quit two weeks later and initiated a disability claim.

A physician examining him then recorded: "There is no question that he had pre-existing venous problems in the right lower extremity prior to the industrial accident. Furthermore he had surgical procedures for this condition and has evidence of a post-phlebetic syndrome as a result."

Nevertheless Mr. O persisted in the medical community. His second office visit resulted in a referral to another doctor who gave nerve blocks which failed to relieve his pain. He was sent to a third physician for another consultation which revealed nothing. This was followed by two additional nerve blocks, and referral to a psychologist for testing. The MMPI and interview did not provide explanation for Mr. O's determined assumption of the sick role. New X-rays were ordered and nerve blocks continued, without avail. During this time Mr. O. had attained prescriptions of vitamin B for nerve tissue damage, Parafon Forte as a muscle relaxant, Valium as a muscle relaxant and tranquilizer, Trilafon for sleep at bedtime, Talwen for pain, Darvocet for pain. Demanding stronger pain medication, he was referred to a psychiatrist. The psychiatrist diagnosed depression based on symptoms of insomnia, anorexia, and (moderate) weight loss. Anti-depressants and psychotherapy were initiated. During the course of psychotherapy, Mr. O continued to present for other medical interventions by various other physicians. He added Sinequan and Percodan to his medications.

Additionally he was referred for physical therapy, obtained a subcutaneous nerve stimulator, crutches, a cane; additional nerve blocks were ordered and surgery twice to remove pieces of vein. The workman's compensation office generated forty pages of correspondence to the various practitioners and patient. Mr. O's alcohol consumption increased notably and his social activities became more tenuous; his wife left him and he changed his place of residence six times in eighteen months. Physicians working with him reported frustration and confusion: "I am nonplussed that the patient gets results from Rolfing, I can't personally recommend it as a specific treatment for venous problems. I can't authorize payment for it."

"My evaluation of Mr. O's condition in his lower extremity has really come to an end."

"His current complaint of disability is above and beyond that which can be accounted for physically."

"I recommend that a 5% disability of the right lower extremity be considered in order to facilitate closing of this case."

Just before his referral to our clinic, the 34th physician to have treated Mr. O in two years wrote, "He has the feeling that the Clinic will be helpful to him and I do not believe that anyone can convince him otherwise". Thus he was sent to us.

This man shows a typical course of illness (but not disease) characteristic of problem patients. His particular complaint of venous leg pain was not ordinary — more than sixty percent of those referred to the clinic complained of orthopedic problems — low back and cervical — and concomitant nerve pain, muscle spasm, and headache. But his progress through the medical system and the degeneration of his extra-medical world were typical. Several paradigms are evident, as we apply the Parsonian model.

(1) The sick person is exempt from other role responsibilities for the duration of the disease. Mr. O was derelict, early in his presentation to practitioners, in his work role. He quickly disqualified himself as capable of physical labor and qualified himself as eligible for monetary compensation for his inability to work. In this attitude, he is normative. The American public has gradually determined that health is a right and its absence is deserving of compensation. The deprivation of health is equivalent to the provision of a substitute, usually in the form of money. One trades wellness for so many dollars: in the disability system, one may trade a percentage of one's disfunction for a formulamatic amount of money. Mr. O entered, with his physicians, into a negotiation about how much his injury was worth. The transactional nature of ill health in our culture is not shared completely by medical practitioners. A general counsel for the American Medical Association said, "when God put you on *' e face of the earth, He did not mean for you to receive compensation for every a. tress that occurs" (New York Times, May 7, 1975). In this area, public and practitioners are not in consensus.

Our exploration with Mr. O revealed that he also had forfeited his marital and sexual roles. Neither had been particularly satisfying to him or his wife: "We got along, but that's all", said his ex-wife. His injury, or his portrayal of it, prevented him from doing the things at home that he and his wife felt he should. She had to assume lawn mowing and carrying out the trash, in full view of the neighbors. It is important to note an ironic contributing factor to Mr. O's relinquishing of home responsibilities. The disability claims led to investigations which included sending investigators to Mr. O's neighbors, to inquire whether they saw him doing "laborious" things that would bely the reality of his ailment. Thus any attempts by Mr. O to counter his ailment or deny it would jeopardize his right to obtain compensation. Sexual impotence and an uncertainty in his masculinity occurred early in his illness.

Previously gregarious and active in a wide range of things, Mr. O became increasingly fixed on illness. His range of activities diminished. His sociability became circumscribed. He shifted from friends to acquaintances, and ultimately to barroom cronies. The men he had previously worked and joked with adopted the view that he was malingering and exploiting his previous employer: they rejected him.

Like many men referred to the clinic, he maintained a rigid blue-collar ethic: men worked, unless disabled. Moreover his entire work history had been physical, as opposed to "mental": he identified work with physical labor. Sedentary employment was "another name for sitting on your duff". His recreational pursuits had also been physical. He fished, bowled, and attended sports events. These were given up and replaced by television-watching and drinking.

Mr. O saw himself the victim of these changes and as unresponsible for the loss

of these role competencies. His sick role perception excused him from the performance of role commitments by virtue of his *illness*: not merely the injury, *but
what it did to him*, was justification of his withdrawal and deserving of compensation. But the medical community excuses people on the basis of *disease*, and
demands that the patient be accountable for what the disease does to them. That is,
the medical community holds the patient *accountable for illness*. In Mr. O's case,
the disease was seen as inadequate to justify his response to it. Mr. O was seen by
the medical community as immoral and aberrant in his willingness to capitalize
on his disease.

(2) The sick person is not responsible for his/her disease. As said, medical practitioners do not hold the patient accountable for most diseases or injuries, unless
the patient admits to willful negligence. Smoking, obesity, alcoholism, drug addiction, and intentional risk taking, as well as suicide attempts, are gradually attaining
the status of kinds of willful negligence. We see ambivalence in their treatment, and
whether they are diseases or abuses, and thus voluntary in their origins and as
causes of other conditions, has not been finally determined. Historically and at
present, these acts have evolved with medical explanations of predisposition,
constitutional weakness, psychopathology — the person "can't help" smoking or
overeating; alcoholism and drug addiction are "diseases". Even malingering is
still sometimes diagnosed as a form of hysteria or hypochondriasis. But this sick
role criterion is undergoing redefinition and may eventually be obsolete for some
ailments. A patient's "compliance" with prescribed treatments is closely related
to the progress and definition of disease, but will be discussed below.

Mr. O was not held accountable for his disease by practitioners, nor were most
of the patients referred to the clinic who had identifiable somatic problems. All
were tacitly held accountable for their illnesses. Practitioners did not make the
distinction well or clearly; but it was implied that any utilitarian objective attaching
to a disease was an illicit and intended secondary gain. Patients, on the other hand,
did not see that distinction at all. They sustained an integrated percept. "I'm
sick" meant "I'm diseased and I'm ill and I can't help it". Mr. O never analyzed
his problem into a condition and his reaction to it. The suggestion that he was
"5% disabled" was to him a testimony to the lack of understanding and competence of his doctors.

(3) The sick person must seek and cooperate with resources to eliminate his/
her illness, and (4) the sick person must be motivated to abandon his/her disease.
These two criteria are related. As we are using the term "illness", it includes the
perceived disease and the sick person's behavioral response to it. Part of that
behavioral response is the patient's enlistment of practitioners to eliminate or
"cure" the disease and hence the illness as well. Motivation to get well is expressed
in these acts.

Mr. O, like most patients refered to the clinic, engaged in zealous seeking and
cooperation. Indeed, most of his time was spent seeking "help". He saw 34 physicians in 24 months and participated enthusiastically in their various therapies. In
his case, the therapies remained relatively conservative, albeit noncurative. Some

of the clinic patients had mobilized more radical (and noncorrective) interventions. They were addicted to narcotic analgesics; they had numerous surgeries. One patient had eleven major abdominal surgeries for an undiagnosed intestinal complaint. Many had spinal surgeries. A large number had been given psychiatric labels followed by unsuccessful psychiatric therapy, causing a vigorous prejudice in them against the possibility of any psychological component in their problems.

The absence of definite organic pathology in most of the patients, in spite of extensive diagnostic procedures, did not rule out organic pathology. False negatives are possible; no negative finding is conclusive. Clinicians doubted the validity of many patient complaints, but could be no less cautious. They must treat. A prevailing rule in medicine is "do something" (Haney 1971: 422).

The patients, either sensing clinical doubt or being told of it, redoubled their efforts to convince the medical community of the reality of their disease. This was done by expanding and elaborating their illness behavior. Of course, the result was paradoxical: the sicker they behaved, in the absence of organic bases, the less sick they seemed to their practitioners. Referral by one doctor to another was as common as the "doctor shopping" done by patients. Mr. O, unsatisfied by the treatment given by one doctor, would promptly seek another. A doctor, unsatisfied by Mr. O's lack of response to his ministrations, would refer him to another specialist.

It is tempting to assume that there exist "imaginary diseases." That is, some people may imagine that they are sick and then proceed to enact with sincerity the sick role, But ultimately the hallucination or imagination of a disease entails severe psychopathology and it is not demonstrable that the majority of patients thought to malinger are so affected, or so uniquely affected by a neurosis or psychosis that imaginary disease is a predictable outcome.

Mr. O's case is shared because he sought rewards for illness on all levels. He is exemplary of a successful instance of illness maintenance. The basis of his disease was a minor injury. The etiologies of his illness were many. The onset of his illness came at a time when his job had become monotonous and unchallenging, his marriage dull and frustrating, his manhood tentative, and he was aging. He was able to detour these problems and excuse his failure to perform well in various roles by virtue of his involuntary sick state. He ultimately gained a 25% disability status and a generous insurance settlement. He blunted his alienation from previous friends and hopes with alcohol and with prescribed analgesics and tranquilizers. He structured his days with wholesome help-seeking self-indulgence. He experienced a renewal in his sense of self and purpose in the intense attentions and concern he gained from the medical community, our clinic included. He claimed a certain superiority in proving himself "right" when 33 physicians implied he was "wrong". (The 34th was instrumental in arranging the monetary rewards.) In the larger nonmedical world of peers, he emerged a winner: "I beat a clumsy, unfair, and over-rated professional system and got what I had rights to get." He wove illness into the fabric of his life, repairing rents and tears. When the patch was done, he reverted to a nonsick role. He was never cured, but he did get well.

It is difficult for the medical community to see that illness maintenance as demonstrated by Mr. O requires ingenuity, wide knowledge of the health care system, and a separate morality. Was Mr. O deviant? If he was, deviance will persist, for its rewards are large. National health insurance is the largest imaginable system of rewards for illness maintenance.

For comparison, the case of Miss M is instructive. She was 18 years old when she began a correspondence with me. At that time she was being treated with hemodialysis at a hospital, after an unsuccessful transplant and six months on home dialysis. Exerpts from her letters follow: We never met.

Marion M

I enjoyed reading your article. It made me re-evaluate my role as a patient. It made me curious as to how relationships can be improved – how patients can become better patients without losing self-esteem or identity . . . The physicians set down rules for the staff to follow. These rules can be flexible if adapted to patient needs (no two patients are alike). But the nurses who have the most closest contact with the patient, only have the authority to carry out the rules in the strictest sense. They feel insecure legally and intellectually. They would rather take the safe side and adhere strictly to the rules. Ultimately the patient suffers . . .

When they feel we aren't cooperative, they react with negative reinforcers . . . Do as you're told and we'll not withdraw you from the renal program. Do as you're told and we won't stop you from preparing your dialysis machine. Do as you're told and we won't treat you differently from the other patients . . .

Patients soon realize that threats to life can't be carried out. They (patients) reject staff dominance and their general attitude that "we are only doing this for your own good" or "we know what is best for you." Patients like to test their environment and they see other patients doing the same thing . . .

Staff try to convince patients that home dialysis is best. They would always say that home is a more relaxed environment, you can arrange dialysis to fit your own schedule, you can get a job, etc. But you didn't trust yourself to go home. It was like being thrown in the water and told to swim. You didn't trust yourself with the treatment, you didn't trust others with your needles . . . Relationships became very strained when you discovered that all your family members were dense, or when they discovered you were an impossible person to please. Then, there's a sense of finality about going home. You are sent there because you are an inconvenience to the hospital, because they want to make room for other sicker people. It seems as if everybody would be completely satisfied if you went home and they would forget about you. But you didn't want everybody satisfied that you were home and adjusting well to hemodialysis because you hated it and wanted them to know you hated it . . .

On the other hand, it was competitive in the hospital. "Older patients" had seniority, "sicker patients" had seniority, "transplants" had seniority. There's a perpetual contest to see who can get hooked up first. Everybody has their own ideas on the best methods for fixing the machines . . . The whole chronic patient story is disgusting. Doctors and staff generally patronize their patients . . . Patients just compare their aches and pains like some pathetic exclusive breed of legitimate hypochondriacs . . . I even find myself looking at the obituary notices, to see if someone I know may have passed away.

In the hospital you soon observed that the other fellow patients all had problems you didn't want to admit to – family problems, unemployed, alone . . . There was a feeling of rejection and failure. You were in the hospital because you were a family inconvenience . . .

Marion read Mann's *Magic Mountain* and Solzhenitzn's *Cancer Ward* during our correspondence. She was explicitly seeking an understanding of the chronic sick role.

Mann emphasized the lack of the time element in the sanitarium. I think it's the opposite here. Time becomes very important to us, measured with care. Long range goals secretly become short-term goals . . .

I must tell you that I like the way you write – very sincere – and that I'm not afraid to write back. This is weird because I don't even know you. Writing always seems easier than talking . . . you can say exactly what you mean, you can be truthful, or what you feel is truthful . . . I keep a diary now. I hope you won't discuss this with anyone. I don't want to get in trouble for what seems like 'complaining'. Already I'm not on the best of terms with them.

Unlike Mr. O, Marion painfully and articulately separated herself from her disease. She self-consciously created her own patient role and monitored its changes. She found she could not resume pre-illness patterns of behavior; she could not go home, resume work, return to school. She had changed, and so had her percepts of those things. Nor could she conform to a prescribed sick role or "good patient" role. She found illness repugnant and demeaning. She could not come to terms with the first Parsonian premise. She describes the adaptations of other patients: they compare ailments, create social hierarchies on the ward, compete with and share medical methodologies. They demonstrate and discuss proper patient comportment. But Marion could not enter into that socializing. The most important pre-illness role she wanted to resume, which was not an option, was her own nonsick status.

You know that sinestrol, female hormone shots, that Kostoglotov (in *Cancer Ward*) had to take, to supress the metastatic process? It reminded me so much of the deca-durabolin, male hormone shots, that kidney patients take to increase red blood cells . . . Kostoglotov's objections to the hormone shots were about the same as mine. P. 385; 'How could you have assured me so strongly that the injections were essential but that I would not understand their significance? What was there to understand? What is so hard to understand about hormone therapy?'

Do you know that none of the staff told me that those weekly deca shots were male hormone shots? One evening one of the staff accidentally left the brochure on deca-durabolin on my bed. Naturally I read it and concluded – so that's why my voice was so low and hoarse – maybe that's why my monthlies stopped – oh, and all the other horrible things I read. Càn you imagine growing a beard? I read it and read it over again. I just know I couldn't take it anymore and I refused to take it that night. That started many problems with the staff. They just couldn't understand and I couldn't explain it to them. I was afraid they would all laugh at me – I couldn't tell them my fears in front of other patients. The staff would repeatedly tell me "you must not be uncooperative . . . you know you have to take those shots to increase your red blood cells . . . it will be just that much harder to get a transplant, and you do want a transplant, don't you?"

I proved them all wrong. My blood count didn't get any lower. In fact at one point it got higher. And I did get a transplant, even though it rejected . . .

Every time I discuss this with someone – be it staff or patient – I get the reaction "don't be uncooperative." Don't get me wrong – I'm not trying to change the system nor does it mean I don't like the staff. I like them a lot. What I am saying is that a patient has the right to express his individuality and if he chooses to, to reject the stereotypic patient image. Just because he chooses to deviate from conventional guidelines doesn't automatically mean he is an "uncooperative and problem patient". He maybe merely trying to retain his self-esteem and self-identity. I'm not afraid anymore.

Marion did not exercise the right granted by the second Parsonian premise.

Her disease was not involuntary. From a practitioner point of view, she was guilty of willful negligence — "noncompliance" — which exacerbated her disease. Yet she expresses for us an explanation for noncompliance not usually encountered in the medical literature on the subject: it provided her a means of asserting her nonsick self.

There are aspects of denial in Marion's rejection of the hormone shots which compare importantly to Mr. O's case. She rejected the therapy itself. Mr. O never rejected a therapy: he always rejected its efficacy. These were important patterns observed in the two groups of chronically ill patients. Noncompliance, denial of disease, and flights into health were regular occurrences among those with organic pathology that could only be palliated. Compliance, compelling arguments "proving" disease, and determined persistent illness behavior characterized those patients thought to be malingering. Mr. O fulfilled the responsibility of the third Parsonian criterion: he sought and cooperated with helping resources, thereby confirming his motivation to get well. Marion M. did not always fulfill the responsibility to seek and cooperate. Thus she also expressed her motivation to be well.

Ultimately Marion elected a second transplant, a poor match, knowing well the risks. She died within four days of the surgery. Her last letter arrived a week before the implant.

I hate the role of patient. I really hate dialyzing. Now, more than ever, I've grown so tired of it. I'm so tired of putting up a front for everybody — the brave, independent soul — I'm tired of fixing the machine for myself, I'm tired of putting in the fistula needles — and they do hurt — I'm tired of cleaning the machine, I'm tired of trying to fit my dialysis schedule to be convenient to my family, I'm tired of becoming friends with patients and some die and they all get sicker, I'm tired of hearing all the problems the patients and staff have, I'm tired of hearing about transplant failures and I'm tired of being envious of transplant successes. I'm tired of hearing about all these hopes for miraculous medical achievements — they'll never come. I guess I'm tired of just about everything. I would never say this to anyone else. But don't be concerned. I tend to get a bit dramatic, and I guess everyone gets tired of things some days. Pax Vobiscum.

DISCUSSION AND APPLICATIONS

Two cases have been reviewed, each representing some of the problems of the chronically ill. Mr. O's case reflected characteristics of those patients who present symptoms in the absence of convincing signs. They have illness, but no apparent disease. Miss M's case expressed some of the problems of those who have incurable and palliated disease. Mr. O demonstrated a kind of adaptation: he used his illness to attain rewards and to avoid onerous and unsuccessful role performances. However his behavior is morally culpable within the context of American medicine. Miss M. did not adapt to her disease. Her illness behavior did not gain her rewards within or without the context of medical care. She ultimately withdrew from the "game which is a segment of 'real' life".

Several objectives guided the development of this chapter. The exploratory and general discussion of chronic illness recommends that far more rigorous analysis is needed. Some directions are hopefully suggested by the cases of Mr. O and Miss M. Certainly simplistic constructs explaining the elaboration of illness, such as "hysteria" and "secondary gain", are inadequate. The application of the classic Parsonian sick role model was not, in my view, particularly informative.

In fact an implicit objective was to test the utility of the Parsonian model against the situation of chronic, as opposed to acute and transient, ailing. The model was adjusted to accommodate the necessary disease-illness distinction, and then it was applied to material about chronic illness. It was employed as the instrument of analysis, rather than the object. I find its descriptive validity for chronic circumstances doubtful, clumsy, and semantically awkward. We can briefly criticize the model on the basis of its use in this chapter:

(1) Chronically ill people are *not* exempted from other role responsibilities for the duration of their disease, or for the duration of their claim of disease. In fact the medical community expects patients to return to "normalcy" once it has decided that the disease is controlled or discredited. Evidence of the success of medical intervention is sought in the patient's resumption of a "normal life style." This is equivalent to the demand that patients abandon their illness, regardless of their disease status. They should go home, be employed, be productive, etc.

(2) Chronically ill people *are* responsible for their disease: disease is not involuntary. The issue of compliance is critical to control and amelioration of disease and the patient's full participation in treatment has become definitional of the disease. A palliated disease, unlike a transient virus, is redefined by the activities that modify it. Miss M. was guilty of exacerbating her condition. Mr. O was suspected of fabricating his.

(3) From the view of the medical community, the Parsonian adage that the sick person must seek and cooperate with helping resources persists as true. From Miss M's point of view, an equally rational perspective, her only means of maintaining a part of herself independent of illness and disease and thus healthy, was to not cooperate fully. Rather she refused an intervention the consequence of which was more heinous to her than the condition it intended to correct. Nor does this criterion stretch to include the patient who seeks and cooperates with *too many* helping agencies, as did Mr. O.

(4) Motivation to evacuate the sick role is sometimes unrealistic, self-defeating, and always ambiguous. If by motivation we mean the patient devoutly wishes to be well, Miss M was highly motivated subjectively. If we mean that we infer motivation from the patient's intense help-seeking and cooperative behavior, Mr O was highly motivated objectively. If less cogently but more generally, we mean that illness behavior can be motivated by extrinsic factors and rewards, as well as by disease, but that it should not be so motivated, we are foolish. When the rewards of illness exceed the rewards of wellness in our society, we should be prepared for its growth and prevalence. In such case, we must make a moral judgment. Such exploitation of the system, in the absence of clear criteria for ruling out organic pathology or disease, is either relatively adaptive and normative:

or it is absolutely deviant and wrong. Again, the required judgment is moral, not medical: and its object is the entire healing-ailing complex in our society, not merely individual patients.

Parsons' sick role concept has value and appropriate applications to the circumstance of acute and transient disease. It has limited descriptive validity in the emerging circumstance of interminable illness. A new American sick role is currently defining itself. It is hoped that social scientists will generate new and sensitive models and constructs to analyze it.

REFERENCES

Alexander, L.

1976   The Double-Bind Theory and Hemodialysis. Archives of General Psychiatry 33: 1353–1356.

1979   Clinical Anthropology: Morals and Methods. Medical Anthropology 3: 61–108.

1981   The Double-Bind Between Dialysis Patients and their Health Practitioners. In L. Eisenberg and A. Kleinman (eds.), The Relevance of Social Science for Medicine. Dordrecht, Holland: D. Reidel Publ. Co.

Bateson, G.

1972   The Cybernetics of 'self': A Theory of Alcoholism. In G. Bateson: Steps to an Ecology of Mind. Chandler Publishing Company.

Carlson, K. and L. Alexander

1978   Crock or Crook? Ambivalence in American Medicine. Paper presented at the American Anthropology Association Annual Meetings, Los Angeles, California.

Chrisman, N.

1977   The Health Seeking Process: An Approach to the Natural History of Illness. Culture, Medicine and Psychiatry 1: 351–377.

Fox, R.

1979   Training for Uncertainty. In R. C. Fox: Essays in Medical Sociology. John Wiley and Sons.

Freidman, M.

1969   Pathogenesis of Coronary Artery Disease. New York: McGraw-Hill.

George, V. and A. Dundes

1978   The Gomer. Journal of American Folklore 91: 568–581.

Groves, J.

1978   Taking Care of the Hateful Patient. The New England Journal of Medicine, April 20: 883–887.

Haney, C. A.

1971   Psychosocial Factors Involved in Medical Decision Making. In T. Milton: Medical Behavioral Science. W. B. Saunders, Co.

Illich, I.

1975   Medical Nemesis: The Expropriation of Health. London: Calder and Boyars.

Kaplan, H. I. and H. S. Kaplan

1957   The Psychosomatic Concept of Obesity. Journal of Nervous and Mental Disorders 125: 181–201.

Kasl, S. and S. Cobb

1970   Health Behavior, Illness Behavior, and Sick Role Behavior. Archives of Environmental Health 12: 246–265.

Kassebaum, G. G. and B. B. Baumann

1965   Dimensions of the Sick Role in Chronic Illness. Journal of Health and Social Behavior 6: 16–27.

Kleinman, A., L. Eisenberg, and B. Good
　1978　Culture, Illness and Care. Annals of Internal Medicine 88: 251–258.
Langner, T.
　1962　A Twenty-two Item Screening Score of Psychiatry Symptoms Indicating Impairment. Journal of Health and Human Behavior 3: 269–276.
Luborsky, I., J. Dogherty, and S. Penick
　1973　Onset Conditions for Psychosomatic Symptoms. Psychosomatic Medicine 35: 187–204.
Mannon, J.
　1976　Defining and Treating 'Problem Patients' in a Hospital Emergency Room. Medical Care 14: 1004–1013.
Mechanic, D. and E. Volkart
　1961　Stress, Illness Behavior, and the Sick Role. American Sociological Review 26: 51–58.
Parsons, T.
　1958　Definitions of Health and Illness in the Light of American Values and Social Structure. In E. G. Jaco (ed.), Patients, Physicians, and Illness. Glencoe, Ill.: The Free Press.
Parsons, T. and R. Fox
　1952　Illness, Therapy, and the American Family. Journal of Social Issues 8: 4: 31–44.
Pflanz, M. and J. Rhode
　1970　Illness: Deviant Behavior or Conformity. Social Science and Medicine 4: 645–653.
Rushmer, R.
　1975　Humanizing Health Care. Cambridge, Mass.: MIT Press.
Szasz, T.
　1956　Malingering: 'Diagnosis' or Social Condemnation? A. M. A. Archives of Neurology and Psychiatry 76: 432–443.
Wooley, S., B. Blackwell, and C. Winget
　1978　A Learning Theory Model of Chronic Illness Behavior. Psychosomatic Medicine 40: 379–401.
Zuckernann, I.
　1977　Pathology, Adversity, and Nursing. Social Science and Modern Society 14: 52–54.

SUE E. ESTROFF

LONG-TERM PSYCHIATRIC CLIENTS IN AN AMERICAN COMMUNITY: SOME SOCIOCULTURAL FACTORS IN CHRONIC MENTAL ILLNESS

INTRODUCTION

Clinically relevant anthropological research began with the psychiatric work of Gregory Bateson (1956), William Caudill (1958), and Jules Henry (1964, 1973). Caudill encountered sociocultural systems among psychiatric patients and staff, documenting their influence on the experience of hospital treatment. Henry focused more on individual patients and their families, exploring the interpersonal and psychodynamic factors which contributed to psychosis and hospital adaptation. Bateson developed ideas about the contribution of paradox, contradiction, and confused communication to schizophrenia from his clinical interactions with patients and their families. Our ancestors set precedents in theory, methodology, finding and application of results which are not only reflected by contemporary research, but legitimate the pertinence and usefulness of such work.

Thus, we find ourselves with access to the clinical psychiatric scene, serving most importantly as descriptive analysts of sociocultural phenomena that effect the content, process and outcome of treatment. We analyze and appreciate psychotic process and psychiatric patienthood in their own terms and as reflective of and contributing to cultural context. The focus is both individual and sociocultural; the method qualitative, investigative, and intensely participatory; the perspective and theoretical orientation relativistic, holistic, and inductive. We seek to identify ancillary sociocultural factors in the illness and treatment experience. We attempt to gain a level of understanding which does not diagnose or intervene but helps in discovering individualistic and systemic factors which impede or facilitate effective alleviation of psychic suffering within a particular behavioral and belief system. Within this tradition, I sought to understand and describe the lives of a group of clients involved in the recent massive de-institutionalization and community treatment movements in the United States.

De-institutionalization and community treatment reflect shifts in ideology and policy regarding the care, treatment, and social place of the mentally ill in our society. Typical of social movements in any complex society, the sources of change have come from many sectors — legal, medical, social, and economic, bringing together both information from research and deeply held beliefs about the causes and cures for mental illness. While not new (Caplan and Caplan 1969), these forces have precipitated unprecedented activity in the past two decades, representing perhaps the most serious recognition American psychiatry has made of the influence of sociocultural factors in mental illness. Patients were removed from psychiatric hospitals largely because social science and clinical research established that the interpersonal relationships between patients and staff, patients and other patients,

369

N. J. Chrisman and T. W. Maretzki (eds.), Clinically Applied Anthropology, 369–393.
Copyright © 1982 by D. Reidel Publishing Company.

patients and their families and significant others, and the sociocultural systems which formed in institutions were not therapeutic, and were in fact detrimental to the overall life circumstances of patients. Parallel developments in the law with the principle of least restrictive alternatives and in medicine with the discovery and widespread use of antipsychotic medication, in particular the phenothiazines and lithium carbonate, also propelled the process.

There is ample need and rationale for clinically applied anthropological research in this area from both clinical and anthropological perspectives. Psychiatric de-institutionalization and community treatment bring together powerful and complex sociocultural and clinical changes, representing especially appropriate arenas for this type of research. These developments present psychiatric clinicians with intimi-datingly large numbers of new treatment problems which are often due to and inseparable from sociocultural factors.

For the anthropologist, interesting and important arenas for research have been created for which there is historical precedent for our involvement. Ethnographic information gathered in psychiatric hospitals proved pertinent in motivating and justifying de-institutionalization. Having pointed out problems in hospital socio-cultural systems, both the invitation and obligation to track the treatment system's responses are significant. It is surprising that relative to the attention paid to the sociocultural worlds of patients in psychiatric hospitals, anthropological research about psychiatric clients in community treatment systems is sparse. In sum, we have a rare opportunity to engage in research which has precedent, pertinence, and abundant application in both anthropology and clinical fields which has yet to be exploited.

THE CLINICAL PROBLEM

During the past fifteen years, the number of persons residing for treatment purposes in psychiatric hospitals in the United States has decreased by more than one-half million. Simultaneously, length of stay for those hospitalized has greatly shortened and out-patient care has increased by 70% (Witkin 1980). These numerical indi-cators reflect the formidable scope of the de-institutionalization and community treatment movements. In human terms, these professional/clinical, social, and philosophical changes have drastically altered the lives and treatment of hundreds of thousands of persons who experience not only acute psychotic episodes, but chronic and often complex problems in living in our society. Persons who used to live in psychiatric hospitals are now attempting community life and many who might have been treated in hospitals ten years ago, find themselves instead as out-patients, responsible for daily living tasks while they receive treatment for often severe behavioral, cognitive, and affective disorders.

Massive de-institutionalization began before anyone except the most innovative and careful clinicians were prepared; before communities could provide adequate support services, and before the needs of patients and their families were known or before they were actively invited to participate in the planning and provision of effective treatment. Now, appropriately, mental health care givers are thrust into the whole of their clients' lives. Traditional clinical psychology, psychiatry, nursing and social work skills and training were devised largely for institutional settings and despite the best intentions, fall woefully short in the community treatment endeavor. Clinicians now must assist with the struggles of fearful, disorganized, often psychotic, and frequently unskilled persons with few adequate coping skills who must manage to survive daily life on the street, not to mention work on deeply experienced emotional and cognitive problems. There are subsistance supplies to be sought, jobs and shelter to be found and kept, simple hygiene and domestic skills to be taught, anxieties, pain and sometimes delusions to be ministered to. There is isolation, bizarre behavior, stigma, violence, and the vicissitudes of public opinion to contend with. And as always, the mazes of agencies and administrative strata to negotiate. Now, the clinician attempts to heal within a context where social factors as often as intrapsychic factors precipitate and exacerbate symptomatology.

The clinical problems facing the providers of adequate community treatment for long term psychiatric patients cannot be simply or briefly stated. In broad scope, the question is how best to help heal, if not prevent, chronic mental illness in our society; how to help those who think and feel differently from the majority of others to live as freely and fully as possible. We now know that compared to persons who experience similar symptoms in some non-Western settings, persons in our society and other Western cultures fare worse over time and have poorer prognoses on nearly every measure (WHO 1979; Sartorius, Jablensky and Shapiro 1977, 1978; Edgerton 1980). Thus, we cannot safely attribute the chronicity of mental illness to a disease process any longer. Clearly, there are as yet unidentified factors that contribute systematically to American psychotics, particularly schizophrenics, improving less than their non-Western counterparts.

The clinical question may be posed as follows: Now that patients are mainly out of the hospital, how can we provide treatment that will facilitate the richest quality of life, foster the most autonomy and self-esteem, without promoting a sense of inadequacy and low self-esteem or dependence and enmeshment in yet another institution − the community mental health system? That is to say, how can (community) treatment succeed in attaining its goals of re-integration into the community, enhancement of clients' subjective and objective experience in living, and management, if not alleviation, of psychotic symptoms? How can we develop a healing system that will not undermine sociocultural adjustment in the process of attaining clinical improvement? Or, in view of the cross-cultural data, we might ask, Why aren't our patients improving as much as others? What are we, they, or all of us doing that contributes to such relatively poor outcomes? In order to answer these questions, it will be helpful first to know more specifically about the outcome of community treatment in the U.S. Next I will report my research and findings in view of these questions, and will conclude with application of these findings to clinical practice.

As I assess and discuss community psychiatric treatment, I will focus on a

particular group of clients — the long-term, severely, complexly troubled.[1] Clinically, these people are described as extremely dependent, deficient in coping skills
and consequently vulnerable to the stresses of daily life, experiencing repeated
difficulty in achieving nurturant, symmetrical relations with others, and often
unable or unwilling to participate in providing for their own subsistence, responding
to problems in any or all of these areas by becoming symptomatic or psychotic
(Test and Stein 1978). Most often these clients are diagnosed as schizophrenic,
but the major affective, character and personality disorders are also represented
(Minkoff 1978).

Anthropologically, these persons can be described as negatively different — that
is, different from most members of our society in ways that are negatively valued.[2]
They experience difficulty and behave divergently in activities such as work and
relations with others that express powerful cultural values and represent carefully
regulated functional facets of our social system. Their dependency and vulnerability
depart from and challenge our values of autonomy, interdependence, competency
in coping, and perseverance in the face of stress. The quantity and chronicity of
their symptoms and needs are in conflict with proper sick role behavior for it is
not clear that they can or want to 'get well'; i.e., behave and feel more like the rest
of us (Erikson 1957; Mechanic 1977). So, not only do these long-term clients
experience internal, psychological difficulties in thinking and feeling, but live in
ways that are negatively valued in our sociocultural system, consequently eliciting
powerful social responses — be these punishing, caring, or attempts at change or
treatment.

Findings from Community Research

Outcome and program evaluation research conducted during the past several years
pertinent to this population yields consistent findings. I will summarize these only
very briefly here and refer the interested reader to comprehensive reviews published
elsewhere (Anthony, Cohen, and Vitalo 1978; Bachrach 1976; Estroff 1981; GAP
1978; Talbott 1978; Test and Stein 1978).

Amount of *time spent in the community* (*community tenure*) has increased
more significantly than other treatment variables since de-institutionalization
began.[3] On the average, long-term clients spend 5–10% of their time, or about four
weeks per year as in-patients. Translated to the individual level, they experience at
least one relapse resulting in hospitalization every three to five years. The number
of patients who *relapse* increases over time after baseline discharge: 25–30% relapse
by 6 months; 35–50% at one year; and 65–75% by three to five years (Anthony
et al. 1980). *Recidivism* then, represents a continuing problem for clients and
clinicians because the ability of treatment efforts and available support services to
prevent relapse seems time limited.

Providing for one's own subsistence in culturally acceptable ways represents one
of the most powerful components of self-esteem and competence in our society.
Therefore, community treatment programs have focused on the employment of
clients and here again have produced temporary and limited success. Within the

first year after discharge, and during active participation in vocationally oriented treatment, 30–50% of clients may work. After one year, 75–80% are unemployed. Jobs in sheltered workshops or competitive employment in custodial or other menial situations typifies the work experience of most of those who are employed. Income maintenance programs ranging from city welfare to federal Supplemental Security Income (SSI) carry the responsibility for providing money for the necessities of life for the unemployed. On the basis of the 1975 figures (Kochhar 1979), I estimate that in 1980, 372,000 long-term psychiatric patients are receiving SSI at a cost of $65 million annually. However, by far the largest costs in monetary terms are in lost productivity in the labor force, estimated in 1971 as approaching $17 billion (Levine and Levine 1975: 50). It is clear then, that the subjective and objective enhancement of personal and social adjustment sought via employment has proved difficult to achieve. The reluctance of employers to risk hiring applicants with such poor work histories and few job skills and the clients' apprehension, apparent inability to tolerate moderate levels of interpersonal stimuli, internal disorganization, and often external differentness in behavior and appearance contribute to this dismal scenario. Costs for providing food, shelter, and treatment remain in the public sector in large part, and the clients remain dependent upon social institutions for subsistence.

Integration or re-integration of the negatively different into American communities has also been a goal of community psychiatric treatment because hospitalization was thought to disrupt social relations and undermine social role performance. Community treatment has meant to restore and retain social networks for clients outside a formal care-giving system where relationships were destined to be asymmetrical and dependency enhancing (Ludwig 1971). However indirect, data about living situation provide the most plentiful available indications of clients' social relations. The majority live alone or with other negatively different persons, in residences which may be supervised (board and care, residential treatment, and halfway houses) or unsupervised (single room occupancy hotels, rooming houses, YM or YWCA's, and apartments). A few have returned to live with their families of origin or procreation, but the numbers have lessened over time (Talbott 1980). Research about the quality of life, clinical condition, and social relations of clients in the above settings suggests that while these living arrangements may provide a sense of security and asylum, they also do not promote personal growth, community integration, or the creation of social networks that are nurturant and autonomy supporting (Lamb 1979a; Segal and Aviram 1978; Reynolds and Farberow 1977; Sokolovsky et al. 1978). Problems with formal, informal, and mutual rejection, avoidance, and disinterest between community members and clients are reflected in both the employment and residential statistics (See also Aviram and Segal 1973; Segal, Baumohl, and Moyles 1980).

Additional qualitative information is sparse in the outcome research. Psychosocial functioning remains relatively low for these persons, but there are some indications that self-esteem, quality of life, and satisfaction with treatment are no worse in the community than in the hospital and higher in some cases (Test and

Stein 1978). Two recent community treatment research projects conducted at multiple sites in the United States confirm that improvement in subjective and psychosocial areas is difficult to achieve. Among other findings, the clients in these studies reported significant levels of agitation and depression (Hogarty et al. 1979) and that they had not changed their negative evaluations of themselves in view of their own aspirations (Linn et al. 1979).

Finally, even when treatment may help and is available in various forms, many persons refuse or do not utilize it. Long-term clients account for less than 30% of all outpatient psychiatric care and nearly 75% drop out of outpatient and aftercare treatment even when it is recommended (Minkoff 1978). Further, psychotropic medication is widely prescribed and believed by many to prevent relapse (Davis 1976), yet fewer than half of the patients take the medication in the desired amount, if at all (Blackwell 1973; Van Putten 1974).

To sum up, thousands of people with chronic and moderate to severe clinical symptomatology are now living and being treated in American communities instead of psychiatric hospitals. However, the vast majority are unintegrated into community life, do not engage in positively valued subsistence activities, avoid or refuse treatment, score poorly on psychosocial adjustement measures, and relapse with stubborn consistency. Talbott (1979) has called the care and treatment of these persons 'a national disgrace'. Lamb (1979b: 201) goes somewhat further writing, "Now suddenly we have discovered that we substituted one kind of neglect for another by shifting these people to an unprepared and unreceptive community where many are living impoverished lives."

In view of this information, the clinician could choose from a long list of problems. For example, why is it so difficult for these people to work? Why do they refuse medication which undeniably helps to reduce symptoms? What contributes to their continued dependence on their families, social institutions, and care givers and lack of ties with the community at large? Why are so many depressed, agitated, and lacking self esteem and coping skills? Or conversely, what treatment modalities can be designed that will be more effective than those of the present which produce such limited success?

THE RESEARCH

In view of the above, the goal of my research was to provide an ethnographic description and analysis of a group of clients who were participating in a community based psychiatric treatment program which is intended as an alternative to hospitalization (Stein and Test 1980). I sought an understanding of the sociocultural worlds of the clients that might address some of the clinical issues raised by the outcomes of psychiatric de-institutionalization thus far.

Forty-three persons were studied for a period of two years, both during and after intensive participation in the treatment program. A majority of the subjects were diagnosed as schizophrenic and were clinically classified as chronic patients (see note 1). There were twice as many males as females in the group and the average age for the entire group was mid-twenties, although the range was from 18 to 56 years old. Except for five who were divorced, all were single and had never married. With regard to previous 'formal' psychiatric history, the group displays a diverse background. Three clients had no prior psychiatric admissions, though the average number of admissions for the entire group is 5.36, averaging 21.34 weeks of total hospitalization per person. The range in number of psychiatric hospitalizations varies from one to fifteen. Eight persons had been admitted only once previous to my encounter with them; seven had had more than ten inpatient episodes. On the whole, there were very few novice patients, and most had lived with problems for quite some time, whether formally involved in treatment or not.

An inductive and participant observer methodology was employed to gather the data. I participated *as if* a client in all feasible treatment activities, including working in a sheltered workshop, taking anti-psychotic medications, and attending group recreational and therapy sessions. Outside the treatment setting, I interacted daily with clients in their homes and my own, in public places, and anywhere we might meet. During the research, I also drew heavily upon information from staff members and anyone else who interacted with the clients. The research was not covert, and my identity and purpose for participation were made known to clients and program staff by me at the outset of the fieldwork. The project was explained in detail to the staff and they were asked for their cooperation, assistance, and any criticism they might have of my conduct while working with them. I told individual clients about my work in private and as I got to know them.

The process of 'placing' myself (Goffman 1971) in a triangular relationship with staff and clients proved to be an essential task for the first phase of fieldwork, but was somewhat isolating and at times conflict-ridden and stressful. I wanted to construct study affiliations and loyalties with the clients that were recognized and respected by staff. At the same time, the support and trust of staff members was imperative. I asked them to participate in a grossly asymetrical relationship with me in which they were vulnerable and open, giving me information about clients, while I would censor any knowledge I had of clients with them.[4] Much to the credit of this treatment staff, we were able to negotiate a happy working relationship with minimal limit testing.

Because of my peculiar and unique position in clients' and staff's worlds and their intersection, ethical and tactical questions abounded. Would I lend money to a client on a strict money contingency program? Should I spend time with a client who was supposed to be at work when the staff wanted to strongly persuade the person to be there? What should I do if the staff were misinformed about a client who was in acute distress? Could I let clients know that I attended staff report and parties; had relationships with staff that they would like to have had? Decisions were made on the basis of my evaluation of their consistency with ethical and strategic principles appropriate for the setting: (1) clients and their sensibilities come first, (2) avoid at all costs undermining or altering the trust of clients or staff in each other or me, (in other words, avoid getting split or caught in the triangle); (3) evaluate how information would flow were I not present and "let the system be"; (4) do not deliberately deceive, misinform, or misrepresent any group or individual — client or staff.

I have raised these issues for they are vital to the conduct of research in clinical settings. It is important to acknowledge how inherently perilous, personal, and complicated is the fieldwork discovery process. The anthropological researcher in the clinical arena needs to balance often conflicting experiences and viewpoints, simultaneously allowing oneself to *participate* as fully as possible. Those moments when I felt as discouraged, desperate, confused, and depressed as the clients, taught me much that I would never have known had I maintained distance and objectivity (if such exists) (see Jules-Rosette 1978).

The clients from whom I learned live in a self and other created world of Catch 22's, paradoxes, and ricocheting realities. It seems that nearly all those measures taken to ameliorate symptoms and problems in living can and do work for *and* against the clients. As I report my findings, I will describe how I think clients learn to live with their psychoses and divergent life adaptations and how we and they contribute to perpetuating and in some cases amplifying their negatively valued differentness even as we reach out to help. Due to the shortage in space, I will confine the discussion to only two areas: subsistence strategies and medications.

Subsistence Strategies

A subsistence strategy represents the means through which a person obtains the necessities of life in our society — food, shelter, clothing, and money. My conceptualization of the clients' strategies is that they are professional patients. That is to say, these persons live within the confines of a cash economy, based on the exchange of labor, goods, and expertise for remuneration. The clients are however, for the most part, either unable or unwilling to participate in a conventional sense in this economic system. What the clients do exchange or provide for their 'wages' are their disabilities, diagnoses, and deficits. Being psychiatrically disturbed permits them to receive money, goods, and services in a similar way that possessing and utilizing the skills of a plumber permits one to earn wages. The clients differ from the plumber for their motivations and intentions are not to engage in such a career, but when we look objectively at what credentials entitle them to income, we find only their symptoms and the resulting deficits in living skills. I put forth this formulation because, with few exceptions, the clients I worked with were enmeshed in a psychiatric disability oriented system wherein most were unemployed and receiving support from federal and local income maintenance programs. Their participation in positively valued subsistence endeavors is restricted by the security and availability of disability related income as well as their feelings of fear and incompetence, lack of training, work skills, and opportunities for employment, and repeated failures with work.

During treatment, the clients participated in four types of employment: Sheltered, Volunteer, Subsidized, and Competitive. Sheltered employment entails paid jobs in workshops that are specifically designed to employ and train persons with developmental and psychiatric disabilities. Volunteer placements are usually unpaid positions in community service organizations for clients who are extremely disorganized or unskilled or for whom other work is unavailable. State vocational rehabilitation services and federal programs such as CETA have subsidized positions for some clients in mainstream work settings otherwise inaccessible. Competitive work consists of jobs obtained by clients without regard to their disabilities in a variety of businesses and services in the community. Over the two year period, 71 to 78% were nearly constantly employed. The vast majority of work that lasted for more than four weeks was in sheltered settings such as Goodwill Industries. Competitive jobs tended to require doing menial tasks such as janitoring and dishwashing. The clients quit jobs somewhat more often than they were fired, but may have left work before they could be terminated. While a total of twenty-six held some type of competitive job during the research period, only twelve of these were for periods of longer than four weeks. Seventeen never had a competitive job, though virtually everyone did volunteer work or had a sheltered job at some time largely because of strong pressures from treatment program staff. In overview, only five of the group engaged in competitive employment with any predictability.

With the exception of two persons, virtually every client received or receives some form of financial assistance based on their psychiatric disability. Twenty-seven receive SSI, four receive Veteran's benefits (three of these also get SSI), three receive other forms of Social Security payments, and others used a combination of city welfare, state unemployment compensation, and covert and overt family support.[5] These figures, however, tell only the most obvious part of the story.

Sheltered employment at the Goodwill Industries workshop and another catering to more severely physically and developmentally disabled persons was the type of employment most readily available for the group and was emphasized by the treatment program staff. Although many clients did work for a time at either or both places, with very few exceptions, they found these to be aversive experiences. It seems that among the negatively different in our complex sociocultural system, a hierarchy of acceptability exists. These clients do not like to be lumped with or categorized with those who are physically and developmentally disabled, though structurally, institutionally, and in the public eye this often occurs. Many explained with the old joke whose punch line is, "I may be crazy but I'm not stupid." Their experience of sheltered employment was that they *were* considered to be like the others working in these places, and most of the clients eventually preferred not working and to receive SSI. In addition, their wages in sheltered employment were quite low and the work dull and repetitive from their perspective. As one fellow put it, "Why should I work there for 50 cents an hour at a pretend job?" Amidst this resistance to the multiple derogatory messages contained in the workshop situation, several clients became deeply involved in social relationships with their co-workers. All the while, however, they expressed ambivalence and distaste for these 'friends' and some despair at their limited choices in companions. The experiences of most clients who rejected the workshops were equally negative; almost none obtained outside employment or were fired or quit; and the rest simply opted for income maintenance programs.

It is not fair to assume, however, that the persons I was learning from were averse to work in general. In response to questions on a social adjustment schedule used to supplement the observational material, most clients reported that they valued work *per se*, unfortunately aspiring to jobs for which they were hopelessly unqualified and unprepared. Most accurately evaluated their present work performance at well below proper levels, but they also felt grossly underpaid. When told that sheltered employment was a step toward more rewarding work, some clients believed this for a time. But the pattern was to leave Goodwill or the other workshop after discharge from the treatment program, or well before discharge, with few options for other employment.

For their part, these clients demonstrated overwhelming reluctance, anxiety, distaste, lack of experience, and inertia regarding work. Part of this aversion stems from prior multiple terminations, the wish to avoid close interaction with other persons, and an inability to cope successfully with the perceived pressures of a work setting. They have substantiated for themselves and others time and time again that they can not or will not work. Many could execute the necessary tasks in a vacuum, but not when other factors are present as they always are. Absenteeism, tardiness, low productivity, and lack of motivation characterize their work performance. A cycle of lack of confidence, failure, termination or quitting, and increased feelings of inadequacy is perpetuated. Clients are caught. If they put heavy emphasis on the social and personal significance of work, they seem destined to experience frustration, failure, and negative evaluations of themselves. If they reject the work ethic, they become alienated even further from community reality by not working, and must seek out other means to support themselves.

But clients alone are not responsible for these gloomy circumstances. Many of the alternatives presented to them by the treatment and sociocultural system are markedly unattractive and seen as humiliating and degrading. Overt and covert discrimination in hiring confronts many clients when they seek outside employment. Some employers simply will not hire clients when they see the poor previous work history, evaluating the person as a poor employment risk. Still others skeptically offer a client a chance at usually menial work, firing them if another choice presents itself or the client's anxiety or differentness becomes apparent. A few employers work in conjunction with the treatment program and so effectively compromise the independence from staff and patienthood sought by some clients.

Income maintenance programs would seem to offer an acceptable solution to this dilemma. The client can obtain a guaranteed income which often exceeds what s/he may make in many other jobs, and in Wisconsin, Medical Assistance and other services customarily accompany SSI. But there are symbolic, social, and ultimately very personal prices to be paid for this option. In order to qualify for SSI and VA benefits, a person must have a medically determinable, medically certified physical or mental impairment of significant duration, culpable for the person's inability to engage in gainful employment. Symbolically, the client must profess his or her disability and have such certified by a qualified physician. Applying for these benefits means formally and symbolically recognizing inability to work, establishing longevity of pattern, and proving that the reason for this circumstance is a mental disorder. In essence, qualifying for income maintenance money means exposing and confronting how disabled and negatively different one really is – or at least presenting to others and self that this is so in order to receive the money. At the same time, the treatment and healing system communicates that in some way, having a psychiatric disorder means that one can not work, and the blame is placed on the disorder. The disability is simultaneously legitimated, predicted, and probably enhanced because the clients then lose many of the motivations they may have had to try to support themselves (Ozawa and Lindsey, 1977).

The paradoxes of disability-connected income are many. In order to relieve pressures that undermine community adjustment, these persons in effect must settle into their disability and lack of social competence. In order to survive outside the stigmatizing sheltered workshop system, they must turn to yet another inadequacy related means of support. These people are asked to socially legitimate their problems in living as a disease and to live a 'sick role' which all agree acts as a deterrent to progress, not an incentive (Lamb and Ragowski 1978).

Another paradox arises from the interpersonal dynamics of income maintenance systems. Among this client group, SSI, VA, and even city welfare represent legitimate sources for subsistence supplies. Yet as a group, the clients consistently express ambivalence: some feel they deserve it, some prefer it to the anxiety of constant money shortages due to sporadic employment, others prefer it to the pressures of work, and still others do not wish to risk the consequences of available alternatives. If one remains within the confines of the social network of other patients and receives SSI just like everyone else, one's esteem and self-value may be less bruised and undermined than if one ventures outside the group to interact with others. Thus, income maintenance money and the attendant feelings about it and self among clients and the community may impede integration into the community at large. In addition, if one does not work in a conventional sense, one may be temporally, spatially, and interpersonally segregated from the community at large and clustered with others such as the aged who are also negatively valued and do not work.

People who work experience time and use space differently. The employed customarily categorize time as either work or leisure; the unemployed cannot share such structure and distinctions. The employed belong in space other than their living space, e.g., offices or plants, and move from one to another, experiencing changes in their roles, identities, and activities. The unemployed often experience no sense of belonging outside their living space or any variety in role, identity, and activity. The unemployed also lack the interpersonal networks that the employed have and develop in the work setting.

Further, without marked and visible physical signs of and reasons for disability, many non-working clients have difficulty legitimizing (to themselves and others) their unemployment and receipt of income maintenance. With very few exceptions, no other group in our society receives long term financial support without the benefit of physical impairment of some kind. These clients then, cannot be consistent with American values about appropriate sick role behavior and dependency legitimated by illness or injury.

Thus, clients are put in the position of consciously or unconsciously proving to themselves and others that they *are* disabled and deserve to be supported in this way. Is it any wonder that self-esteem is low, that many are depressed and see themselves as incompetent? When a system is arranged so that one earns one's livelihood at the expense of low confidence, decreased motivation to change, and negative self-value, is it any wonder that prognosis is poor and that employment rates are low?

Yet what if there were no income maintenance programs? No doubt many of these people would be forced to seek food and shelter in hospitals or burden their families financially and psychologically. The contradictions and paradoxes inherent in this situation are more sociocultural than clinical, yet they influence clinical conditions and create clinical problems.

Antipsychotic Medications

A similar circumstance exists for these clients with regard to the antipsychotic medications that most take. To the outsider, 'meds' represent a vocabulary, set of behaviors and attitudes, and system of feelings and meanings distinctive to the medical, and in particular, psychiatric world. Medications are pervasive in the sociocultural system of clients and staff. Only one of the 43 subjects took no medications at all during the research period. Of the 39 who were consistently receiving meds, 27 were prescribed primarily fluphenazine decanoate, hereafter referred to by its trade name, Prolixin. Six received Prolixin along with lithium carbonate, hereafter referred to as lithium. Three received lithium alone. Two people received phenothiazines other than Prolixin as their primary medication. The other medications prescribed with greatest frequency were side effect medications (Cogentin and Artane), anti-anxiety agents (Valium and Librium), sleeping medications (Dalmane), and anti-depressants. While taking meds represents one of the obvious commonalities among the group, clients differ in their experience with medications, compliance in taking prescribed amounts, and in their attitudes and feelings about 'being on meds'.

Prolixin has an impressive record in controlling clinical schizophrenic symptoms such as delusions, hallucinations, and disordered thinking (Ayd 1975), and a repeatedly substantiated positive influence in prolonging the community tenure of psychiatric patients who comply with dosages (Hogarty et al. 1973; Davis 1975).[6] Lithium likewise has established its efficacy in the treatment and management of major affective disorders (Mendels 1976; Reifman and Wyatt 1980). Both drugs produce side effects among persons who take them. Nausea, diarrhea, general gastrointestinal distress and hand tremor are the most common with lithium, while toxicity and possible renal failure are the most serious. Phenothiazine takers most frequently experience extra-pyramidal symptoms and pseudo-parkinsonian side effects. Pseudoparkinsonism is expressed as akathisia, or general restlessness and jitters, tremor in the limbs, a jiggling or bouncing of the legs when one is seated, or shifting back and forth from foot to foot when standing. The clients called this leg bouncing the "Prolixin Stomp". Other parkinson-like effects are akinesia, or lack of spontaneous facial expressions, feelings of weakness or fatigue; dystonias, or muscle stiffness and spasms, facial grimacing and other involuntary muscle movements, and oculogyric crises or uncontrolled rolling of the eyes up and into the head; general rigidity of limbs, poverty of movement, gait and postural disturbances called by clients and staff the "Mendota Shuffle"; and tardive dyskinesia, a relatively rare, in most cases permanent, irreversible side effect which is expressed as involuntary facial contractions and movements of the tongue, jaw, and mouth not unlike puckering and pursing of the lips, and rolling and flicking of the tongue (Task Force 1980).

In my research group, twenty-nine persons developed side effects, or 85% of those taking phenothiazine medications. One experienced oculogyric crises and three others had developed tardive dyskinesia by the end of the research period. Most of the side effects experienced and displayed by the group are of the stiffness, shakes, and gait disturbance type. It is often hard to distinguish whether the predominant flat facial expression is due to medications or other factors. I observed several occurrences of the eye rolling and had detected the tardive dyskinesia before confirming the diagnoses with the treatment program psychiatrist. Interestingly, none of the clients with tardive dyskinesia mentioned this to me even during our discussions of medications.

In surveying client attitudes and behavior surrounding meds, I constructed four categories (positive, neutral, negative, and ambivalent) which reflect stated feelings and behavior with regard to compliance and side effects, for the two at times conflicted. On the whole, phenothiazine takers were markedly negative to ambivalent about medications and lithium takers were more positive. Phenothiazine takers complained more frequently and bitterly of side effects and were less compliant than those taking lithium. People who most frequently and consistently complied with phenothiazine recommendations thought the medicine actually helped them, did not think the side effects were worse than the benefits of the drug, or simply did not have strong enough feelings in the matter to make a struggle with staff worthwhile. The most non-compliant phenothiazine takers blamed medications for physical discomfort, inability to concentrate or sit still, and did not experience a sufficient alleviation of symptoms to make the side effects worthwhile. Satisfied lithium takers believed (and were told) that they had a biochemical imbalance which caused their problems and which was corrected by taking lithium.

The treatment program staff as a group were deeply convinced of the necessity for medications for their clients, although three staff members had reservations and thought clients should have more freedom in decision making regarding dosage and type of medication. Everyone on the staff was in some way involved in the medication prescribing and delivery system. Client services assistants passed pills, arranged for clients to come in for injections, and at times suggested medications be reviewed for a particular person. Nurses did the same, also giving the injections and setting up packets of daily or weekly self-service medications. The psychiatrist and rotating psychiatric resident did all the formal prescribing and medication monitoring. Negotiations about medications were almost always referred to the physicians, though all staff participated in convincing reluctant persons to take their medications. Families were also enlisted to help as were an occasional employer or landlord. Clients sometimes tried to convince each other to take their medicine; others would urge or encourage refusal. They displayed regular interest in what other persons were taking and sometimes suggested dosage changes based on their companion's behavior. Most of the clients had learned a great deal about medications through years of experience with one or an array of different drugs. I witnessed bitter struggles about medications between staff and clients, and also saw grateful improvement associated with drugs. Every client refused medication at some time during the research period; some in almost ritualistic fashion, voicing the same objections, hearing the same admonitions from staff, and eventually complying with the same ambivalence and resignation.

The multiple paradoxes of medications cluster around their obvious utility in symptom reduction and the attendant side effects and powerful symbolic, personal, and social meanings of the drug (see Amarasingham 1980). The meanings attributed by clients and others to psychotropic medication and the attendant side effects, in my view, contribute to highlighting clients' deficiencies to themselves, and their deficits and differentness to others. The clients are consistently told in multiple ways that they need meds, probably for the rest of their lives, and are also told that they are sick and will probably never 'get well'. The messages they receive are not that with perseverance and care they will be cured. On the contrary, they hear that they will need to take this medicine which makes them feel uncomfortable and will not 'solve' their problems; and that they must take a majority of the responsibility for getting well themselves. Psychotropic medications do not fit neatly into the prevailing medical paradigm of illness – they do not work like antibiotics, resulting in complete or visible cure; they hold out no guarantees, few absolute signs, and require profound effort on the part of the patient in working on emotional and interpersonal problems.

The clients come to see themselves as caught between a non-medicated, positively valued world that is out of reach, and a medicated, conflicting one that identifies them as chronically ill people; people with problems in their heads and lives. Clients may embellish this construction of reality by accepting medications and their disabilities as parts of a permanently crazy self, and then behaving, living, and even thinking like crazy people for they have nothing to lose (see Farina et al. 1978). Other identities and roles being cut off to them, they make the best of it in a passively defiant way by adapting all too successfully to being chronic patients. At times, the same results are achieved when clients like their craziness more than the straight life that they both want and fear or reject (see also Weppner 1973). The reach for another, non-patient identity epitomized by refusing meds and trying to make it on one's own, may be a desire for health, or reveal a wish to be crazy (Van Putten et al. 1976) if that provides an escape from other realities that are negatively perceived and experienced.

The clients from whom I learned are well aware that only crazy people have to take Prolixin and lithium. Normal people do not need to take the meds that they do. The irony is, of course, that in an effort to become more like others — i.e., not take meds — many become more different and psychotic, further removed from non-patienthood and develop more despair and hopelessness about themselves. Nearly all of the clients who refused medications long enough experienced an exacerbation of symptoms and life problems. The admonitions of the staff and others who warned them that they would get crazy if they went off medications were almost always borne out by their own experience. The confusing contradiction is that clients must, if they want to try to get well, carry a badge of illness.

In addition to the above dilemmas, side effects may function as visible markers and badges of differentness to outsiders and of commonality with other clients. Persons who take Prolixin often appear fidgety, flat, nervous, detached, and depressed (See Van Putten and May 1978). Once attention is drawn by these signs, other differences in behavior and comportment are revealed. It is difficult for others to interact with persons who are agitated and depressed (Coates and Wortman 1980), difficult for the clients to sit still and interact with others when they feel the need to move and pace because of akathisia. My experience taking Prolixin confirmed that these are not unimportant factors. I too could not sit through therapy groups and found myself leaving the dinner table, an important sharing and caring place, quicker than usual because I needed to move about. And these are only the minor side effects. What of the person with tardive dyskinesia who had uncontrollable facial grimacing and the woman whose eyes roll up into her head? Again, the paradox is that these drugs that help people to stay out of institutions, may mark, differentiate, and eventually segregate them from large portions of the human community within which they reside because of physical stigmata. Tardive dyskinesia represents a significant risk and cost in sociocultural terms for the thousands of patients who take phenothiazines (See Gardos and Cole 1980; Tepper and Haas 1979).

Another perverse dynamic of meds, similar to the one with subsistence strategies, is the reinforcement of ties with other clients and the impairment of feelings of belonging and comfort with non-clients. This applies not only to side effects such as tardive dyskinesia, but also to medications in general for they represent common ground among clients, like experience, and a topic for mutual commiseration. They tie the most symptomatic with the least symptomatic in association and identity. That is to say, clients who take the same meds often fear or presume that their problems are equivalent to the ones they may observe and disdain in a fellow client. At the same time, one need not be self-conscious about side effects if one remains among others who have them also and will not reject or view you with suspicion on this basis. In these ways, clients may be motivated to confine themselves to social and interpersonal relations with those to whom no explanations or excuses need be made, with those who can understand and share one's discomfort and feelings about meds.

The paradox here is that the group to which one has access and shares similarity is a group of long-term psychiatric clients. The group that one does not perceive as accessible and with whom one has little in common is the presumed normal, non-med taking group. This self- and other-constructed identity and social system perpetuates the patient identity. Those who stay within the network (which can offer positive and helpful factors as well) in relation to meds and also subsistence strategies that put them out of synch with large portions of the community, are exposed not only to the seeming continual failures, problems, inertia, and frustrations of their comrades, but experience their own as well. Taking a symbolic interactionist approach in which reality is negotiated and constructed within and between individuals and groups, it is not difficult to trace the possible sources of enforcement and re-enforcement of chronicity and a chronically crazy life herein. As we see these sociocultural processes revealed, Sapir (1956 [1932] : 151) reminds us that, "The true locus of culture is in the interactions of specific individuals and, on the subjective side, in the world of meanings which each of these individuals may unconsciously abstract for himself from his participation in these interactions." The factors contributing to the birth and healthy infancy of a 'culture of chronicity' in the medications complex just outlined, and the subsistence circumstances discussed previously should startle us all.

I have stressed the differences between clients and the community at large and similarities amongst them. The reason for so doing is to highlight that although community treatment has as one of its primary goals the integration of such persons into community life, the effort has not been terribly successful. I have focused on sociocultural factors among clients and their treaters that are seldom if ever discussed. Clearly, factors that are more external, such as stigma and inadequate funding for services for example, contribute to these processes and situations, but I cannot properly deal with them here.

In a sort of ethnographic overview, I have described how the subsistence strategies and medications experiences of the clients can contribute to re-enforcing their experiences of themselves as negatively different in a community context. These differences are not valued in our sociocultural system — dependency, physical symptoms and stigmata, lack of participation in employment, lack of skill or interest in interaction with others; none of these is held in high esteem amongst us. Yet by virtue of the structure and content of our caring system in part, and the adaptive strategies of clients themselves, the clients are isolated in time, space, and experience from persons who live positvely valued lives. The client who does not work, has no office to go to, no friends at work, and no time schedule to order daily life, does not have an acceptable answer they can offer when a causal acquaintance asks, "What do you do?" They are concentrated spatially, particularly residentially, by their limited incomes, lack of independent living skills, programs designed to help community clients find rooms or apartments, and the reluctance of landlords to rent to persons whose source of income is disability connected and who may appear anxious and different. The client who takes medications may develop visible markers of his or her differentness, may come to feel dependent upon such drugs and thus is perpetually 'sick', never well. The client who rejects the multiple, powerful medications messages often finds him or herself in worse distress than before if medications are ceased.

When I began the research, I sought to describe the lives of the individual clients I encountered through the treatment program. Then, I worked in a sheltered workshop and felt treated as if I were retarded and unreliable. I took Prolixin and got the shakes, felt vulnerable and exposed to those around me as I jiggled my legs, and was unwilling to sit still long enough to really make contact with someone because I felt the need to pace. The daily distresses of my companions and the staff members who worked with such persistent effort and good intentions against such overwhelming factors with so little success, darkened my whole outlook on life. Consequently, I altered my interest to trying to understand how and why it was that the clients I knew were trapped, by themselves and others, into a chronic course of patienthood.

I am convinced that psychosis occurs universally, but do not think that chronicity develops with such frequency, regularity, and great cost as it does within the confines of our sociocultural system (see also Waxler 1977, 1979). Data from the World Health Organization's Follow-Up Study of the International Pilot Study of Schizophrenia (WHO 1979; Sartorius et al. 1977, 1978) confirm this hypothesis. The paradoxical circumstances I have described briefly above are confounding, confusing, and immobilizing enough to me and others who do not experience marked thought and mood disorders. One can imagine their effects upon those whose thinking and reacting capacities are different and limited. Curing or altering a sociocultural system is quite a different task than treating a disease, or doing therapy with individuals and groups. Yet that is what community psychiatric treaters are confronted with, and they and all the rest of us have helped to create the situation, consciously and unconsciously, culturally and clinically.

CLINICAL APPLICATIONS AND IMPLICATIONS OF THE RESEARCH

Short of profound sociocultural change, disconnecting the complex circuits of chronicity I have outlined requires much more research and trial and error in clinical settings, with small steps in focused areas. In this concluding section of the chapter, I will first set down what I believe to be appropriate and successful tactics in doing clinically relevant research. Then I will report both actual and potential clinical applications of this research.

Research Tactics

First and foremost it is important to work in collaboration and not competition with clinicians and mental health professionals in planning, executing, and applying research. The accusations and exposes that typify the history of social science research in psychiatric settings result from research which is biased and poorly

planned from the outset and will not be heard by those who need to listen (see
Weinstein 1979). Careful research which is well documented and clearly communicated will have more impact, even if the findings are not entirely congratulatory to
the treatment system. Participating in the clinical application of results is imperative, if the researcher is able or allowed to do so. Making suggestions that are
directly germane to the particular setting consumate the partnership with the
clinician and convince him or her of the utility of the research. For example, after
participating in social skills groups twice a week for one year, I suggested to the
staff group leaders that some of the social skills they were teaching were not always
relevant to the social settings of the clients. Instead of practicing how to introduce
oneself to someone at a party, we needed to work on how to handle someone who
was aggressively hustling money on the street or in a rooming house. "Assertive"
behavior at times was not appropriate to the setting. The clients needed to learn
how to be heard and respected, even if this meant being aggressive or angry. So we
began to focus on how to say no when someone was constantly bumming cigarettes,
or threateningly asking for money or sexual contact.

   Along the same lines, it is important not to overestimate and oversell the potential findings of this type of research in any given clinical setting. It is not adequately
clear at this time how important sociocultural factors are in the etiology, perpetua-
tion, and recovery from psychic distress and severe disorder. I think it is more
prudent to take an exploratory, inductive stance rather than approaching one's
subject with a strictly social model of mental illness in mind. We need not stake
out professional turf by espousing single cause theories or by paying lip service
to biological theories and then neglecting to incorporate them in our work. I
am impressed with recent advances in work in genetics, neurochemistry, and
biochemistry in tracking down fundamental processes in the major psychiatric
disorders (See Schizophrenia Bulletin 1980). Our utility in the psychiatric arena is
not undermined by these findings. If we expect to be full partners in the psychiatric
research enterprise, and if we expect medical personnel to take heed of *our* perspective, we are obligated to learn equally from them.

   The research period should be as extensive as funding and design allow. One
earns credentials with clinicians and clients and deepens understanding of the
research arena with long-term involvement. At the same time, one needs to resist
becoming too enculturated, losing one's naivete, or fading into a clinical role.
The temptations are strong but need to be resisted. Feeling out of place and that
everyone else has a role or job and is doing something worthwhile and visible, is to
be expected, especially in the clinical setting. But the anthropologists' roles are to
be in and out of the system at the same time, to *not* lose the perspective of the
outsider as we experience the insideness. Identifying too closely with either patients
or staff, unless one group is the focus for research, will obscure sociocultural factors
and lessen the validity of the findings. I found that when I was feeling aligned with
one group against the other, thinking about why I felt that way and seeking events
and processes that led to those feelings helped me to discover important parts of
the ethnographic scene. For example, when I felt angry with a staff person for

pushing medications very persuasively with a client who desperately wanted to refuse, I became aware upon reflection of the plight of both parties and realized that my anger stemmed from the helplessness and powerlessness of any of us to do anything about the dilemma.

Preparation for clinical fieldwork and research in the psychiatric area in particular should include clinical experience with patients in a variety of settings, at best supervised by a clinician, at least combined with reading and discussing current theory and practice in the field with colleagues. Without this prior learning process, one is tempted to react strongly to circumstances which could be integrated into an understanding approach, rather than a reactive one. One cannot, for instance, understand a staff person's perspective and apparent calmness upon having to place a patient in seclusion if this is the first time one has seen such an action taken or is so involved in one's own reactions as to be unable to observe the responses and behaviors of others. Learning about the clinical area is also important because one cannot contribute pertinent research material without knowing the important and complicated issues current in the field. Psychiatric research in particular has attracted a number of insufficiently trained social scientists whose work often needlessly replicates previous findings, neglecting to address itself to newer and more pertinent questions (Estroff 1978).

Research Implications and Applications

There are certainly more implications than easy applications of the findings of my research. Many of the understandings that accompany the ethnographic perspective point to factors that are complexly interwoven and outside the influence of the clinician. Perhaps the most productive, general, and simple application has been communicating the findings to clinical personnel in the field. This initiates their own critical analysis of their roles in creating and perpetuating paradoxes for their clients. Once sensitized, staff members can share with each other and patients a sense of empathy and commonality previously unacknowledged. The same process holds true for teaching residents and medical students. Given this type of view of their clinical behavior and the results, they are more apt to think about cultural correlates and consequences.

More specifically, we have found that educating patients about medication side effects, the actual pharmacologic properties of the drugs, and various interpersonal factors that contribute to refusal helps with compliance. The medication process can also be made more therapeutic by encouraging clients to ask questions about meds, participate actively in determining dosage, and listening attentively as they describe their physical and emotional reactions to meds. In addition, having a medications group where clients talk with each other and staff members about their experiences with and feelings about medications has proved useful. The group can become a social event for clients and many attend and get their Prolixin injections more regularly. Another means of applying the findings has been to work directly with clients to help them gain control of side effects. Many are unaware of how they look and videotaping with role playing and practicing sitting still, responding more fully facially, and relaxation therapy for those with tremor seems beneficial. The general acknowledgement of the power of medications beyond the biological level is extremely helpful.

Subsistence strategies represent a more difficult arena within which to make adjustments because factors within the mental health system are so influential. However, we have explored several possibilities. One of these is job sharing. For clients who can not concentrate or manage the stresses of working eight hours a day at a well paying, interesting job, sharing the job with others so that each works for two to four hours is an option. This requires adjustments and cooperation from employers and coworkers, but opens the door for work that is a worthwhile alternative to income maintenance. On the other hand, group and individual therapy work around the issues of loss of self-esteem, guilt, ambivalence and inadequacy for those receiving income maintenance has proved helpful in diluting some of the negative effects. Conceptualizing income maintenance in more benign ways and directly confronting the social and stigmatizing issues can alleviate anxieties and stress that further immobilize and trouble these clients. Acknowledgment of the legitimacy of clients' feelings about sheltered employment also goes a long way in avoiding power struggles between clients and staff about working in these places. The disincentives built into the income maintenance system will not be removed easily and require efforts at all levels: clinical, legislative, bureaucratic and community.

One of the most paradoxical and detrimental features of the American mental health treatment system is the continuing asymmetry and differential access to power and resources between givers and receivers of help, between staff and patients. Clients cannot achieve independence, positive self-experience, and confidence in their ability to manage their lives when they are consistently and deeply involved on the receiving and from persons who control almost all aspects of the relationship. Patient controlled alternative treatment programs (Chamberlain 1978) offer a promising development. Not all patients are willing or able to participate, but many can take credit for their own successes and failures, experience themselves as both givers end receivers of help, and provide less costly caring when encouraged to manage their own and their fellows' treatment. Short of such a radical departure from the norm, treatment staffs will want to consider giving up some of their power, facilitating the participation of clients in the delivery of care, and the actual equal partnership of clients in the design, management, and change of programs. Clinical personnel need to examine their own investments in maintaining the power differentials and espousing of their own value systems (Lamb 1979b). This task will prove to be perhaps the most difficult for then the clinical subsistence strategy becomes less viable. But as long as there are professional clinicians treating psychiatric clients such as those discussed in this chapter, there will inevitably be professional patients.

The challenges rising out of the implications and applications of this research are clear. Are we willing to dismantle some of the expressions of profound cultural ambivalence toward the negatively different that are so evident in our treatment system? Can we sort out the contradictory indications that confuse and immobilize patients and adopt beliefs and behaviors that are more benevolent and consistent? Surely, the changes will not come easily and there will be more paradoxical and unintended consequences to contend with even as we progress. Without an attempt at this, in the decades to come we will still be wondering why schizophrenics in Nigeria have prognoses so much more promising than those in our midst.

NOTES

1. We may distinguish among four potentially overlapping categories of patients who have been and are affected by de-institutionalization. These are: (1) Long term hospital residents who were discharged, (2) Patients with multiple and episodic hospital admissions and psychotic episodes who sought periodic asylum, support, and subsistence from hospitalization, now treated almost exclusively on an out-patient basis with short, crisis-oriented admissions, (3) Patients who have not had extensive in-hospital experience but who are consistent consumers of out-patient community treatment, and (4) First break or 'one time' acutely distressed persons who may not be hospitalized now when they would have been before, or hospitalized only briefly. The first two groups have been the focus of *de*-institutionization while the second two represent benefactors of *non*-institutionalization efforts. Both groups have been targeted for community treatment.
2. The anthropologist should avoid the wholesale use of clinical classifications in referring to clinical research subjects, especially in the psychiatric area. S/he should be knowledgeable and aware of these categories, but most avoid the ethnographic error of accepting these cultural codifications of the predominant healing-belief system as if they held universal validity. This caution is especially pertinent in the Western medical setting where we tend to forget that Western medicine is but one of many cosmological, behavioral, and belief systems concerned with healing. In order to maintain anthropological and theoretical integrity without becoming 'converted', one needs to develop alternative, socioculturally sensitive and sophisticated terminology.
3. However, this could hardly be attributed solely to successful treatment. Changes in legal commitment standards which set the criteria for involuntary detention very high, parallel alterations in clinical thresholds for ordering hospital admission, and reductions in funding for in-patient services combined with a proliferation of out-patient, crisis, and day care services no doubt account for much of the difference. In other words, social and structural mechanisms are also keeping patients out of hospitals, not necessarily improvements in their clinical conditions. Persons with moderate to severe levels of psychiatric disturbance can survive, albeit questionably, without being hospitalized. But, mental health care professionals may have changed their attitudes and practices and social structural factors may have been altered as much or more than patients have improved.
4. The exception to this rule was the serious possibility of imminent suicide.
5. Due to research design in the treatment program, patients were not allowed to live with their families of origin and contact was monitored and supervised by the treatment program staff. Families were also encouraged not to lend their offspring money or bail them out of scarcities in subsistence supplies.
6. Recently, this view has been challenged by research findings that demonstrate few significant differences in relapse between phenothiazine, in particular fluphenazine, takers and non-takers and persons on placebo. Gardos and Cole (1976) reviewed the maintenance drug therapy research and found that as many as 50% of the people who were taking phenothiazines could survive in the community without them. Schooler et al. (1980) found no significant differences in relapse and adjustment measures between patients taking injectable versus oral Prolixin; the assumption being that the people in the oral group compiled less

well than those in the injectable group where compliance was carefully monitored. Linn et al. (1979) and Hogarty et al. (1979) report that phenothiazines did not significantly alter social adjustment and that agitation and depression, which may have been due in part to side effects, was high among their subjects. Agitated depression as a side effect has been investigated by Van Putten and May (1978) who found that depressive symptomatology decreased when phenothiazine takers were given side effect medication. Thus at present, the utility and necessity of phenothiazines in outpatient maintenance therapy are being questioned.

<h2 style="text-align:center">REFERENCES</h2>

Amarasingham, Lorna Rhodes
   1980 Social and Cultural Perspectives on Medication Refusal. American Journal of Psychiatry 137: 3: 353–358.
Anthony, William A., Mikal R. Cohen, and Ray Vitalo
   1978 The Measurement of Rehabilitation Outcome. Schizophrenia Bulletin 4: 3: 365–383.
Aviram, Uri and Steven P. Segal
   1973 Exclusion of the Mentally Ill: Reflection of an Old Problem in a New Context. Archives of General Psychiatry 29: 126–131.
Ayd, Frank
   1975 The Depot Fluphenazines: A Reappraisal After 10 Years Clinical Experience. American Journal of Psychiatry 132: 5: 491ff.
Bachrach, Leona
   1976 De-institutionalization: An Analytic Review and Sociological Perspective. NIMH Division of Biometry and Epidemiology, Survey and Reports Branch, Series D, No. 4.
Bateson, Gregory, Donald Jackson, and Jay Haley
   1956 Toward a Theory of Schizophrenia. Behavioral Science 1: 251–264.
Blackwell, Barry
   1973 Drug Therapy: Patient Compliance. New England Journal of Medicine 289: 5: 249–252.
Caplan, Ruth B. and Gerald Caplan
   1969 Psychiatry and the Community in 19th Century America: The Recurring Concern with the Environment in the Prevention and Treatment of Mental Illness. New York: Basic Books.
Caudill, William
   1958 The Psychiatric Hospital as a Small Society. Cambridge, Mass.: Harvard University Press.
Chamberlain, Judi
   1978 On Our Own: Patient Controlled Alternatives to the Mental Health System. New York: McGraw-Hill.
Coates, Dan and Camille Wortman
   1980 Depression Maintenance and Interpersonal Control. In A. Baum, Y. Epstein, and J. Singer (eds.), Advances in Environmental Psychology, Chapter 7. New York: Lawrence Erlbaum.
Davis, John M.
   1975 Overview: Maintenance Therapy in Psychiatry: I: Schizophrenia. American Journal of Psychiatry 132: 1237–1245.
   1976 Recent Developments in the Treatment of Schizophrenia. Psychiatric Annals 6: 1: 71–111.

Edgerton, Robert B.
  1980 Traditional Treatment for Mental Illness in Africa: A Review. Culture, Medicine and Psychiatry 4: 2: 167–189.
Erikson, Kai T.
  1957 Patient Role and Social Uncertainty – A Dilemma of the Mentally Ill. Psychiatry 20: 363–375.
Estroff, Sue E.
  1978 The Anthropology-Psychiatry Fantasy: Can We Make It a Reality? Transcultural Psychiatric Research Review XV, October: 209–213.
  1981 Making It Crazy: An Ethnography of Psychiatric Clients in an American Community. Berkeley and Los Angeles: University of California Press.
Farina, Amerigo, Jeffrey Fisher, Herbert Getter, and Edward Fischer
  1978 Some Consequences of Changing People's Views Regarding the Nature of Mental Illness. Journal of Abnormal Psychology 87: 2: 272–279.
Gardos, George and Jonathon O. Cole
  1976 Maintenance Antipsychotic Therapy: Is the Cure Worse than the Disease? American Journal of Psychiatry 133: 32–36.
  1980 Overview: Public Health Issues in Tardive Dyskinesia. American Journal of Psychiatry 137: 7: 776–781.
Goffman, Erving
  1971 The Insanity of Place. In Relations in Public: Microstudies of the Public Order. New York: Basic Books, pp. 335–390.
Group for the Advancement of Psychiatry (GAP)
  1978 The Chronic Mental Patient in the Community. Vol. X, Publication No. 102. New York: G.A.P.
Henry, Jules
  1964 Space and Power on a Psychiatric Unit. In A. F. Wessen (ed.), The Psychiatric Hospital as a Social System, Springfield, Illinois: Charles B. Thomas, pp. 20–34.
  1973 Pathways to Madness. New York: Vintage Books.
Hogarty, Gerard E., Solomon Goldberg, and the Collaborative Study Group
  1973 Drug and Sociotherapy in the Aftercare of Schizophrenic Patients. Archives of General Psychiatry 28: 1: 54–64.
Hogarty, Gerard E., Nina R. Schooler, Richard Ulrich, Frank Mussare, Peregrino Ferro, and Eileen Herron
  1979 Fluphenazine and Social Therapy in the Aftercare of Schizophrenic Patients. Archives of General Psychiatry 36: 1283–1294.
Jules-Rosette, Benetta
  1978 The Veil of Objectivity: Prophesy, Divination, and Social Inquiry. American Anthropologist 80: 3: 549–570.
Kochhar, Satya
  1979 Blind and Disabled Persons Awarded Federally Administered SSI Payments, 1975. Social Security Bulletin 42: 6: 13–23.
Lamb, H. Richard
  1979a The New Asylums in the Community. Archives of General Psychiatry 36: 2: 129–138.
  1979b Roots of Neglect of the Long-Term Mentally Ill. Psychiatry 42: 3: 201–207.
Lamb, H. Richard and A. S. Ragowski
  1978 Supplemental Security Income and Sick Role. American Journal of Psychiatry 135: 10: 1221–1224.
Levine, Daniel S. and Dianne R. Levine
  1975 The Cost of Mental Illness. DHEW Publication No. (ADM) 76-265. Washington, D.C.: U.S. Government Printing Office.

Linn, Margaret W., E. M. Caffey, J. Klett, G. E. Hogarty, and H. R. Lamb
    1979 Day Treatment and Psychotropic Drugs in the Aftercare of Schizophrenic Patients.
          Archives of General Psychiatry 36: 1055–1066.
Ludwig, Arnold
    1971 Treating the Treatment Failures: The Challenge of Chronic Schizophrenia. New
          York: Grune and Stratton.
Mechanic, David
    1977 Illness Behavior, Social Adaptation, and the Management of Illness. Research and
          Analytic Report Series No. 9–76. Madison: University of Wisconsin Center for
          Medical Sociology and Health Services Research.
Mendels, John
    1976 Lithium in the Treatment of Depression. American Journal of Psychiatry 133: 4:
          373–378.
Minkoff, Kenneth
    1978 A Map of the Chronic Mental Patient. In J. A. Talbott (ed.), The Chronic Mental
          Patient, Washington, D.C.: American Psychiatric Association, pp. 11–38.
Ozawa, Martha N. and Duncan Lindsey
    1977 Is SSI Too Supportive of the Mentally Ill? Public Welfare 35: 4: 48–52.
Reifman, Ann and Richard J. Wyatt
    1980 Lithium: A Brake in the Rising Cost of Mental Illness. Archives of General Psychiatry
          37: 4: 385–388.
Reynolds, David K. and Norman L. Farberow
    1977 Endangered Hope: Experiences in Psychiatric Aftercare Facilities. Berkeley and Los
          Angeles: University of California Press.
Sapir, Edward
    1932 Cultural Anthropology and Psychiatry. Journal of Abnormal Social Psychology
          27: 229–242.
Sartorius, Norman, A. Jablensky, and R. Shapiro
    1977 Two-year Follow-up of the Patients Included in the WHO International Pilot Study
          of Schizophrenia. Psychological Medicine 7: 529–541.
    1978 Cross-cultural Differences in the Short-Term Prognosis of Schizophrenic Psychoses.
          Schizophrenia Bulletin 4: 102–113.
Schizophrenia Bulletin
    1980 Conference Proceedings: Schizophrenia and Platelet Monoamine Oxidase, 6, 2.
Schooler, Nina R., Jerome Levine, Joann B. Severe, Benjamin Barauger, Alberto DiMascio,
Gerald L. Klerman, and Vincente Tuascon
    1980 Prevention of Relapse in Schizophrenia: An Evaluation of Fluphenazine Decanoate.
          Archives of General Psychiatry 37: 1: 16–24.
Segal, Steven P. and Uri Aviram
    1978 The Mentally Ill in Community Based Sheltered Care: A Study of Community Care
          and Social Integration. New York: John Wiley and Sons.
Segal, Steven P., J. Baumohl, and E. W. Moyles
    1980 Neighborhood Types and Community Reaction to the Mentally Ill: A Paradox of
          Intensity. Journal of Health and Social Behavior 21: 4: 345–359.
Sokolousky, Jay, et al.
    1978 Personal Networks of Ex-Mental Patients in A Manhattan S.R.D. Hotel. Human
          Organization, Spring.
Stein, Leonard I. and Mary Ann Test
    1980 Alternative to Mental Hospital Treatment. I. Conceptual Model, Treatment Program,
          and Clinical Evaluation. Archives of General Psychiatry 37: 4: 392–397.
Talbott, John A. (ed.)
    1978 The Chronic Mental Patient. Problems, Solutions, and Recommendations for Public
          Policy. Washington, D.C.: American Psychiatric Association.

Talbott, John A.
1979 Care of the Chronically Mentally Ill – Still a National Disgrace. American Journal of Psychiatry 136: 5: 688–689.
1980 Toward a Public Policy on the Chronic Mentally Ill Patient. American Journal of Orthopsychiatry 50: 1: 43–53.
Task Force on Late Neurological Effects of Antipsychotic Drugs
1980 Tardive Dyskinesia: A Summary of a Task Force Report of the American Psychiatric Association. American Journal of Psychiatry 137: 10: 1163–1172.
Tepper, Stewart J. and J. F. Haas
1979 Prevalence of Tardive Dyskinesia. Journal of Clinical Psychiatry 40: 508–516.
Test, Mary Ann and Leonard I. Stein
1978 Community Treatment of the Chronic Patient: Research Overview. Schizophrenia Bulletin 4: 350–364.
Van Putten, Theodore
1974 Why do Schizophrenic Patients Refuse to Take Their Drugs? Archives of General Psychiatry 31: 1: 67–72.
Van Putten, Theodore, Evelyn Crompton, and Coralee Yale
1976 Drug Refusal in Schizophrenia and the Wish to be Crazy. Archives of General Psychiatry 33: 1443–1446.
Van Putten, Theodore and Phillip May
1978 Akinetic Depression in Schizophrenia. Archives of General Psychiatry 35: 9: 1101–1111.
Waxler, Nancy
1977 Is Mental Illness Cured in Traditional Societies? A Theoretical Analysis. Culture, Medicine and Psychiatry 1: 3: 243–254.
1979 Is Outcome for Schizophrenia Better in Non-Industrialized Societies: The Case of Sri Lanka. Journal of Nervous and Mental Disease 167: 144–158.
Weinstein, Raymond M.
1979 Patient Attitudes toward Mental Hospitalization. A Review of the Quantitative Research. Journal of Health and Social Behavior 20: 237–258.
Weppner, Richard S.
1973 An Anthropological View of the Street Addict's World. Human Organization 32: 2: 111–121.
Witkin, Michael J.
1980 Trends in Patient Care Episodes in Mental Health Facilities, 1955–1977. Mental Health Statistical Note No. 154. Washington, D.C.: Department of Health and Human Services, Division of Biometry and Epidemiology, Survey and Reports Branch.
World Health Organization (WHO)
1979 Schizophrenia: An International Follow-Up Study. New York: John Wiley and Sons.

ELIZABETH L. BYERLY AND CRAIG A. MOLGAARD

SOCIAL INSTITUTIONS AND DISEASE TRANSMISSION

We must always keep in mind that medicine is not a natural science, either pure or applied. Methods of science are used all the time in combating disease, but medicine itself belongs much more to the realm of the social sciences because the goal is social. Medicine, by promoting health and preventing illness, endeavors to keep individuals adjusted to their environment as useful and contented members of society. Or by restoring health and rehabilitating the former patient, it endeavors to readjust individuals to their environment. – Henry Sigerist (cited in Clark 1967: 1)

INTRODUCTION

Sigerist's admonition is perhaps more applicable in the present context of public health and preventive medicine than ever before. Since the first volume of Johann Peter Frank's *System einer vollstandigen medizinischen Polizey* appeared in 1779 (Holland and Wainwright 1979), the impetus to examine the impact of the social environment upon the individual, and the individual's adaptation to that environment, has continued to influence the field of public health. Notable in this regard is the most recent edition of the classic *Maxcy-Rosenau Public Health and Preventive Medicine* (1980). This volume now contains seven chapters on behavioral factors in relation to health.

Our perception of the anthropologist's contribution to public health is straightforward. It is in the production of descriptive data to aid problem solving by public health personnel in the specific area of group adaptive behaviors concerning illness. Our emphasis is on the social rather than the demographic aspects of disease occurence in human communities, and therefore pertains to social epidemiology.

The epidemiologist is concerned with the distribution of disease within a population, its causes, and the development of preventive measures. The anthropologist is also concerned with distribution, cause, and prevention, but, in addition, with the cognitive and behavioral patterns of population groups which affect occurrence and transmission of disease or illness.[1] Social behavior and cultural practices frequently function as risk factors in disease process. We will attempt to show that the response of a human group to physical indisposition (real or potential) in terms of prevailing world view and values has as much to do with the pattern of illness in a community as do other environmental components.

During the course of field research concerning the health of migrant farm workers in Washington state, our contact with a rural alternative healing commune coincided with an outbreak of type A, infectious hepatitis among members of the commune. Our data describing the lifestyle, world view, social networks, and travel patterns of this group will be used here to illustrate how one of their social institutions, the New Age "gathering", has a latent function as a risk factor in disease transmission.

N. J. Chrisman and T. W. Maretzki (eds.), Clinically Applied Anthropology, 395–409.

RESEARCH BACKGROUND

Our data were obtained during a three-year (1977–1980) federally-funded investigation of health-related behaviors and decision-making among a multiethnic population of migrant farm workers in north central Washington state. Ethnic groups studied were Mexican, Mexican-American, American Indian, Anglo-American, and New Age counterculture. The focus of this research project was the comparative investigation of health care systems within one delineated occupational group.

The study employed standard anthropological methods of participation and interview, including ethnoscience techniques. These methods were used to discover those points in the belief systems of the target groups where there was choice-making, revealing (1) maximum divergence or contradiction with biomedical beliefs, and/or (2) maximum convergence or overlap of systems. Ethnoscience methods obtained data primarily from the orientation of the informants, rather than from the viewpoints of health professionals.

One goal was to ascertain decision-making pertaining to health-seeking through a formal and cognitive approach to perceptual and classificatory resources in the domain of health. Nursing interventions were later proposed on the basis of these findings. Operationalization of the methods used in the study appear in detail elsewhere (Molgaard and Byerly 1981). In all, over 164 individuals provided some form of data concerning migrant health to the investigators during the period of this project.

Ethnoscience interviews were constructed so as to obtain classificatory data in regard to sickness, causation, healers, therapies, and preventions for each of the ethnic groups. Some questions produced short answers, some long lists of lexemes, and some long narratives. An interview schedule, question-frame elicitation, and the card-sort procedure provided sufficient structure to obtain data in areas of interest, but also to allow flexibility for validating responses by relevant inquiry and participant observation.

Sample

The group of New Age people discussed in this paper (N=17) were migrant and seasonal agricultural workers employed in various aspects of orchard work. They had organized a New Age healing center (pseudonym "Agni Circle") in a small rural town, and offered a variety of holistic healing classes and therapies for themselves and for more transient members of their subculture. Medical philosophies of this subculture include aspects of Ayurvedic, Chinese, Native American, homeopathic, naturopathic, and chiropractic medicine. The emergence of the New Age groups from the earlier counterculture, the New Age emphasis on communalism, spiritualism, and healing as a lifestyle *per se*, and the unifying motif of "energy" or spiritual force have been discussed elsewhere (Molgaard 1979; Molgaard, Byerly and Snow 1979; Byerly, Molgaard and Snow 1979; and Molgaard, Golbeck and Byerly 1979). Interpretations of New Age health beliefs and behavior presented here are based on one and one-half years of research with members of this healing commune.

Social Environment

Of particular importance to our interpretation of the hepatitis outbreak are three elements of the New Age environment: the network of New Age communities in the Pacific Northwest, the value placed on mobility by these people, and the New Age healing gathering circuit.

The network of New Age communities. New Age subculture in the Northwest consists of an interconnected and intercommunicating network of rural and urban communes dedicated to a spiritual life-style and holistic healing. During the course of the field work with Agni Circle healing center, we became aware of the existence of over one hundred separate New Age communities scattered throughout British Columbia, Washington, Oregon, Idaho, and Northern California. There were undoubtedly many more of which we were not aware. Although these communes were diverse in terms of group focus and overlapped in function, members of the groups were involved at the most general level with the integration of somatic, spiritual, and psychological healing systems.

Communication among the New Age communities in the Northwest was maintained in three ways. One was through an exchange of newsletters, bulletins and announcements; some groups maintained mailing lists for such purposes. A second means was the result of travel of individuals between communes; and a third consisted of new and renewed contacts made at New Age gatherings.

The value placed on mobility. The value placed on physical transiency was expressed by New Age people in two ways: (1) in-state and out-of-state occupational travel, and (2) avocational travel. In the Northwest, many New Age persons earned a marginal living from migrant and seasonal farm work. Occupational travel within Washington, for example, consisted of a search for organic or near-organic orchards in which to work. Occupational travel out-of-state, by individuals temporarily without communal ties, often followed migrant paths along the West Coast similar to those of Hispanic, American Indian, and other Anglo farm workers. Beginning in California in early spring, they traveled north into Oregon and Washington, and sometimes into Idaho and Montana, for field and tree fruit harvests. Some worked for part of the summer on coastal fishing boats, then moved to eastern Washington in early fall for the apple harvest. Many headed for the warmer climate of California and the Southwest at the onset of winter, although a few remained in Washington to work in packing sheds or at pruning and other miscellaneous winter jobs in agriculture.

Avocational travel occurred during the "off-season" and was often a pilgrimage to other New Age healing centers, schools, or recognized "masters of healing" for continued instruction in the spiritual and healing arts. During the course of this research, different members of Agni Circle journeyed in search of such instruction to Oregon, California, New Mexico, Colorado, Massachusetts, and Canada; and one member traveled to Great Britain.

The fluidity of the subculture in the Northwest was largely dependent on the fact that healing communes such as the Agni Circle fulfilled a number of vital functions for the individual transient. Aside from providing food and shelter and a personal support network, they functioned as a communication center for this widely dispersed and mobile population. As one member of Agni Circle said:

I mean, we are mountain people, migrant people. And we don't collect together very often, so you kind of lose track of being part of a bigger thing. But when you come to Agni, for instance, and you read our letters, and you see how much mail comes in and how many people are all over, or you hang out here for a month and you see how many people come through the door, it gives you an identity of being a part of something that is bigger than yourself. It's kind of reassuring to know that there are other folks doing the same type of things that you are doing, and that you are in somewhat the same headspace. You don't feel so lonely, even though you are isolated and alone where you happen to live your life. You are still part of a greater whole. Unless there is some way of that whole communicating with itself, you don't know about it.

The subcultural focus on alternative medical and religious systems was also structured in terms of the value placed on transience by New Age people. The ideal healing commune, as with all New Age institutions, was conceived of as being extremely short-lived, so that any sort of organizational inertia inhibiting personal and spiritual movement would not have a chance to limit personal growth. The life span of Agni Circle *per se* was approximately three years, although members still remain in contact.

The gathering circuit. The New Age gathering is an important social institution of this subculture. In general, a gathering is a festival of variable size sponsored by one or more communes, with the purpose of exchanging information, ideas, therapies, spiritual practices, or commodities currently in vogue in the New Age milieu. Gatherings are usually held in isolated rural settings, last from one to five days, and may be attended by anywhere from twenty-five to several thousand people. More established communes hold them every year; one group in New Mexico had done so for five years and another in Colorado for three years. Other groups in British Columbia sponsored them on an annual basis. The Agni Circle organized three such events during the period of our research. One, which we attended, took place in May of 1978, and two others were held during the springs of 1979 and 1980. All three were healing gatherings and were heavily attended, with an average of about one thousand participants at each.

Most pilgrims to the healing gatherings come from New Age communities. It is not unusual for people to travel over one thousand miles to attend. Participants travel alone or in small groups. Many hitchhike; others drive or share rides.

In the Northwest, the usual gathering circuit covers a period from mid-March to late October and consists of several annual events, plus other less well-known and spontaneous gatherings which have potential for evolving into annual events. The 1977 circuit began with the Spring Festival of Awareness in early March in British Columbia. This was followed by the Agni Circle Gathering of Healers in May in central Washington, the Rainbow Gathering of Healing in July in southern Oregon, the Mid-Summer Gathering of Healing in Idaho, the Ashtanga Yoga Retreat during August in British Columbia, the October Bonner's Ferry Midwife and Birthing Gathering in Idaho, and the Northern Washington Barter Fair held during October.

The gatherings varied in focus, but all were spiritually oriented. Some, such as the Spring Festival of Awareness and the Mid-Summer Gathering, combined spiritual and healing interests with celebration of changes in seasons. Others, such as the Agni Circle and Bonner's Ferry gatherings, were more heavily oriented toward exchange of information via workshops, lectures, and demonstrations of holistic health therapeutic lore.

The Barter Fair was a festival observing the end of apple harvest in Washington and celebrated barter as a valid means of economic exchange. Fair participants traded craft products, herbs, garden produce, and other food without the aid of money, in simulation of an economic system which, it is believed, would exist during the coming spiritual "new" age. It was at such a fair in 1977 that three members of the Agni Circle contracted infectious hepatitis.

HEPATITIS

Viral hepatitis is a major public health problem in the United States today, with over 55,000 cases reported to the Center for Disease control in 1975. In that many cases are not diagnosed, diagnosed but not reported, or asymptomatic, the annual incidence is actually much higher. We discovered the incompleteness of these morbidity rates when we attempted to determine the incidence of hepatitis A for late 1977 and early 1978, the time period when Agni Circle people were sick. Neither state nor county epidemiologists could give us complete statistics for this period; the local migrant health project had none at all. We knew, of course, that only one of our informants had contacted a physician when she became ill, and then only to confirm what the remainder of the group had already diagnosed as hepatitis.

Two epidemiologically distinct types of viral hepatitis have traditionally been recognized: type A, commonly known as infectious hepatitis, and type B, or serum hepatitis. Evidence continues to accumulate that a third type of viral hepatitis (non-A/non-B hepatitis) also exists (WHO Chronicle 1980). The primary mode of transmission of type A is through the fecal-oral route, usually food-borne from an infected food handler. In situations where sanitation is a problem and/or water has been contaminated, occasional outbreaks of infectious hepatitis may occur. Children and young adults, particularly males, are most common victims. Type B, or serum hepatitis, is commonly believed to be transmitted parenterally, but there is evidence of occasional person-to-person transmission. Tests for Australian antigen, a viruslike particle in the blood of victims of type B, help differentiate hepatitis B from A (Luckmann and Sorensen 1980: 1495).

Infectious hepatitis has a short incubation period; jaundice appears approximately one month after exposure and lasts about three weeks. The infectious period lasts roughly from three weeks prior to development of jaundice to three weeks after. Standard gamma globulin, if it is to provide immunity to persons known to be exposed, must be given within two weeks of exposure to the virus. Symptoms commonly observed are jaundice, clay-colored stools, darkened urine, rash or pruritis, right-upper-quadrant pain, fever, anorexia, nausea and vomiting, fatigue and weakness. Although prolonged bedrest is often prescribed, the best guide to activity restriction appears to be avoidance of fatigue. Dietary recommendations include an adequate caloric intake, taking into consideration problems of nausea, vomiting, and anorexia. A balanced diet is encouraged. Recovery is usually complete, and immunity specific to type A hepatitis is conferred.

The New Age episode. In October 1977, immediately prior to our first contact with the Agni Circle, members of this commune journeyed to the Barter Fair, held that year in north central Washington. While there, three (two men and one woman) of the seventeen members of the commune were apparently infected by hepatitis type A viruses, probably present in food or water from the communal eating and drinking facilities characteristic of New Age gatherings. At the close of the fair, they and other members of Agni Circle returned to the commune. One of the infected men, however, left immediately to attend a holistic healing school in a west coast city. Within a month, recognizable symptoms of hepatitis had developed to some degree in all three adults and in the five-year old daughter of the woman. The commune of seventeen persons was soon the site of a minor epidemic of hepatitis, and another New Age community, the healing school attended by the above young man, was exposed to the illness. At the height of the hepatitis episode in Agni Circle, eight of the fifteen adults and the two children became ill. In all, ten of the seventeen members were victims of the illness. Three appeared to have contracted it at the fair and, in turn, infected other commune members after returning home.

Therapeutic response to the illness by persons in the healing center was characteristically varied. Following a tentative diagnosis by Circle members that the malady in question was hepatitis, one young woman sought and received confirmation from a local physician. Standard medical referral was then made to a public health nurse, who contacted the group to offer preventive gamma globulin for those who had been exposed, and to suggest rest and dietary prescriptions (a high caloric diet) for those who were ill.

Those who refused the preventive injection relied instead on a New Age therapy called the "liver flush", a prophylaxis composed of citrus juices, garlic, olive oil, and cayenne. This was said to cleanse the liver of toxins and to heal it. Still others made use of both biomedical (gamma globulin) and New Age (liver flush) alternatives. Interestingly, some of the group were working part time in a nursing home at the time they became ill. After discussing the high caloric diet with some of the nurses, they came to the conclusion that such a diet meant food with a high sugar content. Because sugar is a major avoidance in the New Age view, the people assumed this dietary recommendation was another example of poor medical prescription and resorted instead to fasting with fruit and vegetable juices and herbal teas. After some time the symptoms of the sickness lessened and the people began to recover. Within a few weeks all had returned to their normal activities, although some complained of weakness and recurrence of some symptoms for some time afterward.

As a result of the hepatitis outbreak, this New Age commune became the target of considerable censure by members of the majority culture in the small town where the healing center was located. The small girl who became ill had treated her kindergarten class with cookies baked by her mother just a few days prior to appearance of symptoms in both child and mother. As word of this spread (the regional news media made much of the affair), it caused considerable consternation among the local townsfolk and resulted in some thinly-veiled verbal threats against the commune. It was noted, however, that no members of the local community developed hepatitis A, despite the usual patterns of social interaction between Agni Circle and local townspeople during the period between exposure at the Barter Fair and the course of the illness spisode. For this outbreak, the disease episode was essentially subculturally specific.

One of the women reported the experience in the Circle's newsletter, noting their response to the illness and warning of care needed while traveling and attend: ing gatherings:

What a blessing it was to get hepatitis as an early Christmas present this year! First, there was the chance to fast for a week. It was easy – no appetite! Second, there was bedrest and taking it easy for another few weeks. And then, there was the diet given by a naturopathic doctor – 75% raw fruits and vegetables, 25% protein. That's real close to the diet we want to follow anyway. So having hepatitis gave us the incentive to make our desire for a raw food diet into a reality.

Hepatitis is very infectious, even during the two weeks before any symptoms develop. For those of us with few contacts and hygienic personal habits, this is no problem, but among larger gatherings and on the road, or in unsanitary kitchen and bathroom conditions, the risks can be very great. A person remains infectious for about a week after the appearance of jaundice. The recovery period can extend from a few weeks to six months.

So stay clean this winter. Wash hands after trips to the toilet and before eating. Consider having a personal bowl, cup, and spoon. And keep your liver healthy with raw food, plenty of rest and exercise, and a loving heart. 'Give me, O God, ears to hear the flute of the universe which is played without ceasing and its sound is love.' (Agni Circle 1978)

COGNITIVE ADAPTATION

The reaction of this group to the hepatitis episode is illustrative of the distinction between socially-defined and physically-defined illness. As Kleinman has noted:

Clinically-oriented investigations tend to undervalue the importance of health beliefs, health maintenance, preventive practices, the role of popular understanding of normal bodily functioning in the social construction of the illness experience, and the non-treatment-related psychological and social function of illness. (Kleinman 1977: 11)

For Agni Circle people, physical maladies such as hepatitis were conditions caused by spiritual imbalance, and symptoms or signs of physical distress were considered to be the objectification of such imbalance. Figure 1, a taxonomy produced by a commune member after the hepatitis episode, illustrates how such a biomedically-labeled illness reflects the New Age notion of imbalance. In this case the informant was using a sickness classification system based on humoral theory from Eastern medicine. In Figure 2, another informant used an alternate means of categorizing by labeling hepatitis as a "purifying organic infection".

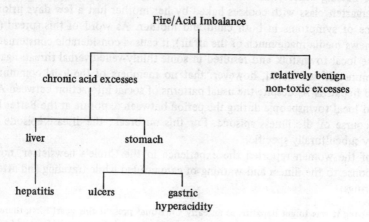

Fig. 1. New Age taxonomy of sickness: Relationship between humoral imbalances and bio-medically-labeled illnesses.

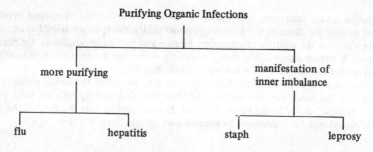

Fig. 2. New Age taxonomy of sickness: Examples of "purifying" disease.

Such cognitive reading of the multitude of biomedically-defined sicknesses was a common strategy in this group. Signs and symptoms of physical distress were commonly relabeled as either a "purification" or a "healing crisis". A "purifying disease" is one in which a specific organ in the body is believe to contain a very high level of toxicity, and where some causative agent (a "germ", for example) triggers the organ to discharge the toxicity. Such conditions are thought to purify the body and spirit, and are attributed positive value in that they remind one of spiritual realities.

A "healing crisis" is a condition in which every organ of the body is thought to expel toxins simultaneously. Symptoms of previous purifications return, as the body releases retained toxins. Such events happen only to those who are relatively healthy at the time; they are of short duration, and indicate that the individual is on the road to perfect spiritual and somatic existence. In essence, the healing crises is conceived as part of a lifelong process in which toxins deposited during a previous life-style in the majority culture are removed by the body as a result of the newer life-style.

Prophylaxis and remedies for either purifying disease or healing crises are consistent with beliefs about cause and disease process. They are selected to help eliminate toxicity, restore balance, and assure progression to a higher state of spiritual and physical health.

SOCIAL RESPONSE

The Spring Gathering of Healers

As mentioned earlier, we did not attend the 1977 Barter Fair. We did, however, attend the 1978 Spring Gathering of Healers. Description of this gathering emphasizes its position as a social institution predicated on the mobility of the New Age population. It illustrates how an anthropological interpretation of subcultural beliefs, behaviors and institutions can lead to improved understanding of disease transmission and to subcultural response to potential or actual illness.

Plans for the 1978 event began during late winter when Agni Circle issued invitations to its third annual spring healing gathering. Because the previous gathering had been large and unwieldy, and had presented health problems as a result of difficulties in providing fresh water and toilet facilities, letters were sent out on a selective basis in an attempt to limit attendance. The gathering was scheduled May 19–21, but other groups were invited to send a few members one or two weeks in advance to help prepare the site for the event. The invitation included travel directions to the meeting location, a map detailing the general layout of the area, a preliminary schedule of events, and other general information. Emphasis was placed on "no tobacco, alcohol, drugs, and please, no dogs".

The village

The gathering village, when complete, covered an area of about twenty-five acres in a relatively secluded organic orchard in the Naches Valley near Yakima, Washington. The village consisted of four main sections: workshop area, parking, camping sites, and a large assembly area. The latter included children's playground, first aid tent, tea kitchen, communal kitchen, garbage pit, hot tub, equipment shack, teepees for formal meetings, bulletin board, and a spacious open area for activities of the gathering "circle".

Permanent toilets were scattered throughout the orchard. Limited handwashing facilities with running irrigation water were near the assembly area. Fresh drinking water was trucked in large tanks and positioned near the kitchen. Agni people, still sensitive to their experience with hepatitis, had made a decided effort to avoid some of the hygienic problems of the previous gatherings.

The workshop area, which was within the confines of the orchard proper, consisted of a grid of approximately sixteen numbered sites, at which various lectures or demonstrations pertaining to holistic health were held. Times and locations for each day's events were posted the evening before on the bulletin board. Format of the schedules resembled that of a day's schedule of college classes, with which many of the participants were very familiar. Five workshop sessions were held each day, each of about two hours' duration; they were offered on a voluntary basis by persons who believed they had something of interest to share.

The activities

The day's activities were partly structured. Each morning a sunrise circle was held, characterized by chanting of the Om (an incantation consisting of the sound "ommm . . . "used in contemplation of ultimate reality) and designed to focus the sun's energy at the site of the gathering. Then workshop sessions took place until approximately 8:00 a.m., at which time a general group meeting and gathering circle occurred. Here people stood or sat in a large double-concentric circle while organizers and lecturers announced late changes in scheduling of workshops, asked for cooperation in solving current organizational problems, and imparted other information of general interest. Following the general meeting, members of the gathering stood, held hands or clasped arms, and danced in a circle while chanting and singing. Circling involved, usually, nearly 250 people.

Circling represented the spirit of the gathering, brotherhood and sisterhood, and the generation and direction of power and healing energies from the universe to The Mother, that is the Earth. The primary goal was to help The Mother become balanced so that all life on Earth could also be balanced and live in harmony with it. As circling progressed, energies were directed to specific persons in the New Age network who were known to be ill. Someone either in or out of the circle might shout, "We have a very sick sister in one of the tents. Let's all help her". The chanting and circular movement would then increase in volume and tempo as energy was sent to this person. Or someone might shout, "So-and-so in Portland is very sick and needs our help." After attention had been drawn to several persons in this manner, the circling would continue for some time, ending in time for breakfast.

The communal kitchen, organized and coordinated by Agni Circle people, served mostly raw foods: fruits and vegetables, sprouts, nuts, dried foods and some grains. Participants brought foods which were given to the kitchen people and prepared by them. Agni Circle provided a continuous supply of various kinds of sprouts and wheat grass juice for everyone. Following breakfeast, workshops were held until late afternoon, at which time the evening circle and the second and final meal occurred.

Social interaction at the gathering was that of joyous celebration and closeness. Singing, music, and dancing were unrestrained and lively. Greetings of old friends, playing with children, gossiping, praying, and meditating coexisted in a milieu in which both sexes discarded various items of clothing in order to achieve a more perfect union with the natural environment.

Similarly representative of the spirit of the gathering were the holistic healing lectures and demonstrations. A sample of topics during the 1978 workshops included healing leprechauns, guardian angels, rebirthing, hatha yoga, tai chi, first aid, home birthing, various forms of massage, polarity therapy, healing hermeneutics, color healing, color visualization, fasting, herbal tincture-making, nutrition, clay therapy, iridology, astrology, psychic healing, Oriental medicine, Bates method, shiatsu, centering on God, acupressure, Bach's flower remedies, chakra balancing, naturopathy, and herbology.

Workshops and demonstrations began with an informal lecture by the leaders, followed by an extended question-answer session. As the day progessed, people moved from one station to another for presentations of interest. The unifying motif for the disparate healing and religious concepts presented was that they represented alternative ways of manipulating or using "energy." New Age people define energy as a spiritual force emanating from God, and as the single reality of the universe. They consider all other physical manifestations to be illusion.

Observations at the Gathering

Our observations at the healing gathering provided an opportunity to consider both the environment and human activity from an epidemiological as well as anthropological view. Due to the experience of Agni Circle with the aforementioned hepatitis in 1977, organizers took added precautions in selecting a site in which they could avoid previous sanitation problems. Choice of a well-established, though old, orchard meant that some wooden toilets were available among the rows of trees; other temporary ones were erected. The owner had diverted running water from an irrigation system which was used for washing hands. Portable tanks of drinking water were brought in. Food preparation and distribution seemed fairly well controlled.

In spite of these arrangements, we noted some potential for transmission of infection. Irrigation water, though running, is a well-known source of intestinal and other infections, and although it was not intended for drinking, some persons did so. The orchard toilets were insufficient in number to accommodate the unexpectedly large crowd, and seats were sometimes wet and soiled. Containers of sprouting seeds were placed within three feet of the open garbage pit. The end of the hose for drinking water lay on the ground behind the kitchen tent.

Participants enjoyed the social, psychological, and physical benefits of the gathering. We know of no illnesses which resulted; but once the people had dispersed, there would have been little chance in follow-up, given the indeterminate nature of paths of movement to other areas of the country. There were plenty of therapeutic options among the group medical belief system had anyone become seriously ill; and, if one became sick, it would have been a purification, something to be welcomed in the progression to a higher plane of existence.

DISCUSSION

Epidemiologic Implications

Description of the frequency and distribution of disease in a population typically revolves around characteristics of person, time and place — who is affected, when and where (Austin and Werner 1977; Lilienfeld 1976). The hallmark of descriptive epidemiology is the use of such information comparatively — e.g., the frequency of disease occurrence in different populations and in different segments of the same population, in order to formulate hypotheses relating disease frequency to population characteristics or exposures. Of necessity, most formal epidemiologic measures, such as incidence, prevalence, morbidity, and mortality, require known population figures to which age- and sex-specific case rates can be applied. In the present situation, the New Age subculture presents problems not usually encountered with a defined population. With the latter, data from both affected and control groups are more readily obtainable, especially where a medical records-linkage system exists or cases have been seen in a hospital or a physician's office. Major factors which impede the epidemiologic method among New Age people are their extreme mobility, extensive and sometimes complicated networks, and their unique interpretation of physical indisposition of any kind. New Age diagnoses and determination of the causes and processes of physical distress take alternate forms to those of biomedicine. As a result, some illnesses not only do not come to the attention of epidemiologists, they are relabeled by New Age people in ways that are meaningless to health workers without knowledge and understanding of the world view, values, and life-style from which they derive.

SUMMARY

The type of observations we have offered lack contextualization in a systematic experimental design. Virtually every bias that haunts an epidemiologist's worst nightmares exists in this analysis: sampling bias, selection bias, and response bias, to name but a few (Sackett 1979). Controls are absent from this presentation because the overall research design consisted of general descriptive comparisons across major ethnic groups. Yet it must be remembered that in this discussion we are not conducting a scientific test of a hypothesis or a therapy. The potential of ethnographic research lies in: (1) assessing risk factors for disease which supplement age, sex, occupation, socioeconomic status, marital status, and other traditional and relatively available epidemiologic variables; and (2) providing information on the degree to which cultural milieu and cognitive frame may constrain health care planning, intervention, and prevention for social groups that operate with very different conceptions of the significance of biological events. As Syme and Berkman (1976: 1) noted,

... preventive approaches must involve community and environmental interventions rather than one-to-one preventive encounters. Therefore, we must understand more precisely those features of the environment that are etiologically related to disease so that interventions at this level can be more intelligently planned.

A number of techniques of popular health culture in use by New Age people are also being implemented in some medical and (especially) nursing circles. In fact, visualization, acupressure, laying on of hands, and various other holistic health-related concepts and constructs are now being taught in some schools of nursing. The objective of such techniques is *care* rather than *cure*. The New Age commune, as a care unit staffed by non-professionals, is a lay example of a prevention and care modality in the approach to disease. As one alternative model to costly and understaffed biomedical delivery systems in rural settings, it deserves consideration by health planners.

The continued existence of social class gradients of mortality, morbidity, and life expectancy, whether in the case of farm workers or other less fortunate members of our society, requires social assessment of risk factors for disease and of cultural strengths for intervention. In support of this thesis, we have argued that (1) medicine is not applied biology, but preeminently a social science dealing with human adaptation; (2) one of anthropology's contributions to public health services and epidemiology lies in the documenting of those risk factors for disease transmission that develop from group-specific patterns of adaptation to the environment; (3) the New Age gathering, a social institution predicated on the mobility of a subcultural population, carries the latent function of spreading disease; and (4) the New Age healing commune, as a type of popular culture community clinic oriented to transience, is a cultural unit which can complement public health intervention for migrant workers. In an era in which, as Barrett *et al.* (1980) have pointed out, the migrant farm worker is a marginal issue among competing priorities for public health service resources, non-professional staffing of less-than-traditional (yet monitored) care units may be a viable approach to health management. The healing commune, while specific to the New Age subculture, does have such potential, for it embodies two characteristics of the occupational group of migrant farm workers: limited financial resources and an emphasis on self-care.

NOTE

1. Because we move between biomedical and non-biomedical discussion in this paper, we have not attempted to differentiate between "disease" and "illness", although we generally assign the former term to abnormal and pathological conditions of the body which are usually treated by physicians. "Illness" we consider to be a broader term having social and psychological meaning and representing conditions which may be treated by non-medical healers or by the use of popular and folk remedies. We use the term "sickness" in our research study because it is often considered an even broader term encompassing both "disease" and "illness". Some of our New Age informants, however, told us they preferred the term 'dis-ease" because to them it represented more precisely their state of being when ill.

REFERENCES

Agni Circle
    1978 Newsletter, 1: 3.
Austin, Donald F. and S. Benson Werner
    1977 Epidemiology for the Health Sciences: A Primer on Epidemiologic Concepts and
          Their Uses. Springfield, Illinois: Charles D. Thomas.
Barrett, Stephen E., John Gillespie, and Richard L. Call
    1980 Migrant Health Revisited: A Model for Statewide Health Planning and Services.
          American Journal of Public Health 70: 10: 1092–1094.
Byerly, Elizabeth L.
    1981 Health Care Alternatives of Multiethnic Migrants. Final Report of the I.C.N.E.
          Rural Health Research Project. Washington, D.C.: National Technical Information
          Service System (NTIS).
Byerly, Elizabeth L., Craig A. Molgaard, and Charles T. Snow
    1979 Dissonance in the Desert: What to Do with the Goldenseal? In Madeleine Leininger
          (ed.), Transcultural Nursing '79. New York: Masson Publishing USA, Inc., pp. 97–
          113.
Clark, Duncan W.
    1967 A Vocabulary for Preventive Medicine. In Duncan W. Clark and Brian MacMahon
          (eds.), Preventive Medicine. Boston: Little, Brown and Company, pp. 1–11.
Holland, W. W. and A. H. Wainwright
    1979 Epidemiology and Health Policy. In P. E. Sartwell (ed.), Epidemiologic Reviews,
          Vol. I. Baltimore: Johns Hopkins University Press.
Kleinman, Arthur
    1977 Lessons from a Clinical Approach to Medical Anthropological Research. Medical
          Anthropology Newsletter 8: 4: 11.
Last, John M. (ed.)
    1980 Maxcy-Rosenau: Public Health and Preventive Medicine. New York: Appleton-
          Century-Crofts.
Lilienfeld, Abraham M.
    1976 Foundations of Epidemiology. New York: Oxford University Press.
Luckmann, Joan, and Karen G. Sorensen
    1980 Medical-Surgical Nursing: A Psychophysiological Approach. Second edition. Philadel-
          phia: W. B. Saunders Company.
Molgaard, Craig A.
    1979 New Age Hunters and Gatherers. Doctoral dissertation, Department of Anthropology,
          University of California at Berkeley.
Molgaard, Craig A. and Elizabeth L. Byerly
    1981 New Age Health and Healing: Applied Ethnoscience in Rural America. In Donald A.
          Messerschmidt (ed.), Anthropologists at Home: Toward an Anthropology of Issues
          in America. Cambridge, England: Cambridge University Press.
Molgaard, Craig A., Elizabeth L. Byerly, and Charles T. Snow
    1979 Bach's Flower Remedies: A New Age Therapy. Human Organization, 38: 1: 71–74.
Molgaard, Craig A., Amanda L. Golbeck, and Elizabeth L. Byerly
    1979 Prototypes of Internal Category Structures: Fuzzy Sets in Nursing Research (Ab-
          stract). Communicating Nursing Research 12: 83–84. Boulder, Colorado: Western
          Interstate Commission on Higher Education.
Sackett, David L.
    1979 Bias in Analytic Research. Journal of Chronic Disease 32: 1/2: 51–63.
Sigerist, Henry E.
    1951 A History of Medicine, Vol. I: Primitive and Archaic Medicine. New York: Oxford
          University Press.

Syme, S. Leonard and Lisa F. Berkman
  1976 Social Class, Susceptibility, and Sickness. American Journal of Epidemiology 104: 1:
        1–8.
World Health Organization
  1980 Non-A/Non-B Hepatitis: A 'New' Disease. News and Notes. WHO Chronicle 34: 12:
        495–496.

AUTHOR INDEX

411

SUBJECT INDEX

Acculturation
  to Western diet and lifestyles
    and obesity problems, 154, 156
Action style
  of clinicians
    vs anthropologists styles, 16
Actuarial tables
  criticism of
    and obesity problem, 160–61
Adaptation
  behavioral
    and culture/nutrition relationship, 146
  as central concept
    in nursing, 117–18, 123
  to chronic mental illness
    and medication, 382–83
Adaptive advantages
  of body shape
    and obesity background, 154–55
Adherence
  and treatment relation to everyday life, 195
  see Compliance; Compliance/noncompliance
Adoptive/nonadoptive
  definition of concept
    in Mexican-American study, 331
Advertising industry
  in U.S.
    and obesity problems, 164–66
Affect
  as part of illness, 101
Agni Circle
  see New Age healing center
Alcoholism
  anthropological approaches to, 38–39, 51
Alternative coping strategies
  elective seminar in, 41–47
Alternative healing commune
  and disease transmission study, 395–407
Alternative health care systems
  and changing explanatory models, 301
  and health/illness ideology, 290

Alternative psychiatric treatment
  for chronic mental patients
    research on, 374–85
Alternative theoretical options
  and clinical teaching, 88
American folk medicine
  as cultural belief complex, 125
Analytic models
  use by anthropologists, 16
Anglo view
  of supernatural assistance
    vs Mexican-American view, 333
Anthropological strategies
  clinically applied, 99–106
Anthropologist roles
  in health science settings, 18–24, 369
Antipsychotic medications
  of chronic mental patients
    and sociocultural factors, 380–85, 387–88
Anxiety
  and patient/practitioner communication, 337–38, 345
Appropriate
  illness behaviors as
    and chronic illness, 358
Asian Americans
  and doctor-patient relationship expectations, 97
Attitudes
  of anthropologists
    toward medical culture, 87
  and health
    sick role model, 355

Bahamians
  in Miami
    health beliefs and practices of, 206, 212, 235
Bales' Interaction Process Analysis
  and patient compliance studies, 299
Basic concepts
  in teaching clinical behavioral science, 71–74
Bedside manner
  confused with cultural sensitivity, 182

417

The Culture, Illness, and Healing Book Series

Editor

Arthur Kleinman

1. Leon Eisenberg and Arthur Kleinman (eds.), *The Relevance of Social Science for Medicine*, 1981, x + 422.

2. Arthur Kleinman and Tsung-yi Lin (eds.), *Normal and Abnormal Behavior in Chinese Culture*, 1981, xxiv + 436.

3. Carolyn Fishel Sargent, *The Cultural Context of Therapeutic Choice*, 1982, xii + 192.

4. Anthony J. Marsella and Geoffrey M. White (eds.), *Cultural Conceptions of Mental Health and Therapy*, 1982, xii + 414.